ESSENTIALS

for the

ACTIVITY PROFESSIONAL

in

LONG-TERM CARE

SUSAN E. LANZA, ACC, LNHA

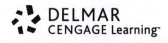

DELMAR
CENGAGE Learning

Australia • Brazil • Japan • Korea • Mexico • Singapore • Spain • United Kingdom • United States

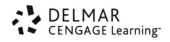

DELMAR
CENGAGE Learning™

Essentials for the Activity Professional in Long-Term Care
Susan E. Lanza

Publisher: Susan Simpfenderfer

Acquisitions Editor: Kimberly Davies

Project Development Editor: Coreen Rogers

Production Coordinator: John Mickelbank

Art and Design Coordinator: Vincent S. Berger

Editorial Assistant: Donna Leto

Marketing Manager: Dawn Gerrain

Cover Illustration: Sergio J. Sericolo

Cover Design: Vincent S. Berger

For product information and technology assistance, contact us at
Cengage Learning Customer & Sales Support, 1-800-354-9706
For permission to use material from this text or product,
submit all requests online at **cengage.com/permissions**
Further permissions questions can be emailed to
permissionrequest@cengage.com

Library of Congress Control Number: 96-19631

ISBN-13: 978-0-8273-7387-7

ISBN-10: 0-8273-7387-2

Delmar
Executive Woods
5 Maxwell Drive
Clifton Park, NY 12065
USA

Cengage Learning is a leading provider of customized learning solutions with office locations around the globe, including Singapore, the United Kingdom, Australia, Mexico, Brazil, and Japan. Locate your local office at:
international.cengage.com/region

Cengage Learning products are represented in Canada by Nelson Education, Ltd.

For your lifelong learning solutions, visit **delmar.cengage.com**

Visit our corporate website at **www.cengage.com**

Notice to the Reader

Publisher does not warrant or guarantee any of the products described herein or perform any independent analysis in connection with any of the product information contained herein. Publisher does not assume, and expressly disclaims, any obligation to obtain and include information other than that provided to it by the manufacturer. The reader is expressly warned to consider and adopt all safety precautions that might be indicated by the activities described herein and to avoid all potential hazards. By following the instructions contained herein, the reader willingly assumes all risks in connection with such instructions. The publisher makes no representations or warranties of any kind, including but not limited to, the warranties of fitness for particular purpose or merchantability, nor are any such representations implied with respect to the material set forth herein, and the publisher takes no responsibility with respect to such material. The publisher shall not be liable for any special, consequential, or exemplary damages resulting, in whole or part, from the readers' use of, or reliance upon, this material.

Printed in the United States of America
19 20 21 22 23   13 12 11 10 09
ED156

T A B L E   O F   C O N T E N T S

P R E F A C E

As a licensed nursing home administrator and former activity director, I have seen the activity field change and grow tremendously over the last sixteen years. The professional growth has led to the need for high-caliber materials for the new and working activity professional. A textbook of this type has been long overdue to assist activity professionals in gaining the edge they have been seeking for years.

This book is designed to be a comprehensive text with clear references (some very old!) to professional facts and studies. The text is not meant to be a list of specific program ideas, such as "101 special events" or the "best craft projects." Many books exist with unique ideas for programs. Instead, this textbook is a compilation of the major subject areas of which activity professionals should have knowledge in order to perform effectively.

My opinions as an administrator and activity director guided the organization of the text and the type of material I felt was relevant. The chapters and sections have been organized according to my ideas of information flow; my organizational choices may not agree with those of other instructors.

Sections I, II, and III divide the material into three distinct areas. The chapters in Section I contain basic facts and initial information that an activity professional may need immediately in a new position. This material is especially important for the newly hired director who is also enrolled in a basic education course and may be exposed to this information for the first time. The topics covered in this section, such as the history of long-term care, the origins of the activity profession, aging and the needs of residents, getting to know residents, and management and work space/environmental issues are all subjects I have found to be relevant to the first weeks or months on the job. The only exception is the necessary exposure to the information covered in Chapters 12 and 13.

The chapters in Section II represent areas related to program development. Chapters 8, 9, and 10 flow in order because each chapter builds on the previous one. Chapter 7, "Budgeting," was placed before these chapters because most activity professionals are presented with a budget at the time they are hired and are expected to do their program planning knowing their budget in advance. Figure 7-2 shows a sample payroll budget, but may not be reflective of actual salaries in your area. Chapter 11 is important to include in this section on programming because group leadership and marketing impact the successful delivery of programs. Documentation and medical records, presented in Chapter 12, have a direct relationship to program planning and must be presented in this section for clarity.

The chapters in Section III could be presented in any order; however it is important to note that these chapters concern evaluation and enhancement. To me, this information logically flows after initial job training and program development. Some instructors may say, "Why would you put regulatory compliance in the third section instead of the first?" The answer, in my view, is that regulatory compliance is a form of evaluation of the overall program. Earlier chapters discussed OBRA regulations, quality of life, assessment, where an activity department fits into a facility, which regulations guide budgeting, documentation, and so forth. The chapter on regulatory compliance discusses the survey process by putting in perspective the fact that every facility has a regulatory agency to which they are accountable. The primary focus of all professionals should be to meet the standards of practice for their position as well as the needs of the residents; all within a regulatory framework. The other chapters in Section III can be taught in any order because they do not necessarily build sequentially on each other. Program planning from Section II, however, should be understood first. The information from Chapter 19 is important to present last because career advancement is not something that should be considered before the basics are learned. Some of the material from Chapter 19, concerning professionalism and the standards of certain organizations, are applicable to presentation at any stage in an instructor's course.

The Review Questions can be used for class homework, and the On Your Own sections for either class exercises or between class projects. The Further Reading sections at the end of each chapter offer additional opportunities to study particular subject areas. The Self-Assessment Exam in Chapter 20 is provided for the student's use to gauge progress with the material. The appendices are meant to stimulate thinking and provide resource opportunities. Some controversial areas, such as the professional debate between therapeutic recreation and activity professionals, have been discussed briefly, although satisfactory resolution of this will certainly bring further changes to an already changing industry.

Instructors of the basic and advanced activity courses, seminars, and related courses will find that the key subject areas have been addressed in the material presented in this text. Along with this text, instructors may still wish to present supplemental texts or articles in the teaching of this course. The amount of paperwork (articles, handouts) that teachers will have to distribute or students will have to collect from libraries or their facility, however, should be significantly reduced by the use of this text. Because most instructors have individual teaching styles, the text presents opportunities to teach these comprehensive chapters in any order chosen to meet instructor needs and mandated course guidelines.

From my research into studies conducted about activity programming and related issues, it is clear that more experiments and research are needed in areas such as management, orientation, environmental aspects, quality of life, community issues, and professional standards. If you are experimenting with special programs, please write to me in care of the publisher of this text. I hope you will take the initiative to continue the research so that the revised edition of this text will be even more informative. Remember, as you grow, so will the activity profession.

Susan E. Lanza

To Jerry, who always believed in my ideas and encouraged me with love and patience;

To Elizabeth, for her love, her help, and great sense of humor.

ACKNOWLEDGEMENTS

Although one author is listed on the cover of this book, it would not have been possible to complete this project without the generous help of the many people I would like to acknowledge here.

A big thank you to Jerry Lanza and Berkeley Hall Nursing Home for allowing me to use their office resources. Pat Kotyuk, Bonnie Ricker, and Helyne Nathan deserve praise for their expert and last-minute assistance.

A super thanks to Joan and Jim McSpiritt who gave up their free time to help with volumes of typing, book pick-up and deliveries, and miscellaneous support. They even made house calls!

Special thanks go to Marcy McSpiritt for her efforts in making library visits to locate books and other clerical support.

Commendations to Rosemary Allen who came out of "retirement" to share her valuable perspective and help with the research process.

I appreciate the following facilities and staff members for opening their doors to me to observe their programs, and for allowing me to take the original photographs used in this text: Shelley Wyatt and Lynne Wilkesman of Absecon Manor; Robert Piegari, LuAnn Smith, and Carol Burt of Francis E. Parker Memorial Home; Leonard Trager and Pat Whilden of Lakewood at Voorhees; Maggi Gannon and Pam Scharpf of Mainland Manor; Noel Swan and Lisa Reidinger of Valley View Care Center; and Christopher Gillies and Kristine Rutherford of Victoria Manor.

A hearty thank you to all our models who allowed themselves to be photographed: Absecon Manor: Lynne Wilkesman, Helen Jamison, Catherine Bernard, and Margaret Grote; Francis E. Parker Memorial Home: Rosemary Allen, Lillian Bayne, Roger Bernier, Margaret Biel, Kathleen Fidecaro, Nancy Galiardi, Harold Gobble, Barbara Golias, Susan Hall, Kim Hauff, Maude Hoffman, Florence Molineux, Bob Piegari, Betty Priest, Bonnie Ricker, Walter Russi, Jennifer Small, Lu Ann Smith, Jeanne Snell, Frank Viola, and Theresa Wertheim; Lakewood at Voorhees: Michael Dickman, Roger Royer, Pat Whilden, Margaret Wood, and Ed Schrieber; Mainland Manor: Caroline Endicott, Faith Crouch, Debbie Hommel, Dot Jasper, Lillian Lihn, William Petrino, Pam Scharpf, Emma Thielking, Emma Thompson, and Mabel Wagner; Valley View Care Center: Ellen Sabo, Lisa Reidinger, Kathleen Williams, Kaitlin Sabo, Kellie Reidinger, and Elizabeth Lanza; and Victoria Manor: Dorothy Freas, Kristine Rutherford, Betty Beheler, James Roser and Harry Crouse.

Thanks also to the following activity consultants: to Debbie Hommel for support, introductions, and innovative techniques that she piloted, and to Marylou Schnurr for generously giving her valuable opinions on the project.

Supportive friends and colleagues who helped in many ways include: Maggi Gannon, Debbi Reid, Ruth Bannon, Mari Muriayma, Marge Caglianone, and the crew from Logan Drive.

A special thank you to all the libraries that assisted me in obtaining materials:

Hunterdon County Library in Flemington, NJ; North Branch Library in Annandale, NJ; South River Public Library in South River, NJ, and the Nolan D.C. Lewis Library of The Carrier Foundation in Belle Mead, NJ. Lynne Cohn of Carrier Foundation Libraries deserves special praise for locating many difficult-to-find books and articles.

For early exposure to writing for the health care professions, thanks to the late Alan E. Nourse, author and family friend.

Thanks to Dr. Roger Alan Shell of Cardiology Associates of New Brunswick for some technical assistance.

For their foresight and support during this project, thanks to David Gordon, Kim Davies, Cori Rogers, Vin Berger, Dawn Gerrain, John Mickelbank, Donna Leto, and the entire editorial and production team at Delmar Publishers.

Special thanks to Bob Piegari for giving me my first job in activities and allowing me many additional learning opportunities in long-term care.

I would also like to acknowledge the reviewers and thank them for their input into this project: Debbie Hommel, Karen Land, Natalie Davis, Jane Martin, and Susan Rauch.

And finally, to all the activity and other professionals around the world, who sent me information or responded to questions, a big thank you for helping to shape this book.

INTRODUCTION

According to *Roget's Thesaurus*, an introduction is "a short section of preliminary remarks," and I will attempt to abide by this definition.

I take pride in writing this introduction because the author and I have been associated with each other, over the years, in several different capacities: first, in an employer/employee relationship, then as professional colleagues, and finally, as friends.

Essentials for the Activity Professional in Long-Term Care covers the basics for the aspiring professional or student, as well as more advanced information for activities professionals or those employed in the field. The administrator-in-training and the working administrator would also benefit from reading this text. The book would be of great benefit to activities instructors and those leading seminars, as well as educators teaching classes in college.

The general format is a well-organized and balanced presentation covering both historical and factual perspectives. The author uses her diverse background to cover the "basics," and has successfully presented a plethora of varied topics and useful information for the '90s.

The author has used her dual background (Activities Director and Nursing Home Administrator) to full advantage and has given the reader an opportunity to learn from another's experiences. I recommend this book to those in the long-term care field and its use as a text and reference book, as well as its usefulness as a resource book.

I particularly enjoyed reading *Essentials* because the scope of the work is so comprehensive—everything one needs to know is right here! Health care is changing almost daily; new technologies enter our door, but the hands-on approach that all disciplines enjoy in long-term care will not disappear. The changing population in nursing homes (a higher percent today of residents with dementia) dictate that activity professionals gear their programs to different and demanding behaviors.

The author has effectively used her management skills to present budgeting and quality assurance in an interesting manner. She has used her activities background to cover topics dealing with programming, planning, and implementation.

I was struck with the completeness of this text: it is progressive; it is thorough; it is well written; and it is well organized. *Essentials* belongs in your long-term care library.

Robert M. Piegari, LNHA
President
Francis E. Parker Memorial Home
Piscataway, NJ

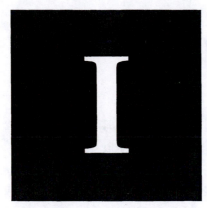

SECTION I

Establishing Yourself and Understanding Your Residents and Department

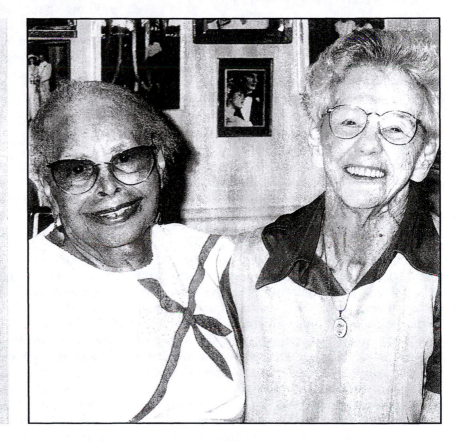

CHAPTER 1
History, Definitions, and Qualifications

OBJECTIVES ....

After completing this chapter, you should:

- be able to define an activity and describe how activities came into the hospital or long-term care setting.
- know about the categories and classifications of long-term care.
- have a background of the differences between activity staffing requirements according to the federal program and the many state-level laws.

INTRODUCTION

Your decision to become an activity professional in a long-term care setting is commendable! You are joining a growing group of individuals committed to improving the quality of life for long-term care residents on a daily basis. Learning how your line of work originated and the kinds of long-term care settings in which you might be working will have implications for the full understanding of all aspects of your job.

Delivery of activity services to long-term care residents is a thriving profession in a growing industry. Understanding the definition and elements of an activity program, coupled with the components of a long-term care setting, provide the building blocks for acceptable practice in the field. Noting the diversity in current state-level activity staffing requirements illustrates the continued need to work on nationalized requirements for coursework, continuing education, and standards of practice in the activity industry.

What is an Activity ....

The cornerstone to understanding your job is to consider how an activity is defined and what the historical view of the profession has been.

Definitions

Many definitions of an **activity** exist, but they have originated from within a framework of the recreation and leisure industry. In their research text, Leitner and Leitner (1985) define **leisure** as ". . . free or unobligated time, time during which one is not working or performing life-sustaining functions," while they consider **recreation** to be an ". . . activity conducted during one's leisure." Additionally, Edington, Compton, and Hanson (1980) define recreation as ". . . a process that restores or recreates the individual . . . from the Latin word *recreatio*, which means 'to refresh'." More than just a definition, recreation relates to the values of an individual, before consideration is made of their medical challenges or chronological age. Sessoms, Meyer, and Brightbill (1975) discussed the link between recreation and personal identity and found that personality factors such as happiness and satisfaction are strongly influenced by recreational pursuits. Additional aspects of life such as emotional balance and mental capacity for learning were also noted to be improved when activities were a part of life. The authors went on to conclude, "Values not only determine the kinds of activities people pursue, they also shape our attitudes toward those activities. . . ."

Because our focus in this text is on services delivered to an individual in long-term care, we have to consider the definition of recreation as residing within a medical context. Speaking of recreation as a professional area of service, a view of **therapeutic recreation** might be the one agreed on by field professionals and referenced by Peterson and Gunn (1984) as ". . . a process which utilizes recreation services for purposive intervention in some physical, emotional, and/or social behavior to bring about a desired change in that behavior and to promote the growth and development of the individual." Leitner and Leitner (1985) identify therapeutic recreation as ". . . leisure activity designed to facilitate an improvement and/or maintenance of one's physical and/or mental functioning and/or promote developmental growth."

So where does the term "activity" fit into this background? It appears that the term activity has roots in the recreation and leisure field, but first took hold in the long-term care industry (then nursing homes or convalescent homes) as a result of legislation in the 1960s that mandated specific services for clients in these facilities. Although there is not an industry-wide acceptable definition for the word "activity," some professionals refer to the one given by Peckham and Peckham (1982) which states that activity in a long-term care setting is ". . . all the action and interaction the resident experiences during a day."

In thinking about the word "activity," it is wise to remember that when using the word to refer to anything, *activity* is the singular form of the word and *activities* is the plural form. When you refer to a department devoted to this service, you use the term "activity department" instead of "activities department." You are an *activity professional*, *activity assistant*, or *activity director*. Using the plural form of the word in this manner is similiar to saying "nursings director." Please use caution in representing your industry correctly.

Origins of Activities and History of the Profession

According to research conducted by Frye and Peters (1972), the concept of using activities in a medical setting has origins in history as far back as Greek and Roman times. Frye and Peters report that there is a small amount of evidence to show that some recreational activity was used at that time for combating illnesses. They also mention that many years later, in the late 1700s and into the 1800s, a number of medical practitioners began to see the benefits of using exercise, occupa-

tional pursuits, or "amusement" to treat many conditions. Some of the records of the late 1800s mention reports of therapeutic games, and even a facility description of an asylum in 1843 which offered "recreational" programs. Their exhaustive research on the start of recreation programming enabled Frye and Peters to discuss the impact that Florence Nightingale had in late nineteenth-century Europe with her notable publication, *Notes On Nursing*. In this work, Nightingale (1860, 1946) makes numerous comments on simple ideas that have current applications to delivery of activities today. Some of her advice to nurses included:

- "Variety of form and brilliancy of colour in the objects presented to patients are actual means of recovery."
- "Volumes are now written and spoken upon the effect of the mind upon the body. Much of it is true."
- "A little needle-work, a little writing, a little cleaning would be the greatest relief the sick could have . . . "
- ". . . we must admit that light has quite as real and tangible effects upon the human body."
- "Always sit down when a sick person is talking business to you, show no signs of hurry give complete attention and full consideration . . . ."

Nightingale also mentioned the importance of using soft musical instruments and even bringing in small animals for comfort at times. Frye and Peters state their opinion of this important work to recreation personnel by saying, "This small volume should be reviewed by all recreators who serve the ill or the disabled and particularly by those who work in a hospital or clinical setting."

According to Frye and Peters (1972), by the first quarter of the twentieth century, recreation programs started to appear in hospital wards and other centers that were needed because of the large number of patients recovering from war injuries. They also cite a milestone in medically-oriented recreation history of the first department of recreation that was established and recognized in 1929 in Illinois to devote study to recreation programs for handicapped children. In addition, the needs created by the two world wars propelled recreation further into the arena of legitimate study when the **Veterans Administration (VA)** added recreation as a functional service of their programs in 1945. As reported by Frye and Peters, the formation of the hospital segment of the American Recreation Society in 1949 eventually led to the publication of *Basic Concepts of Hospital Recreation*. A number of other groups with recreational interests were formed, and were merged into the National Recreation and Park Association in 1965.

Frye and Peters mentioned that around this same time, studies were already indicating that requirements for those making a formal study of recreation were not consistent. The specialty field of therapeutic recreation blossomed out of the recreation profession with practitioner criteria and standards. Between that time and today, numerous other specialty groups have joined the challenge of meeting recreation needs in medical settings and include therapists devoted to music, art, poetry, occupational, and drama, just to name a few.

As the field of therapeutic recreation developed in hospitals and other settings, this technical field was less known in the nursing homes and convalescent centers that are now called long-term care facilities. The most obvious reasons for this phenomenon were lack of awareness about the therapeutic value of the services, the limited resources of facilities trying to hire recreation personnel, and the key fact that until the early 1970s, facilities were not mandated to hire recreation personnel as part of their core staff.

The field of activity direction was born out of a need for diversional and other activity programs for clients who would be residing in nursing homes or convalescent centers. By the beginning of the 1970s, the federal regulations required an on-staff person assigned to directing an activity program whose background included therapeutic recreation or occupational therapy, or who had prior experience working in an activity program. The regulation stated that prior experience was acceptable in lieu of a specific degree, and a whole new subset of the traditional recreation programming in a medical environment was formed. In order to find an apt description for the work of individuals who assisted residents in recreational activity and other functions, but were not degreed in a specialty area, an activity employment position was created with guidelines for an Activity Coordinator, or a similiar sounding job title.

Long-Term Care ....

According to the General Accounting Office (GAO) (1994), the long-term care industry today is serving over twelve million Americans whose medical needs range from physical or mental disabilities to assistance with **activities of daily living (ADLs) skills.**

Definition and Background

An industry definition, reported by the American Health Care Association (1993), states that **long-term care** is "health or personal services required by persons who are chronically ill, aged, disabled, or retarded, in an institution or at home, on a long-term basis. The term is often used more narrowly to refer to care provided in nursing homes." Another point of view, as stated by the American Association of Retired Persons (AARP) (1992), defines long-term care as ". . . a comprehensive range of medical, personal, and social services developed and coordinated to meet the physical, social, and emotional needs of chronically ill and disabled persons."

According to the extended research of the Committee On Nursing Home Regulation (1986), the origins of regulation in long-term care began as early as 1935 when the Social Security Act was adopted. Although this new act set the stage for government assistance to the elderly who are poor, it did not provide for residents in institutional settings. In response to this, the private sector of nursing homes was born. The Committee On Nursing Home Regulation states that the first official survey of nursing homes was held in 1954, after changes were made to the Social Security Act to accommodate payments to health care institutions. The study of the Committee reveals that legislation such as the Hill-Burton Act of 1954 and the Kerr-Mills Act of 1960 aided in providing funds to agencies and the medically needy who required care.

The quality of care provided in nursing homes was called into question as far back as 1956. In 1986, the Committee On Nursing Home Regulation reported that standards for care in the fifties were lacking, and care, in general, was poor. Following a report by the Special Subcommittee On Problems Of the Aged and Aging in 1959, which cited these overwhelmingly substandard conditions, a guideline was drafted and issued in 1963 called the Nursing Home Standards Guide. The advent of Medicare and Medicaid in 1965 broaded the scope of standards, but implementation of the standards was difficult. The Committee On Nursing Home Regulation reported that during his administration, President Nixon began the passage of many enforcement guidelines to streamline and correct the system that included specific training standards for staff in nursing homes. Since 1974, the regulations for nursing home survey process have changed to address the varying differences in the way facilities meet standards, including implementation of the first **skilled nursing facility (SNF)** regulations in 1974, and followed by the intermediate care facility regulations in 1976. A SNF is defined by the American Health Care Association (1993) as a facility or part of an organization ". . . which provides skilled nursing care and related services for patients who require medical, nursing, or rehabilitation services." In 1990, intermediate care facility guidelines were eliminated but replaced with the term **nursing facility** which the American Health Care Association 1993) defines as "facilities other than hospitals which provide nursing care maintenance and personal care to individuals unable to care for themselves due to health problems.

Quality care was again part of more recent legislation, such as the 1984 *Smith vs. Heckler* legal decision, cited by the Committee On Nursing Home Regulation (1986). This case involved a group of residents in a Colorado nursing home who successfully sued the owners of their facility, as well as government agencies (such as Medicaid), for substandard care, disregard of their rights as facility residents, and for acting as a body that failed to properly monitor their problems. Initially won, the case was reversed on appeal, but it impacted changes in the survey process which directed nursing homes to focus their efforts on improved patient care. Surveys by state and federal agencies to monitor compliance with regulations were called Patient Appraisal Survey and Care Evaluations (PACE), evolved into Patient Care and Services Surveys (PACS), and are now called Omnibus Budget Reconciliation Act (OBRA) surveys. The OBRA surveys have a strong focus on resident outcomes and quality of life. More information on the survey methods used today are discussed in Chapter 13.

The United States General Accounting Office (1994) reported that of the twelve million long-term care clients who needed minimal to moderate help with daily functioning, approximately one-sixth actually required institutional assistance such as a nursing home, specialty hospital, or other facility. The surprising majority of the long-term clients, a number totalling over ten million, can live at home or in monitored community settings, and receive the necessary support services to maintain independence in areas such as housekeeping, meals, or infrequent nursing care. The GAO also reported that over 57 percent of all long-term care clients in any setting are elderly, with working age adults comprising 40 percent and children comprising only 3 percent of the total mix.

According to the GAO report (1994), the need for long-term care services among clients ranges in severity from those requiring minimal task assistance to those who are severely disabled and require full assistance and supervision. Assessment of needs and proper placement within the **continuum of care** system usually begins with a view of the limitations of the client in the area of self-care tasks. The continuum of care chart shown in Figure 1–1 illustrates the stages of need across the caregiving continuum, with lower levels of assistance required on the left side up through the highest level of care needed on the right side. Additionally, a report by state agencies to the GAO (1994) showed that the need for services was most frequently determined by a client's ability to perform activities of daily living. Other methods of ascertaining need were based on cognitive skills and support or care provided by family or friends.

Types of Long-Term Care

There are three primary classifications for long-term care services: **home-care services, community-based services**, and **institutional care**. Home-care services are provided by either informal caregivers (such as family members) or professional caregivers ranging from home-health aides to professional therapists. Community care is offered in a variety of settings that include adult day care programs and senior centers. Institutional care is handled around the clock in a facility which provides nursing services, rehabilitation, activities, room and board, housekeeping services, and administration of medication.

Providing services at home helps an individual maintain a high sense of independence. A report by the U. S. Department of Health and Human Services (1994) states that the type of care provided by an informal caregiver (such as family and friends giving unpaid assistance) or formal caregivers (staff in an institution or community-based care center) usually depends on the level of a person's disability, and if he or she has family nearby.

The American Association of Retired Persons (1992) isolated the kinds of home-care services that a client may require on a long-term basis. The research showed that assistance was most needed in areas such as chore and personal care services, repair of items in the home, meals, reassurance, and transportation services. A specialized service such as hospice care can be delivered effectively at home. The more services that can be brought into the home situation, the more a client can be **"aging in place."** This term, used among the providers in the long-term care com-

INCREASING DEPENDENCY NEEDS →

	HOME-BASED SERVICES		COMMUNITY SERVICES			INSTITUTIONAL SERVICES		
HOUSING OPTIONS	OWN HOME ALONE	OWN HOME WITH ASSISTANCE	SENIOR HOUSING COMPLEX	PERSONAL CARE/ ASSISTED LIVING	CONTINUING CARE RETIREMENT COMMUNITY	NURSING HOME	REHAB HOSPITAL OR CENTER	SUBACUTE CARE UNIT
SERVICES PROVIDED	meals transportation	personal care reassurance calls chore/ maintenance adult day care senior center meals transportation home health aide	assistance in ADLs personal care services adult day care/senior center security activity participation room and board fee additional charges for services nursing care available assistance with financing, etc. meals transportation			twenty-four hour nursing care room and board fee charges for additional services security assistance with multiple ADLs transportation all support services available on site: dietary, housekeeping, maintenance, social services, personal care, laundry, activities		

Figure 1–1   The long-term care continuum.

munity, connotes an ideal scenario where a long-term care client can remain in his or her own home or other living arrangement for as long as possible when needed services and support are safely and properly provided. The other objective of the aging in place idea is to keep clients at the lower ends of the continuum of care for as long as possible. Callahan (1992) states that aging in place has become an important issue recently because of higher numbers of homeowners as well as a lingering misconception that many elderly clients are being forced into nursing homes for lack of any other alternative. Other researchers argue that aging in place is an important concept which opens up many opportunities for clients at the beginning of the continuum of care.

The long-term care client also has many options in the community-based service arena. Some of the selections that are available have to do with housing choices while others concern support services. The housing alternatives range from **senior centers** and **adult day care centers** which may be part of a housing complex to **personal care homes, boarding homes, assisted living facilities,** or **continuing care retirement communities (CCRCs)**. Each of these settings offers a different array of services and dependency levels to their clientele. The objectives of the senior center is to provide socialization and meals. Adult day care is normally a supervised experience for clients in need, such as those individuals with early stages of Alzheimer's disease. The assisted living facilities or personal care/boarding homes (there are many dif-

ferent names for almost the same services around the country) usually offer meals, twenty-four hour supervision by staff, and assistance with one or more activities of daily living. The continuing care retirement communities were created to offer clients a range of services within one complex from independent apartment living through skilled nursing care services in an on-site facility.

Support service alternatives in the community for long-term care clients include programs such as a nutrition project that offers meals daily to local residents in need. Caregivers of long-term care individuals also might find counseling and other stress-relieving alternatives through community offerings.

The research of community care in long-term care situations, conducted by Kemper, Applebaum, and Harrigan (1987) argues that for frail elderly clients (those who may be in most need of services), the nursing home system provides more required services than that of the community. One reason for this is the cumbersome procedures that clients must go through to acquire services, which could force them into a nursing home by default. Another issue is that funding for long-term community care is not as readily available. One of the community programs that has been researched to bridge this gap of community long-term care services that are so needed by the frail elderly population is the On Lok Model of managed long-term care, discussed by Steenberg, Ansak, and Chin-Hansen (1993). Focusing deliberately on the frail elderly clientele in their community, the On Lok Model was set up as a **case management system**, which effectively brought together services for clients. By including all types of medical, rehabilitative, and support services for clients that allow them to continue to live in the nearby community, the researchers found the use of traditional nursing home and hospital services was significantly reduced.

Institutional Long-Term Care

When we hear the words "long-term care," our traditional image is of the nursing home and rehabilitation center's delivery of services. In either setting, the care that is rendered is classified as **skilled nursing care**, which refers to facilities delivering twenty-four-hour care under the supervision of a registered nurse for those residents needing medical, rehabilitation or nursing intervention.

According to the GAO (1991), the demand for elderly use of formal long-term care services is expected to grow rapidly because of client longevity and increasing levels of disability. As shown in Figure 1–2, the elderly comprise the majority of our resident mix (note the switch here from the term client to resident) with working age adults and children as other receivers of care. Additionally, because of the growing elderly population, the risk of entering a nursing home and staying for a period of time over one's lifetime has increased significantly, as noted in a report by Kemper and Murtaugh (1991). Other factors that effect the lifetime usage of institutions for traditional long-term care were researched by Kemper, Murtaugh, and Spillman (1991), and include the cost of care, existing health care options, and the availability of services.

Types of Institutional Long-Term Care. Nationally, there are many categories of residents under

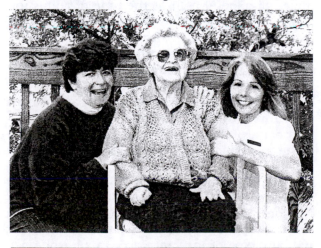

Figure 1–2 Institutional long-term care is one of many methods of delivering health care services to the elderly.

the umbrella of institutional long-term care. For dignity and ease of service delivery, many facilities have made efforts to separate distinct age groups. If admission guidelines in a facility are broad enough to include the range of ages from children through the elderly, planning should be implemented to ensure living arrangements that take the different needs of these distinct age groups into account. By designating a separate unit for each age bracket, the requirements of each group can be addressed. For instance, the dietary and activity needs of pediatric residents are very different from those of working age adults.

Other facilities have experimented with placing residents in separate spaces within the same facility based on their medical needs. For example, there are now specialty areas called **subacute care units**, which the American Health Care Association and the Joint Commission on Accreditation of Healthcare Organizations (1994) define as ". . . goal-oriented treatment rendered immediately after, or instead of, acute hospitalization to treat one or more specific active complex medical conditions. . . ." The kind of subacute care categories that might qualify for placement on a specialty unit include **head trauma**, **AIDS**, **ventilator care**, **wound management**, **cancer**, and **intravenous therapy**. Other nonsubacute specialty wings might include cognitively impaired residents or developmentally disabled older adults.

A common practice of facilities is to house multiple levels of care requirements within one building or complex. A facility might be comprised of a **skilled nursing facility (SNF)** and an assisted living unit. The benefits to the residents of either section would be the ability to transfer to another area should a different level of care be required. Some hospitals and other **acute care** settings are organizing sections for skilled nursing care beds. This approach is successful when the staff members have the time and the flexibility to deliver the required services to each category of resident.

Ownership Structure. Within the institutional framework, a variety of ownership options exist. There are **proprietary facilities** that operate their organizations to make financial profit each year. There are **nonprofit facilities** that are operated on a tax exempt basis. Matthews (1990) reminds us that although proprietary facilities account for approximately seventy-five percent of all nursing facilities, the majority are aware that running a profitable business does not equate with ignoring the principles of good resident care. Within the nonprofit arena, there are individual facilities that are part of a religious parent organization, such as the Quakers or the Presbyterian Church, that may have minimal philosophical or religious connection to the parent organization, or may strictly follow religious guidelines for all residents. Other nonprofit organizations are established for **philanthropic** or charitable reasons and operate at a loss to meet humanitarian goals. A proprietary facility can be owned by an individual, a small corporation, or a large company, and operated through direction from ownership through a licensed administrator. The nonprofit facilities are owned by religious or other organizations and are chiefly operated by a board of directors working through an administrator or executive director.

A third category exists for ownership that is **government owned**, usually on the city, state, or county level.

Payment Sources. Unfortunately, another way we classify residents is through their **payment source**, or the method by which the facility receives its funding in exchange for the residents' care. The facility fee for care services usually includes at minimum room and board, nursing care, meals, housekeeping and laundry, and activity programming.

According to the Health Care Financing Administration (1992), **private pay** sources (or out-of-pocket expenses) comprise an average of forty-three percent of the total nursing home income.

Medicaid (called **Medical** in California) is a state executed but federally administered program for those individuals who are disabled, blind, or medically indigent. Medical and financial eligibility requirements vary from state to state. Medicaid makes up approximately forty-four percent of the payers for long-term care services.

Medicare, a federally administered insurance program for individuals over the age of sixty-five and for those who have been disabled or suffer from other specialized medical conditions, has two parts: Part A and Part B. **Medicare Part A**, called hospital insurance, covers some portion of an individual's hospital stay and skilled nursing facility stay, based on the patient's ability to meet certain criteria. The eligibility requirements for Part A coverage in a long-term care facility include:

- admission to a skilled nursing facility that participates in the Medicare program through a **provider agreement**
- a three-day hospital stay
- transfer made to the long-term care facility within thirty days of discharge from the hospital

- initial and continued verification from the attending physician and the monitoring committee (often called **utilization review committee**) that skilled nursing or rehabilitative care is required on a daily basis.

When a person meets eligibility qualifications, Medicare Part A pays for room and board at the skilled nursing facility, for skilled rehabilitation services, skilled nursing care under the supervision of a registered nurse, drugs, supplies, equipment, and other related health services for a limited period of time (up to 100 days in a benefit period). The responsibility for Medicare Part A payments during the first 100 days breaks down as follows:

- day 1 through day 20—Medicare pays for qualified stays
- day 21 through day 100—Medicare pays a portion of the costs while the resident pays a co-insurance daily rate amount, which is a standardized figure for all providers in this country.

Medicare Part B, called medical insurance, pays for a limited amount of physician visits, other medical practitioners services, and some outpatient care to those enrolled. Individuals entitled to Medicare Part A may also enroll in Medicare Part B. If a patient is not enrolled, he or she can enter the program during one of the enrollment periods. A premium is charged quarterly or automatically deducted from an individual's social security check.

One of the most difficult concepts to understand for new residents and their families is that Medicare does not cover many long-term care facility expenses, if it covers any at all. There is much disappointment at the time of admission when new residents discover the limitations of the coverage. The Health Care Financing Administration (1992) reports that Medicare payments represent approximately five percent of the total financing of nursing home care.

A catch-all category called **third party payers** accounts for another payment source for facilities. Some of the alternate sources include **private insurance, medi-gap insurance, long-term care insurance, welfare** or **general assistance, supplemental security income (SSI)**, and **Veterans Administration benefits**.

None of these sources has made a great impact on the long-term care payment situation. Thus far, any type of insurance accounts for one percent or less of the total financing of care. Some private insurance companies have limited coverage for skilled nursing care and other companies have developed specific policies to address long-term care financing needs. The medi-gap insurance was formulated to fill the gap in payments by paying what Medicare does not.

Welfare or municipal assistance programs are available in most states to help clients pay for some room and board at a skilled facility under certain conditions. A resident applying for admission to a facility may be eligible for welfare or municipal assistance funding if his or her monthly income level is above the required level for Medicaid funding, but not high enough to allow for payment of the care fees. For individuals in this situation, an application may be made to the town where they reside. There may also be contributory requirements for grown children of the resident.

Supplemental security income (SSI) is not usable toward room and board payment in a skilled nursing facility; however, it can be used in some states as payment for personal care homes, boarding homes, and assisted living facilities. The supplemental security income is a federal program established to assist the aged and those with other disabilities such as blindness.

Payment of services by the Veterans Administration (VA) for a veteran's receipt of long-term care services occurs infrequently, since according to Matthews (1990), most veterans are cared for by facilities operated directly by the VA. Rich and Baum (1984) discuss the changes within the VA that focus on allowing some hospital beds to be made available while some veterans are placed in proprietary facilities on a contractual basis. Some facilities may have a contract with the VA to provide care for veterans in their long-term care facility in exchange for payment of a daily rate.

Obviously, different health care plans exist in other countries, and the varied health delivery systems have a direct bearing on what the activity service and staffing requirements are.

Regulatory Framework. All facilities, whether proprietary, nonprofit, or government owned, need to comply with regulatory mandates. It is important to understand certain broad areas of the regulatory system such as the **certification process**, **state licensure**, and the **survey and inspection process**.

The Medicare and Medicaid programs that are part of the payment system for many facilities are both federal programs. Medicaid, although federally organized, allows each state to administrate its individual program. To participate in either Medicare or Medicaid, facilities have to enter into a contractual

arrangement called a provider agreement, with the government. The provider agreement states that in exchange for the facility providing services at an acceptable standard, the federal government will reimburse the facilities at a daily rate for each participant in the program within their facility. Daily rates for Medicaid and Medicare vary by facility depending on many factors.

To monitor the adherence of a facility to the standards set down in the provider agreement, the federal government has established **regulations**, which are written guidelines for conducting appropriate practices to ensure that residents are properly cared for. The federal government makes an agreement with each state to handle its survey and inspection process, which measures the level of **compliance** with the regulations. Additionally, in each state, another set of laws on the state level, dictate the standards of practice that must be followed to provide quality services to long-term care residents. The regulations vary from state to state. Between the federal and state regulations, however, a state agency (usually the Department of Health), conducts a **survey** that is comprised of a visit by one of their employees to determine compliance. At the time of the survey, an **inspection** takes place that involves the viewing of care methods, and speaking to the residents over a period of time. If the findings of the survey are good, the facility becomes eligible to have its provider agreements continued and its state license renewed. Private facilities that do not participate in the Medicaid or Medicare programs are inspected by a regulatory agency based on the state laws only.

The Future of Long-Term Care

The long-term care client base is expected to grow and possibly double in size within the next twenty-five years. According to the GAO report (1994), much of the anticipated increase may be due to the aging baby boomer population. Factors such as significant medical research advances and fluctuating mortality rate, however, may also affect changes.

The General Accounting Office (1994) also reported that other future implications for long-term care include a unification of administration of services for long-term care that makes access of services easy for clients. This model, often referred to as the **single point of entry** approach to long-term care, is being tested in some states across the country.

Delivery of Activity Services in Long-Term Care ....

The service delivery arena that activity professionals are probably the most familiar with is in the area of traditional nursing homes or rehabilitation centers. As mentioned previously, the institutional segment of long-term care participants is the smallest one, but because of its extensive service delivery requirements, all areas of specialty, such as activity programming, are very important to meet the total needs of the resident. Also, the majority of all long-term care clients are elderly, with children and working age adults comprising the other segments.

The home-care setting has not yet offered many opportunities to the activity professional. In the area of community programs, the activity professional can be a part of the staff in facilities such as personal care homes, assisted living facilities, senior centers, and adult day care as regulations are developed and implemented. Wilhite (1987) discusses the upcoming need for recreation professionals to provide services to the home health care client, and concludes "Home delivered recreation does hold promise as a cost-efficient and effective mechanism for expanding long-term care support services. . . ."

Throughout this text we make reference from time to time to these other settings, but the primary focus is to understand the activity professional in the institutional long-term care scene, hereafter referred to as "long-term care."

Qualifications for Staff

Reaching the needs of long-term care residents must be made by qualified staff members. The requirements for staff members who work in a Medicare or Medicaid certified facility are set by federal regulations. The regulations, according to the Federal Register (1991) state the following standard:

"483.15 Quality of Life
(f) Activities.
(2) The activities program must be directed by a qualified professional who—
(i) Is a qualified therapeutic recreation specialist or an activities professional who is—
    (A) Licensed or registered, if applicable, by the State in which practicing; and
    (B) Eligible for certification as a therapeutic recreation specialist or as an activities professional by a recognized accrediting body on October 1, 1990; or

(ii) Has 2 years of experience in a social or recreational program within the last five years, 1 of which was full-time in a patient activities program in a health care setting; or
(iii) Is a qualified occupational therapist or occupational therapy assistant; or
(iv) Has completed a training course approved by the state."

Standards on the state level may require less in terms of qualifications and experience than the federal regulations. An overview of the current activity staffing regulations within the United States and some foreign countries is presented in Appendix A. The rule of thumb for determining which staffing qualifications to adhere to in a facility where both state and federal regulations are followed is to use the more stringent rule: if your state requires a specialty degree above and beyond the federal regulations, you should comply with your state standard.

Viewing the differences between the state and other mandated requirements in Appendix A should raise issues concerning nationalization and reform that favors education and standardized training requirements. You can see the variances in staffing requirements in private facilities (no provider agreements for Medicaid or Medicare) and those in federal programs in states that have no state-level requirements. These variances are not helpful when professional staff members are attempting to deliver consistent programs with diverse staffing backgrounds.

Along with the confusion about state staffing qualifications comes the issue of which professional staff group is truely qualified to manage the responsibilities of the position. At times, members of the three main professional groups involved—the therapeutic recreation community, the activity professionals (who now have professional certification available), and the occupational therapists— have each felt that clearer, more defined regulations would end some of the confusion. One of the issues that has often been raised by activity professionals has been, "Why can an occupational therapist do my job but I can't do his?" Other concerns have to do with lobbying for exclusivity of job title use in certain states. The only way to solve these issues is for the forces to join and present reasonable options to the decision-makers to adequately represent all professions. This topic is controversial, but without addressing these professional problems and unifying the groups, there will continue to be dissension.

Singleton, Makrides, and Kennedy (1986) demonstrated how the three professions of physiotherapy, occupational therapy, and therapeutic recreation were able to compare and contrast their services, and arrive at effective communication for the best delivery of services. With help from the national organizers of the three major professions that are responsible for current activity programming in long-term care facilities, we are hopeful that this issue will be resolved.

Aside from the controversy, there are many other specialty majors and areas of training that bring professionals to the activity industry. Some of the other training modes include music therapy, art therapy, dance therapy, drama therapy, and poetry therapy. A chart illustrating some of the current training requirements for the activity professional and other fields of study is shown in Figure 1–3. For a list of contacts in any of these areas, see the information sources in the back of the book.

FIELD OF STUDY	CERTIFICATION BODY	CREDENTIALS	SUMMARY OF QUALIFICATIONS			
			DEGREE	INTERNSHIP OR CLINICAL	WORK EXPERIENCE	EXAM
Activities	National Certification Council for Activity Professionals (NCCAP)	Activity Assistant Certified (AAC)	BA w/req. courses	—	2,000 hrs. plus 30 CEUs	—
			60 college credits	—	6,000 hrs. plus 30 CEUs	—
		Activity Director Certified (ADC)	BA w/req. courses	—	2,000 hrs. plus 30 CEUs	—
			60 college credits	—	6,000 hrs. plus 30 CEUs	—
			60 college credits or NAAP basic/ adv. course, + 12 coll. crdts.	—	10,000 hrs. plus 30 CEUs	—
		Activity Director Provisional Certified (ADPC)	Meet 3 of 5 NAAP basic/ adv. crse. + 12 coll. crdts.	—	10,000 hrs. plus 30 CEUs	—
		Activity Consultant Certified (ACC)	MA w/req. courses	—	2,000 hrs. activity exp., 40 CEUs, 200 hrs. consulting	—
			BA w/req. courses	—	4,000 hrs. activity exp., 40 CEUs, 200 hrs. consulting	—
Art Therapy	American Art Therapy Assn. (AATA)	Art Therapist Registered (ATR)	MA in AT or equiv.	600 hrs. (60 hrs. supervis.)	1,000 hrs (100 hrs. supervis.)	Yes
	Art Therapy Certification Board (ATCB)	Art Therapist Registered Board Certified (ATR-BC)	ATR	—	—	Yes
Dance Therapy	American Dance Therapy Assn. (ADTA)	Dance Therapist Registered (DTR)	MA (48 credits in dance/music)	700 hrs. + 200 hrs. field exp.	—	—
		Academy of Dance Therapists Registered (ADTR)	DTR	48 hrs. supervis. w/ ADTR	2 yrs. paid clinical exp. in approved setting	—
Drama Therapy	National Assn. of Drama Therapists (NADT)	Registered Drama Therapist (RDT)	MA/MS in drama therapy or related field	300 hrs. supervis. w/RDT 300–700 hrs. supervis. w/ mental health	1,500–2,000 hrs.	—
Horticultural Therapy	American Horticultural Therapy Association. (AHTA)	Horticultural Therapist Technician (HTT)	2 equiv. pts. or combo of coursework/ degree in hort. in related or unrelated field	—	2,000 hours paid employment or 4,000 hrs. combo paid/volunteer —	—

Figure 1–3 The background and training of activity professionals are varied (*continued on next page*).

FIELD OF STUDY	CERTIFICATION BODY	CREDENTIALS	SUMMARY OF QUALIFICATIONS			
			DEGREE	INTERNSHIP OR CLINICAL	WORK EXPERIENCE	EXAM
		Horticultural Therapist Registered (HTR)	4 equiv. pts. or combo of degree in hort. therapy	1,000 hrs.	2,000 hrs. paid employment as horticultural therapist	—
		Master Horticultural Therapist (HTM)	6 equiv. pts. or combo MA in hort.	—	4 years paid employment or 8,000 hrs. in HT.	—
Leisure	National Recreation & Park Assn. (NRPA)	Certified Leisure Professional (CLP)	BA/MA from accredited program	—	—	Yes
			BA/MA from non-accredited rec/leisure prog.	—	2 yrs. exp.	Yes
			BA/MA related field non-accredited prog.	—	5 yrs. exp.	Yes
	National Certification Board (NCB)	Provisional Professional	↓ education than CLP level	—	↓ exp. than CLP level	—
		Certified Leisure Associate (CLA)	AA degree in rec/leisure	—	—	—
			AA degree in related field	—	2 yrs. exp.	—
			Diploma/ Certification	—	4 years exp.	
Music Therapy	American Assn. of Music Therapy (AAMT)	Certified Music Therapist (CMT)	BA/MA in MT	900 hrs.	—	—
		Advanced Certified Music Therapist (ACMT)	MA plus CMT	w/CMT	2 years	—
		Certified Music Therapist—Board Cert. (CMT—BC)	CMT	—	—	Yes
Occupational Therapy	American Council for Occupational Therapy Education (ACOTE)	Occupational Therapist (OT)	BA	Supervised clinical	—	Yes
		Certified Occupational Therapy Assistant (COTA)	2-yr. degree or certificate	Supervised clinical	—	Yes
Poetry Therapy	National Assn. for Poetry Therapy (NAPT)	Certified Poetry Therapist (CPT)	BA/related field	440 hrs. w/100 hrs. supervis.	—	—
		Registered Poetry Therapist (RPT)	MA/related field	1,000 hrs. w/175 hrs. supervis.	—	—
Therapeutic Recreation	National Council for Therapeutic Recreation Certification (NCTRC)	Certified Therapeutic Recreation Specialist (CTRS)	BA in TR or recreation w/specific coursework	360 hrs./ 10 week field placement	—	Yes
			BA accredited school w/specific coursework	—	5 or more yrs. full-time paid therapeutic recreation exp.	Yes

Figure 1–3 The background and training of activity professionals are varied (*continued*).

SUMMARY

The evolution of the activity professional in long-term care began many years ago, but the noticeable importance of the profession has blossomed recently. Understanding the origins of activity concepts as well as the structure of the long-term care industry prepares you to face all the challenges that your new profession has to offer.

R E V I E W   Q U E S T I O N S

1. What is the difference between the definition of an activity as given by Peckham and Peckham and the definition of therapeutic recreation as given by Peterson and Gunn?
2. Define the continuum of care.
3. What are the three components of long-term care services?
4. What are the differences between the Medicare and Medicaid programs?
5. What is the definition of subacute care?

O N   Y O U R   O W N

1. If you work in a facility with skilled nursing services as well as assisted living residents, how can you use activity programming to help the residents age in place?
2. How can the institutional long-term care activity professional share his or her expertise with the community or home-based programs?
3. What are some tactics for helping to nationalize the activity staffing standards between states?

R E F E R E N C E S

American Association of Retired Persons (1992). *Staying at home: A guide to long-term care and housing.* (PF 4936 [1092]. D14986) Washington, DC: author.

American Health Care Association (1993). *American health care association: Glossary of long-term care terminology.* Washington, DC: author.

American Health Care Association & Joint Commission on Accreditation of Healthcare Organizations (1993). *American health care association: Glossary of long-term care terminology.* Washington, DC: author.

Callahan, J. J. (1992). Aging in place. *Generations,* Spring, 5–6.

Committee on Nursing Home Regulation—Institute of Medicine (1986). *Improving the quality of care in nursing homes.* Washington, DC: National Academy Press.

Edington, C., Compton, D., & Hanson, C. (1980). *Recreation and leisure programming: A guide for the professional.* Philadephia, PA: Saunders College/Holt, Rinehart, Winston.

Federal Register (1991). Vol. 56, No. 187, *Part 483—Requirements for long-term care facilities.*

Frye, V., & Peters, M. (1972). *Therapeutic recreation: Its theory, philosophy and practice.* Harrisburg, PA: Stackpole Books.

Health Care Financing Administration (1992). *Report of the office of the actuary.* Washington, DC: author.

Kemper, P., Applebaum, R., & Harrigan, M. (1987). Community care demonstrations: What have we learned? *Health Care Financing Review,* Vol. 8, No. 4.

Kemper, P., & Murtaugh, C. (1991). Lifetime use of nursing home care. *The New England Journal of Medicine,* Vol. 324, No. 9.

Kemper, P., Murtaugh, C., & Spillman, B. (1991). Nursing home use after age 65 in the United States: Differences in remaining lifetime use among subgroups and states. *Agency for Health Care Policy and Research,* Publication No. 91-0047.

Leitner, M. J., and Leitner, S. I. (1985). *Leisure in later life: A sourcebook for the provision of recreational services for elders.* Binghamton, NY: Haworth Press.

Matthews, J. (1990). *Elder care: Choosing & financing long-term care.* Berkeley, CA: Nolo Press.

Nightingale, F. (1946). *Notes on nursing: What it is, and what it is not.* Facsimile edition, New York, NY: D. Appleton-Century Co.

Peckham, C. W., & Peckham, A. B. (1982). *Activities keep me going.* Lebanon, OH: Otterbein Home.

Peterson, C. A., and Gunn, S. L. (1984). *Therapeutic recreation program design: Principles and procedures.* Englewood Cliffs, NJ: Prentice Hall.

Rich, B. M., & Baum, M. (1984). *The aging: A guide to public policy.* Pittsburgh, PA: University of Pittsburgh Press.

Sessoms, H. D., Meyer, H. D., & Brightbill, C.K. (1975). *Leisure services: The organized recreation and park system.* Englewood Cliffs, NJ: Prentice-Hall, Inc.

Singleton, J. F., Makride, L., & Kennedy, M. (1986). Role of three professions in long-term care facilities. *Activities, Adaptation and Aging,* Vol. 9(1), 57–69.

Steenburg, C., Ansak, M., & Chin-Hansen, J. (1993). On Lok's Model: Managed long-term care. In C. M. Barresi & D. E. Stull (Eds.) *Ethnic elderly and long term care.* (p. 179–190). New York, NY: Springer Publishing Co.

U.S. Department of Health & Human Services (1994). *Long-term care: Diverse, growing population includes milions of Americans of all ages.* (GAO Publications No. 95–26) Washington, DC: author.

U.S. Department of Health & Human Services (1994). *The disabled elderly: Informal versus formal long-term care.* (AHCPR Publication No. 94-0130). Rockville, MD: author.

U.S. General Accounting Office (1991). *Long-term care: Projected needs of the aging baby boom generation.* (GAO Publication No. 91-86). Washington, DC: author.

U.S. General Accounting Office (1994). *Long-term care*

reform: State's review on key elements of well designed programs for the elderly. (GAO Publication No. 94–227). Washington, DC: author.

Wilhite, B. (1987) . REACH out through home delivered recreation services. *Therapeutic Recreation Journal,* 2nd quarter, 29–38.

F U R T H E R   R E A D I N G

Matthews, J. (1993). *Beat the nursing home trap: A consumer's guide to choosing and finding long-term care, 2nd edition.* Berkeley, CA: Nolo Press.

McKanzie, N. (1994). *Beyond crisis: Confronting health care in the United States.* New York, NY: Meridian Books.

U.S. General Accounting Office (1993). *Long-term care reform.* (GAO Publication No. 93-1-SP). Washington, DC: author.

C H A P T E R 2
Your Part in the Facility

OBJECTIVES ....

After completing this chapter, you should:

■ understand your job description and the responsibilities of an activity professional within
  a facility.
■ possess knowledge of health care issues and
  practices that provide a safe working environment for you and your residents.
■ learn about some facility specific areas that will
  help you succeed.

INTRODUCTION

As an activity professional in a long-term care setting, you are expected to assume a number of employment functions within your facility. The two
primary roles are activity department head and
health care worker in a long-term care setting.
Success on the job depends on mastery of each
area.

Your Role as an Activity Professional and Department Head

The facility administrator has charged you with
the important task of providing a full range of activity programming for your residents. This crucial department head position requires a great
deal of dedication and resourcefulness on your
part to make it successful. The following are components of your job.

Your Job Description

A written account of all your job duties, known as
a **job description**, establishes your areas of re-

sponsibility within the facility. Some duties are
almost standard within any activity position
whereas other required functions may be specific
only to your facility. If you are working with activity assistants or a consultant, you should receive a delineation of duties within each of your
job descriptions. All activity job descriptions
should contain a section outlining your primary
responsibility, which is to provide activity programming to meet the spiritual, intellectual,
physical, emotional, and creative needs of your
resident population. Other required tasks, entitled
"essential duties," should also be listed under this
section. Clear guidelines on the physical and
mental requirements of the job, such as the
amount of lifting you may encounter in your duties, is also necessary. A proper format for your
job description is important because of the compliance conditions of the **Americans With
Disabilities Act (ADA)** (1992). In his article concerning staff employment issues and the ADA,
Heller (1992) discusses the importance of having
". . . a detailed job description that is not biased
against the disabled . . . yet spells out the essential
functions of the position." Before you accept an

activity professional job, you should request a written job description. After accepting the position, review the job description with your administrator again to eliminate any areas of concern or confusion. A few of the subjects you should clarify with your administrator include:

- employee activity programs
- fund raising

- coverage for other departments
- weekend work responsibilities, if required.

Job descriptions are most effective when they are reviewed by both the supervisor and the activity professional, and then signed. Similarly, you should review a job description with your activity assistant. A sample job description for an activity department head is shown in Figure 2–1.

SAMPLE JOB DESCRIPTION

JOB TITLE: ACTIVITY DIRECTOR OR DIRECTOR OF RECREATION

Essential Duties:
- Plans, develops, implements, and monitors a full activity program to meet the social, spiritual, intellectual, creative, physical, and emotional needs of the resident population, seven days a week.
- Supervises the Activity Assistant and volunteers. Assures that quality standards of practice are maintained.
- Understands the physical and emotional needs of the long-term care resident and plans appropriate programming based on recreation theories and the needs of the resident population.
- Develops and maintains written objectives, policy and procedure manual, and an organizational chart for the activity department.
- Plans and posts an activity calendar monthly in visible locations around the facility; encourages participation by all residents.
- Maintains interest inventories on all residents and updates these records as needed.
- Attends weekly interdisciplinary team care plan meetings and provides necessary medical record documentation to the Minimum Data Set and care plans. Documents in progress notes when necessary.
- Assesses each resident's needs individually, and provides programming in group or individual settings.
- Attends department head meetings and other facility meetings as assigned.
- Recruits, selects, trains, counsels, and terminates employees according to facility policies and procedures.
- Participates in the facility budget planning process and maintains staffing ratios, activities expense budget, petty cash, and capital expenditures.
- Functions as a resident advocate in formal and informal settings.
- Plans and holds in-service education programs for activity department staff and general staff according to a schedule.
- Plans and holds family and community educational programs as required.
- Assists in planning and implementing employee activity programs.
- Transports residents around the facility to group or individual settings as required.
- Plans the activity staffing schedule and works weekends, holidays, and evenings as required. Handles administrative weekend coverage as assigned by the administrator.
- Other duties as assigned.

Physical/Mental Requirements:
- Communicates orally and in writing with residents, employees, family members, volunteers, and the public.
- Performs tasks which require eye/hand coordination and simple manipulation skills (i.e., crafts, operation of audio/visual equipment, using the telephone).
- Frequently lifts, pushes, and carries supplies weighing 50 pounds or less.
- Frequently stoops, twists, or bends to reach, move supplies, conduct activity programs, or to hang calendars or decorations.
- Discriminates colors and sounds to respond to fire alarms and other emergency equipment.
- Interacts with hostile, confused, or emotionally upset residents on a regular basis.
- Frequently reaches at, above, or below shoulder height.
- Concentrates on details with numerous interruptions.
- Understands and relates specific ideas to a number of situations.

Figure 2–1 A job description outlines the responsibilities of a particular position (*continued on next page*).

- Is exposed to seasonal conditions for outside programming and trips.
- Articulates continuously and clearly.
- Operates and drives the facility van.
- Continuously deals with multiple tasks, noises, and interruptions, and works cooperatively with diverse populations.
- Sits twenty-five percent of work day, stands seventy-five percent of work day, walks, and performs physically challenging movements to conduct programs.
- Spends ninety percent of work day indoors and ten percent outdoors.
- Pushes residents in wheelchairs and gerichairs. Assists ambulatory residents.
- Communicates effectively with residents, staff, families, and the public.

Education/Training Experience:
- Activity Director Certified (ADC) or Certified Therapeutic Recreation Specialist (CTRS), or
- College degree in recreation, occupational therapy, music therapy, creative arts, psychology, sociology, social work, or art therapy, and is experienced in working with long-term care clients.
- Meets the facility requirements for managing an activity program on the state or federal level.
- Valid drivers license in the state where the facility is located.

Machines/Tools/Equipment/Work Aids:
- Audio/visual equipment, craft tools, various program supplies, typewriter, copying machine, telephone.

Career Level:
- With skills, education, and training, can advance to Assistant Administrator or Administrator.

Supervised By: Administrator

I have read and understand my job description. I agree to accept the responsibilities of the position.

Employee Signature   Date

Figure 2–1 A job description outlines the responsibilities of a particular position (*continued*).

The Organizational Chart

Every facility, whether large or small, has an internal structure of authority which can be depicted in a diagram called an **organizational chart**. The chart outlines the **chain of command** which is the reporting structure for all positions within a facility (see Figure 2–2). In this textbook, an assumption has been made that the activity department head reports directly to an administrator, but you may work in a facility where an administrator is not your direct supervisor. In Hunter's research (1984) it was found that most activity department heads do have direct reporting responsibility to an administrator. Your facility, however, may place the activity staff in a larger, combined department, such as "resident services." The **job title** or name for your position may vary from one facility to another, based on different types of responsibilities. Hunter (1984) found that fifty-seven percent of activity professionals used the job title "Activities Director" or "Director of Activities." It is important for you to be aware of your position in relation to other positions in order to understand your realm of authority, and your limitations. Clarify to what extent you are expected to represent administration in matters within the facility. As a department head directly under an administrator, do you have the authority and permission to counsel a nursing assistant if you are the only department head working on a particular weekend? Although the organizational chart provides a rough structure, these and other delicate questions that concern the interrelationships of other departments must be discussed with your administrator to ensure there are no misunderstandings.

Mission Statements and Objectives

A **mission statement** guides your position and those in other departments within the facility or larger company, and outlines briefly the purpose and goals of the organization. A mission statement is normally developed by the **governing body** (board of directors or ownership group) of the organization to reflect the reasons for its existence, future objectives, and goals. In discussing

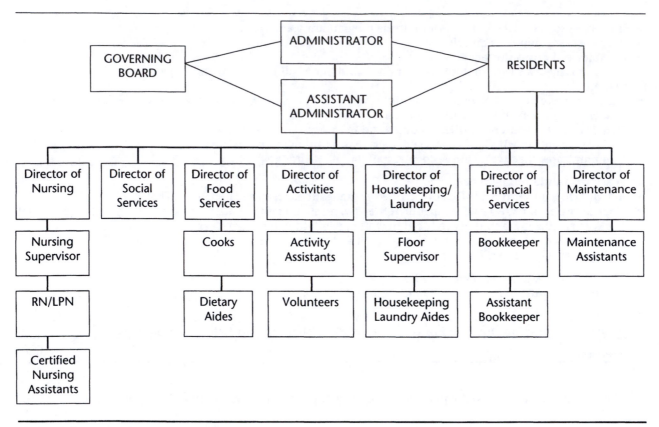

Figure 2–2 A sample organizational chart.

planning within long-term care groups, Goldsmith (1994) states that "In order for the mission statement to have any significance, it must be understandable to the employees of the organization and the market it serves". It is important that your administrator provides you with a copy of the mission statement for your facility to assist you in understanding the philosophy and challenges of the company for which you work.

Working With Other Departments

A successful activity program can be accomplished only with a support system of help from all the other departments. Building and maintaining that system should be a priority for you throughout your career. Getting acquainted with your fellow department heads is the first step toward gaining cooperation. A brief synopsis of other key departments and their responsibilities includes:

1. *Administration:* a licensed administrator (and possibly an assistant administrator) responsible for the full operation of the facility.
2. *Nursing:* Director of Nursing, registered nurses (RNs), licensed practical nurses (LPNs), and certified nurses aides (CNAs) provide nursing care round the clock.
3. *Dietary:* Dietary Manager or Supervisor, cooks, dietary aides and/or servers, and dishwashers, who together prepare and serve three meals daily, plus snacks.
4. *Housekeeping/Laundry:* Housekeeping/Laundry Supervisor, housekeepers, porters, laundry aides, responsible for cleaning all areas of the building and who process facility linen and personal clothing.
5. *Social Services:* Social Worker functions as resident advocate and ensures that the basic needs of residents are met.
6. *Maintenance:* Maintenance Director and maintenance assistants ensure that facility property and equipment is in good working order.
7. *Business Office:* Office Manager, clerical staff, and bookkeepers handle facility communication and correspondence, financial services, and employee payroll.
8. *Admissions Director:* handles tours, inquiries, marketing, and the placement process for all new admissions.
9. *Pharmacy:* an outside provider or an internal department, fills physician orders for residents' medications.

10. *In-Service/Quality Assurance and Improvement:* designated person(s) who handles general staff education and monitoring of quality issues in the facility.
11. *Medical Director:* a consulting physician responsible for planning and directing the overall medical care in the facility.
12. *Rehabilitative Services:* physical therapy, occupational therapy, and speech therapy.

What kind of people will you be working with? What are their issues? How is the activity department viewed by other departments in the facility? The answers to these questions should direct your beginning relations with the other departments. For more information on how to get to know your colleagues, please refer to Chapter 4.

After you have had an initial meeting with some of your co-workers, you may want to consider these general tips to establish harmony:

1. Set up specific times for meetings that reflect both your schedule and theirs. Vary the location of the meeting place whenever possible.
2. If there are negative or preconceived ideas about the role of the activity department, try to change those opinions.
3. Talk to an individual in person whenever possible. Written notes, although a good management tool, can be barriers to developing relationships, especially in the beginning stages.
4. Seek a co-worker's advice on general issues when another opinion might be helpful.
5. Keep sensitive information confidential. You are working with professional people, and this courtesy should be reciprocated.
6. Realize that there will be conflicts and disagreements at times among you and other workers. You may also be faced with having to make unpopular decisions. Conflict is a normal part of the work environment; how you handle it is the key.
7. You do not have to like your co-workers; you do have to work with them. After your best efforts, you may find that you do not enjoy the company of some of them. The feeling may be mutual, but you should not let your feelings interfere with your job performance. The relationship is a working one, not a personal one, and resident welfare must override your personal feelings.

When you see that a relationship with a co-worker has changed in a negative way and your programs are effected, try to resolve the issue. Depending on the outcome, you may need to involve your administrator.

Your Administrator's Expectations

Management styles vary from one administrator to the next. Learn how your administrator views your role and the programs within the facility. You have already covered your job description and your place on the organizational chart, but what does your administrator require from you as an employee? You can ask him or her directly, but the following are some points that most administrators agree are important:

1. Keep your administrator informed! All information is important, and prompt notification about problems is crucial. Date all notes you write and keep copies for your records.
2. Bring in problems for discussion *only after* you have considered some solutions for them.
3. Determine the frequency of contact that your administrator prefers. Is daily, on an informal basis necessary or will a bi-monthly, formal meeting be adequate?
4. Come prepared to all functions and meetings. This means that you have brought a pad, pen, your opinions, and, if needed, a presentation that was planned in advance. Lack of readiness on your part is a poor reflection on you and your department.
5. Express your opinions but respect a decision that your administrator has made. She or he has many difficult issues to resolve on a daily basis, and your understanding is important.

Recognizing Yourself as a Professional

You are not automatically prepared for your new role as activity department head simply because you have the training to manage resident activity programs. You must feel confident in your abilities, as a professional, in your field and as a supervisor, to succeed in dealings with your administrator and co-workers.

In an article concerning departmental roles for the activity coordinator, Halberg and Waters (1991) equate effectiveness as an activity department head with the development of a positive self-image. They assert that many activity professionals do not have confidence in their abilities, and may actually contribute to a lack of approval by colleagues or the administrator by not behaving as supervisors. In a general study of the perceptions that activity professionals have of their abilities, Maypole (1985) agrees in part by suggesting that the average activity person does not see himself or herself in the role of department head or supervisor.

Acceptance of your role as a supervisor in the facility can be enhanced by a number of factors. First, realize that you are an important member of your facility and a partner with all the other activity professionals throughout the world in providing services to your residents. Second, feel more connected to others with similar concerns by plugging into one of the many activity, recreation, or other organizations mentioned in this book. Third, as an additional confidence booster, take every opportunity to develop your management skills. You may find a suitable coach within your facility, or you may prefer a more formal education to gain these vital skills. Finally, realize that recognition of yourself as a department head will increase as you experience initial job orientation, and participate in necessary employee in-service training. Information on in-service training is given in Chapter 18.

Initial Orientation

Because you have acquired the position of activity director or activity assistant, there is an assumption that you have been properly **trained** in your field as required by the state or federal regulations to which your facility adheres. Supplemental to your training is the necessary **orientation** to the following three subject areas:

1. Activity department policies, procedures, and guidelines
2. Administrative policies and procedures
3. Overview of key health care worker issues

Jerris (1993) suggests that all successful employee orientation programs should also include an overview of crucial procedures, an understanding of the expectations of the relationship between employers and employees and a recap of the benefits that employees can expect.

The orientation procedure for all new activity employees can be handled by use of an **orientation checklist**, provided by the supervisor and reviewed with the incoming employee. All listed items must be explained to the activity employee. Once the employee has reviewed the information and appears knowledgeable, the sheet is signed off by both the employee and the employer handling the orientation. A sample orientation checklist is provided in Figure 2-3.

Halberg and Waters (1991) illustrate "An Orientation and Training Checklist . . . " that adequately outlines an orientation sheet for activity assistants. The checklist they propose includes specific departmental practices for new activity professionals. Keller (1984) refers to the importance of activity professionals in developing "certain basic interpersonal relating skills" as part of their training as professionals in a predominantly helping field. Keller uses the model developed by Egan (1975) to illustrate the four basic skills (listening, responding, exploring and/or understanding, and acting) needed by activity professionals to assist their residents.

Additionally, within their work Halberg and Waters mention the significance of providing orientation to other departments for understanding the role of the activity department. The concept of initial orientation for all staff members on the workings of the activity department is sound, and can be accomplished by the activity staff's briefing of groups of new orientees. Another method of reaching general staff members is the making of presentations at general staff meetings by the activity staff. Chapter 18 provides more information on this topic.

All of the general subject areas that an activity professional needs for orientation in a facility are covered in this textbook. A specific list of critical activity areas that you think should be covered with new staff members during orientation needs to be prepared. The sample orientation checklist provides a proposed list of core activity areas.

Your Role as a Health Care Worker in Your Facility ....

Along with supporting your orientation specific to the activity department comes the crucial orientation and training you should receive as a health care worker in your facility. Some of the subject matter you should be exposed to varies among states (i.e., fire codes, safety), but many of the critical educational issues are federally mandated and must be adhered to by every facility. As shown in Figure 2–3, there are key issues for health care workers as well as administrative policies and procedures on which you must be skilled.

Key Health Care Issues

Areas for health care workers can be classified as either state or federally mandated, or facility specific. The following section outlines some of the primary training issues in both categories, and give a brief explanation of the training that you and all of your facility's co-workers should receive on each topic.

ACTIVITY DEPARTMENT ORIENTATION CHECKLIST

I. Activity Department Policies and Procedures
   A. General
      ___review of job description
      ___acknowledgement of hours
      ___activity department work schedule
      ___review of departmental policies and procedures
      ___policy on reporting absences, latenesses
      ___communicating with other departments
      ___requesting time off
   B. Assessment and Documentation
      ___therapeutic assessment
      ___MDS
      ___care planning
      ___quarterly reviews
      ___interdisciplinary progress notes
      ___interdisciplinary care plan meeting
   C. Program Planning
      ___start on time
      ___room usage
      ___use of calendars, newsletters, reminders
      ___emergency activity plan
      ___special events planning
      ___function request form
      ___use of equipment
      ___review of programming based on resident needs
      ___room activities
      ___working with special populations
      ___working with volunteers
   D. Miscellaneous
      ___feeding of residents
      ___therapeutic diets
      ___exercise/range of motion policies
      ___lifting/transferring residents
      ___in-service/seminar attendance policy

II. Administrative Policies and Procedures
      ___facility history/ownership information
      ___facility mission statement/objectives
      ___fire/disaster plan
      ___organizational chart
      ___payroll procedures/payday
      ___time clock use
      ___employee entrance
      ___resident security system
      ___employee benefits explained
      ___transporting residents
      ___facility meetings schedule
      ___incident report
      ___I-9 Form completed
      ___absenteeism policy
      ___abuse reporting

Figure 2–3 The orientation checklist should be completed within the first few days of employment (*continued on next page*).

___confidentiality
___quality assurance/improvement program
___use of facility van or vehicles
III. Overview of Health Care Issues
___resident rights
___OSHA
___bloodborne pathogens
___hazard communication
___Tuberculosis exposure plan
___infection control
___handwashing
___nosocomial infections
___universal precautions
___review of specific infections (i.e., MRSA)
___sharps/location of sharps containers
___Americans With Disabilities Act
___facility modifications to provide access
___advance directives/living wills
___ethics committee
___medical device reporting
___medical waste
___chemical and physical restraints

I have been fully oriented on the aspects of my position.

_____   _____
Employee Signature   Date

_____   _____
Supervisor   Date

Figure 2–3 The orientation checklist should be completed within the first few days of employment (*continued*).

State or Federally Mandated Programs. Requirements in this training category come from either federal or state laws that govern the operation of either health care facilities or businesses. Rulings or regulations have been introduced that guard you as a worker or protect the residents within your facility. You should become familiar with the necessary program elements from this list that are required in your facility.

Occupational Safety and Health Administration (OSHA) mandates a number of regulations that involve a worker's protection from occupational risks and hazards. There are four areas of the OSHA standards on which you should be oriented: **bloodborne pathogens, hazard communication, tuberculosis exposure,** and **ergonomic rules.** Bloodborne pathogen rulings in the Federal Register (1991) were put in place to protect potentially exposed workers from diseases such as **Hepatitis B virus (HBV), human immunodeficiency virus (HIV),** and others which can be transmitted through contact with blood. Each facility is required to develop an **exposure control plan** that outlines the specific employees within your facility who are covered by the standard, lists procedures that employees must follow to minimize the risks of exposure, and mandates the guidelines that must be adhered to for any incident of accidental exposure. In order to protect employees from exposure, the OSHA standard also requires adherence to specific procedures such as following **universal precautions,** practicing good handwashing techniques, managing contact with needles and other **sharps,** wearing protective gear when needed, and receiving an HBV vaccination against possible exposure. The importance of developing very specific facility policies for handling diseases such as AIDS was stressed by Eschelman (1994). Practicing universal precautions means that you, as an activity professional working in the long-term care environment, must treat each contact with a resident as a potential exposure to a bloodborne illness. Therefore, you must reduce your risk by exercising good handwashing practices before and after each exposure to a resident. You should also be aware of contact with needles or other sharps, although you should not have direct contact under normal circumstances. Another method of practicing the concepts of universal precautions is to use personal protective equipment such as gloves, masks, eyewear, and so forth, if you know that you may be exposed to a potentially hazardous situation. Determine if your position has been identified as being covered by this standard in your facility's exposure plan, and if you have access to the HBV vaccination that is offered free of charge to all potentially exposed employees. Most facilities are realizing that activity professionals, with their high level of interaction with residents, staff, and all areas of the building, should be routinely considered as potentially at risk for exposure to bloodborne diseases.

The second OSHA requirement that effects you as an activity professional is in the area of hazard communication, reported in the Federal Register (1987). As a reaction to concerns about health care workers and other employees who potentially may be exposed to unknown chemicals on the job, OSHA set up a method for ensuring that workers were aware of, and able to protect themselves from, chemical hazards and injuries. Employers and employees are responsible for identifying potentially hazardous materials in the workplace and providing detailed information on the hazards they contain, along with notification and training for employees who come in contact with them. In the activity area, the kinds of potentially hazardous chemicals are items such as adhesive, glue, paint, stains, inks, varnishes, shellacs, wood preservatives, paint thinners, strippers, sealers, insecticides, herbicides, and detergents. Because this list contains only general categories, you should check each product in your supply closet and any new items you purchase. After determining the list of potentially hazardous chemicals with which your employees and residents may come in contact, talk to your supplier or the manufacturer of the products to obtain a copy of the **Material Safety Data Sheet (MSDS)** for each product. The data sheets, required and supplied by the product manufacturers, conform to uniform reporting standards that include the name of the product, the name and address of the manufacturer, the technical and common name of each hazardous ingredient, any known health hazards, safety precautions for handling, and emergency procedures for first aid, spills, and clean up. Your responsibility to the activity department requires that you obtain your MSDS sheets for identified hazardous materials and,

once received, hold in-service training with your staff to ensure that all chemicals are used properly. As new products are purchased, it is your responsibility to obtain the new product sheets and inform your staff. As we will discuss in Chapter 6, it is recommended that you maintain your activity-related MSDS sheets in your office and in any primary work area, such as an activity room. Your facility may also require that a master binder of all MSDS sheets be kept in the administrator's office. Be sure to update all binders when new MSDS sheets become available.

A third important area of information you should obtain from OSHA concerns the exposure guidelines for tuberculosis (TB), as noted by the United States Department of Labor (1992). The directive, which follows the **Centers for Disease Control and Prevention (CDC)** (1990) guidelines, was set up in response to employee notifications concerning possible tuberculosis exposure. The measure describes the method of transmission for tuberculosis as ". . . generated when a person with infectious TB disease coughs, speaks, sings, or spits." It is easy to see why activity professionals and other health care workers need proper education and protection from exposure. The guideline also discusses the employer requirements for long-term care facilities for the elderly which has been identified in the report as one of the ". . . workplaces where CDC has identified workers as having a greater incidence of TB infection." Some of the required employer protection strategies for handling and preventing tuberculosis exposure include free medical screening and tests for all employees at the pre-employment stage, and annually thereafter. A more frequent schedule has been established for any worker who has had exposure. Additionally, there are procedures for early diagnosis of active cases, assistance for employees with positive test results, isolation protocol, protective equipment for any possible or determined case, and most important, educational and training information for all workers. Consult with your administrator to ascertain if there are any further requirements in your particular state.

In her article, Spindel (1995) discusses the last area of rules that may effect you as an activity professional. The draft of the OSHA ergonomics rules, if passed, will pertain to personnel with employment responsibilities that involve **signal risk factors**. These signal risk factors include repetitive motions, awkward postures, or handling by lifting or pushing.

During your initial orientation, be aware of the compliance standards of the ADA, as referenced in the Federal Register (1990). This is a civil rights law that was developed to protect qualified individuals with disabilities from discrimination during application, hiring, discharge, compensation, and other employment-related processes. The law details five areas called "titles," that outline specific compliance criteria. Although each title is important, titles I, II, and III have the most applications to the long-term care industry. Title I specifically prohibits an employer from discriminating against disabled individuals in any hiring practices, and directs that reasonable accommodation be made to adapt existing positions to disabled workers. According to Heller (1992), employers have a responsibility to ". . . make the existing positions accessible and may use: . . . job restructuring . . . job reassignment . . . part-time or modified schedules . . . unpaid leave . . . modification of equipment . . . qualified interpreters . . . reassignment of qualified persons to another job . . . appropriate modification of hiring practices." Before the hiring process begins, ensure that the activity department job descriptions comply with the standards of Title I in terms of listing essential job duties, mentioning physical capabilities required, measurement of technical skills needed, and recommendations that can be made for accommodating the position to an applicant. Also, ensure that a hiring procedure is in place that addresses the ADA guidelines and does not permit certain inquiries to be made such as the mental or physical disabilities of a particular applicant. Title II further protects the disabled by making it illegal for participants in government programs (i.e., Medicare or Medicaid) to discriminate against disabled persons. This title is applicable in your initial and on-going training of activity staff on sensitivity to the handicapped, and adaptability of programs for all persons. Title III outlines environmental modifications that must be made by a facility owner to provide access to all services in a particular building. Familiarize yourself and your staff during initial orientation as to how your facility specifically accommodates disabled residents, staff, and visitors through its use of items such as ramps, wide hallways, braille symbols, and so forth.

Learning about **advance directives**, defined as ". . . a written instruction, such as a **living will** or **durable power of attorney** for health care. . . " is a crucial part of your initial health care training in a facility, and is referenced in the Federal Register (1992). Although the mandate is federal, each state addresses the issue of advance directives under its particular state law, usually contained as a ruling in the state administrative code. Understand how the laws in your state interpret the defi-

nitions of advance directive, living will, and durable power of attorney. Both the living will and durable power of attorney are written documents. The difference between them, however, is that the living will describes the residents' wishes for health care under terminal conditions whereas the durable power of attorney designates a person or **health care proxy** (a substitute who has the authority or power) to make health care decisions under circumstances when a resident is unable to do so. Although similar in sound and sometimes appearance, a durable power of attorney is very different from a power of attorney document that normally stipulates authority over the financial aspects of a resident's care. In some cases, attorneys put the two documents together in one form. The admission director or social worker should analyze these forms closely as the resident enters the facility to avoid confusion in the future.

Each facility normally sets specific policies for handling advance directives that are written with state and federal guidelines. As an activity professional, you are not as directly involved in the interpretation of an advance directive to a resident as some of your colleagues, such as the director of nursing, but you should be aware of both the federal and state guidelines. If your facility is large, you may, as part of your duties, become a member of the **bioethics committee**, which gives you exposure in handling problems concerning death and a resident's right to die. The committee usually meets on a quarterly, or more frequent, basis to ensure that resident issues are being managed correctly. One of the hardest tasks that many facility staff members face in honoring the guidelines of the advance directive ruling, particularly those in nursing, is to grant a resident's medical wishes by not rendering aggressive medical care. Interpreting and following advance directives for physicians, family members, and staff can often be a draining experience. Check your facility's policy on the witnessing of advance directives and other official documents. Most facilities inform their staff to *never witness or sign* any documents to avoid possible conflict of interest problems at a later time. As a health care worker and activity professional, you should receive annual in-service training on the subject of advance directives to keep you current.

Understanding the principles of bioethics is important to you as a professional on the bioethics committee. Shank (1985) feels that there are four main bioethical principles: "autonomy, beneficence, non-malfience, and justice." Autonomy is defined as the act of allowing "unconditional regard" for a patient's worthiness and his or her ability to choose his or her own fate. Beneficence and non-malfiicience are related: beneficence is the commitment of health care professionals to "act in ways that benefit patients" and non-malficience requires that professionals cause no harm. Principles of justice ask that fair guidelines be used so that treatment is appropriate and deserved. Shank feels that these principles govern our interpretation of not only advance directive issues, but also our general approach to care.

Another federal law that you should be aware of is called the **Medical Device Reporting Act** as reported by the Federal Register (1991). This regulation of the Food and Drug Administration (FDA), was established to track the reporting of injuries, illness, or death that are a direct result of faulty medical equipment so that manufacturers can be contacted and held accountable. Since medical equipment covers a broad range of everything in a facility from wheelchairs to feeding pumps, any staff member may be a witness to, or participant in, an incident that involves a defective piece of equipment. Learn about the procedure in your facility for filling out an incident report following staff or resident injury. If there is any question that a medical device was involved in an injury, you must include it in the incident report, and notify the administrator immediately. In order to track this information more easily, many facilities have updated their incident report forms to include an area which asks the question "Was the injury or accident a result of a faulty medical device or manufacturers' defect?" The administrator, or another designated staff member, has the responsibility of reporting to the FDA any determined injuries that were attributed to faulty medical devices.

A federal ruling that should be part of your initial staff training is the verification of employment eligibility through use of an **I-9 Form**. The United States Department of Justice, Immigration and Natural Service (1991) issued the Immigration and Reform Control Act that requires employees to verify they are hiring only United States citizens and aliens authorized to work. This verification process occurs through the use of an I-9 Form. The form requires the applicant to complete a written section and produce physical proof of citizenship or alien registration. The employer is responsible for reviewing the paperwork submitted by the applicant, and making photocopies. If the paperwork meets the guidelines for legal employment, the applicant may be considered if she or he also meets the qualifications for the specific job function. You should complete an I-9 form at the time of your initial employment, and will be required to handle I-9 paperwork for any activity assistants you wish to consider for employment in the future.

Compliance with federal laws for programs outlined under OSHA standards, ADA, Medical Device Reporting Act, and the Immigration Reform Act are strict, and hold varying degrees of monetary penalties for facility noncompliance. For more information on how investigations are conducted and penalties assessed, refer to the specific ruling documents listed as references for this chapter.

Adherence to federal and state rulings for advance directives for residents in your individual facility is monitored by your state **Ombudsman** office, an agency created to handle reported acts of complaints or abuse. Ombudsman offices are subdivisions of each state's Office on Aging, mandated originally by the Older Americans Act of 1981. Questions concerning interpretation of advance directives in a state is usually handled by the attorneys in this office. The penalties for noncompliance are not monetary. The potential for liability and malpractice, however, exists for such participants as the attending physician, facility administrator, and nursing personnel in the handling of the advance directive. Contact your state Ombudsman office or an attorney for more information.

Facility Specific Programs. There are many initial orientation topics that have specific guidelines for your particular facility. The information may be presented to you by your administrator or such co-workers as a department head or formal in-service coordinator. The following is a list of some areas that should be included in your facility orientation:

Absenteeism. To maintain the level of services that residents receive, most facilities have a policy as to how absences should be reported. The procedure includes the minimum amount of time needed to call the facility before your scheduled work time, who should be notified, what type of validating information about an absence is required, and how a pattern of absences is handled.

Reporting Abuse. Each state has guidelines for **abuse reporting** to the proper agency if resident abuse, either verbal or physical, is noted by staff members. Your state Department of Health office has a hot-line for the public to report complaints or suspected abuse of the elderly. Chapters 2 and

3 of the Older Americans Act, Administration on Aging (1992), and Title VII also provide "vulnerable elder rights protection" through The Long-Term Care Ombudsman program and Programs for Prevention of Elder Abuse, Neglect, and Exploitation. The ombudsman program provides a forum for resolving complaints made by, or on behalf of, residents of health care facilities whereas the programs for the prevention of elder abuse provide training and education to area agencies that care for the elderly.

Administrative Policies and Procedures. Members of administration have already established policies on many topics that you must be familiar with to do your job properly. Some of the policies and procedures may include smoking in the facility, personal phone calls, appropriate areas for consuming food, uniforms and/or proper attire, name tags, package inspection, responsibility for keys, and so forth.

Committee/Meeting Participation. In your role as activity professional, you are expected to attend a number of meetings that convene on a normal schedule. The number and type of meetings vary among facilities, but the following is a sample list of what you might expect based on your position:

Activity Director (department head)

1. *Ad Hoc Committee:* formed to study or resolve a particular problem (i.e., choosing a new logo for the facility).
2. *Budget Committee:* meets at least yearly with the administrator and other department heads to discuss the facility budget.
3. *Department Head Meeting:* meets weekly, bi-weekly, or monthly to discuss interdepartmental issues with the administrator. Hunter (1984) found that at least seventy-five percent of all activity professionals attended department head meetings on a regular basis.
4. *Ethics Committee:* members usually assigned by the administrator, and may include the medical director, social worker, other department heads, and clergy. May meet monthly, quarterly, or on an as-needed basis to resolve or monitor resident issues regarding ethics (i.e., advance directives, living wills, and so on).
5. *Interdisciplinary Care Plan Meeting:* usually meets at least once a week to handle joint care planning between nursing, social services, dietary, activities, and other rehabilitation services (i.e., **occupational therapy, speech therapy,** and **physical therapy**).
6. *Quarterly Quality Assurance/Therapeutics Meeting or Quarterly Board of Directors*

Meeting: meets four times a year with representatives from all disciplines to review facility progress. Some facilities may have other committees to handle unique concerns such as resident behavior issues or specialty wings.

Activity Assistant

1. *General Staff Meeting:* attended by all staff members, this meeting is held on a regular basis, usually monthly or quarterly. The administrator makes announcements, then opens the floor to questions and comments from all attendees.
2. *Safety Committee/Risk Management Meeting:* usually attended by a representative from each discipline and shift, this committee reviews incident reports, safety issues, and prevention measures on a quarterly or monthly basis.

Confidentiality. Adherence to the policy of not disclosing information about a resident's care except in situations where it is required is an important part of a resident's rights.

Equipment Use. It cannot be assumed that all new staff are familiar with the proper operation of wheelchairs, gerichairs, or other equipment. Murphy (1994) states that the parts of a wheelchair are important to understand, and illustrates the different methods of handling and adjusting a wheelchair for maximum comfort and safety of the resident. Other modes of mobility (i.e., walking aides) are described with details on their use.

Feeding. Many activity staff members routinely participate in the resident's dining regimen by helping design interdepartmental dining situations or feeding residents. Although cross-training of all staff is definitely an administrative advantage, the proper techniques of feeding residents must be taught to staff members by either the nursing staff or the speech therapist. Residents who require feeding assistance should be referred to by staff members as "**enhanced diners**" rather than by the derogatory term "**feeders**."

Fire and Disaster Planning. Every facility must have a written plan for handling fire and disasters. The plan must include a procedure for contacting fire and disaster workers, designating an "in-charge" person, specific responsibilities for every staff member, setting up of a **triage** area (if injuries have occurred), evacuating the facility, and preserving medical records of residents. In addition to a written plan, facilities are required to post an **evacuation plan** in a number of prominent places that describes the exit routes from the building by using a floor plan of the facility.

Another part of the disaster planning process includes the securing of transfer agreements between the facility and one or more local health care facilities. A **transfer agreement** is a written statement of intent between two or more facilities to transfer and house residents temporarily in case of emergency. Fire drills are normally conducted monthly, and disaster drills that involve fire and rescue workers are conducted once or twice a year. If you are unclear on any aspect of your facility's fire and disaster plan at the time of your orientation, or at any time during your employment, make it your responsibility to obtain clarification of your role in a disaster.

Incident Reports. All facilities are required to keep track of, and follow up on, resident and employee incidents and accidents, but how these occurrences are monitored is specific to each facility. An **accident** is an event where injury has occurred whereas an **incident** has a broader meaning, including such circumstances as an accident (an employee slips on a wet floor), or possibly a more unusual occurrence (a resident attempts to elope from the facility). Most facilities require that incident reports be completed on a standard form by either supervisory personnel or department heads within a reasonable period of time (twelve to twenty-four hours) after the actual incident. Your facility should have separate procedures for handling resident incidents and employee incidents. All incidents should be reviewed by administrative personnel for immediate follow-up, and by the safety/risk management committee for acknowledgement of any positive or negative trends (i.e., the number of resident falls on the 7–3 shift decreased during the last three months). Some resident incidents, as well as a few facility incidents, are reportable to either the state Department of Health or the state ombudsman. Employee incidents should be monitored due to OSHA guidelines; procedures are in place for reporting employee injuries and any loss of work time to the facility's **worker's compensation** insurance carrier.

Infection Control. Preventing and controlling the spread of infection in any facility is the responsibility of all employees. Cross-contamination can occur between objects, surfaces and through resident contact without proper monitoring. The infection control program at your facility most likely has three components:

■ identification of infections and education for employees and residents
■ good handwashing techniques, and the use of universal precautions during care

■ data collection and monitoring of infections within the facility to prevent spreading.

Traditionally, the nursing department has been responsible for establishing an infection control program for the facility. As a new employee, you should learn about proper **handwashing** techniques and universal precautions. Garner and Favero (1985) published a study on handwashing, defined as ". . . a vigorous, brief rubbing together of all surfaces of lathered hands, followed by rinsing under a stream of water." They provide specific guidelines on how and when to utilize proper handwashing techniques, and state that "handwashing is the single most important procedure for preventing **nosocomial infections**." Nosocomial infections are acquired in a hospital-like environment through contact with equipment or personnel. During orientation, you should also learn about some specific infections (i.e., **Methicillin-resistant *Staphylococcus aureus* [MRSA]**) that are becoming more common to the long-term care environment. MRSA is a prime example of a nosocomial infection of which long-term care employees from every department must be aware. Because of its resistance to traditional antibiotic therapy, and the fact that transmission is made from hand to hand contact, according to Boyce et al. (1994), MRSA infections can be spread easily throughout a facility unless a strategy and an infection control plan are in place. Continual monitoring of any existing infections within the facility through laboratory testing and close surveillance of specific areas of employee contact (i.e., table tops and faucet handles) should be undertaken on at least a quarterly basis.

Lifting. The lifting of residents, or any lifting for that matter, should only be undertaken after proper training. Your facility may have a policy to identify staff who are permitted to lift. Because of your close association with residents who may need assistance, you should clarify your responsibilities and abilities in this area.

Medical Waste. The collection, tracking, and proper disposal of medical waste (sharps, blood products) has been regulated in recent years by the Environmental Protection Agency (EPA) and OSHA for the protection of health care workers. Each facility follows the guidelines for collection and disposal in their state by keeping detailed records of the date and quantity of medical waste that left the facility, and which designated waste management company was used to remove it. You will probably not be involved with medical waste to any great extent, but you should be aware of how medical waste is defined within

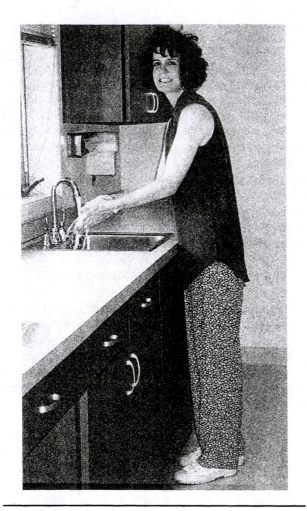

Figure 2–4 Frequent handwashing is crucial to prevent the spread of infection.

your facility, and how to handle any contact or disposal problems should they arise.

Quality Assurance. In Chapter 14, information is provided on how to establish a quality assurance program, a written accounting measure of the outcome of your programs against standards that have been predetermined for the activity department. The quality assurance program for the activity department is part of the larger facility program that you heard about during your orientation. Your progress in quality assurance should be reported quarterly to the committee.

Residents' Rights. Each new employee should become familiar with the rights of residents in your facility. These rights are part of the regulations of the OBRA guidelines, Federal Register (1991) guidelines, and include information on the following resident topics:

- exercise rights as a citizen

- be provided with notice of rights and services
- be notified of any changes
- have funds protected
- have free choice in physician and care
- expect privacy and confidentiality
- air grievances
- view survey results
- work or not work as one chooses
- receive mail and other communications
- have access and visitation rights upheld
- use the telephone
- have personal property protected
- share a room as a married couple
- self-administer drugs if determined appropriate
- refuse certain transfers.

Additionally, the facility must uphold these quality of life factors for residents:

- dignity and self-determination
- participation in resident and family groups, and in other activities
- accommodation of needs
- provide care that is fair and free from abuse.

Updates to the initial OBRA mandate include guidelines on quality of life and acknowledges participation in facility administration, and personal and privacy rights of residents. The large amounts of time that you spend with residents allows you to become a greater advocate for maintaining these rights.

Restraints. By OBRA regulation, residents must be free from any chemical or physical restraint that inhibits or controls behavior. The "least restrictive" environment is sought by the nursing department for each resident in the facility on an individual basis. At the time of orientation, the facility approach to restraint usage should be explained to you so that you can understand your resident, and know your responsibilities in protecting them when they attend a program in the activity room or are visited by an activity director in an individual room. If a restraint is in use on a particular resident in your care, you must understand the release schedule for the restraint, what interventions have been tried prior to restraint use, how the restraint is applied and maintained, and what expected behaviors may occur in the particular resident. You should report the results of the resident's participation in your program and your participation in restraint release and reapplication to the charge nurse or supervisor. Having the nursing department delegate the responsibility for temporarily monitoring a restraint to another member of the care giving team such as yourself can only be done if you are properly trained in this procedure.

Security. Many facilities opt for security systems to protect confused residents from wandering into unsafe areas. If your facility has such a system, learn about its operation during your orientation. Obtain a list of residents who should be monitored against unsafe wandering so that you and your staff can be aware of potential problems (i.e., residents who are noticed in an unsafe area or residents who are seen without an alarm mechanism, if required). Some facilities have found it useful to keep a dignified notebook in the main office of pictures of residents who might wander out of the facility through a main entrance with visitors. In addition to resident safety, you should also be briefed on employee security, use of lockers, exit and entrance doors, safe parking for evening workers, and so forth.

Therapeutic Diets. Residents in long-term care settings are placed on an array of diets, ordered by their physicians and based on their medical needs. Diet options may include "regular," changes in consistency of food such as "chopped" or "pureed" (strained or put through a blender), or diets based on calories or nutrients such as "diabetic" or "1500 calories." A list of individuals with serious diet restrictions should be obtained from the dietary department and updated regularly. Know the dietary restrictions of your residents to avoid safety and emotional issues during activity programs that feature food. Substitutes for forbidden foods should be provided to those residents who are unable to have them.

Transfers/Transporting Residents. Resident transfers from bed to chair or chair to wheelchair are normally made by trained professionals (nurses and certified nursing assistants). Occasions will arise, however, when you must transfer a resident to assist them to an activity. You should receive initial training on how to handle a transfer safely. The information presented earlier on proper use of equipment (a wheelchair coupled with some hints on proper lifting and body mechanics) is necessary to prepare you. Transporting residents to program areas is best done by a combination of activity staff, nursing staff, and assistance from all other available staff. Each facility is unique in approaching this issue. See how it is handled in your facility, and if changes are required, speak to the appropriate departments.

Summary

Receiving a thorough orientation on activity procedures, health care worker issues, and training information on specific facility policies provides a solid ground for your work as a full member of the health care team. Ongoing in-service programming and your own educational interests will help you continue your knowledge about health care and your residents.

R E V I E W   Q U E S T I O N S

1. What is the name of the diagram that depicts the lines of authority within the facility?
2. What is an exposure control plan, and how does such a plan relate to the activity department?
3. Where can you find the written expectations for your department in case of a facility emergency?
4. Define a nosocomial infection and give an example.
5. What type of document should be completed for a facility accident or unusual occurrence?

O N   Y O U R   O W N

1. What are six other activity specific items that can be added to your orientation checklist for new employees in your department?
2. What are some of the ways that you, as an activity professional, can contribute at an ethics committee meeting?
3. Describe how you can effectively uphold residents' rights during routine programming.

R E F E R E N C E S

Administration on Aging (1992). *Vulnerable elder rights protection: Older Americans Act.* DHHS Publication: Elder Facts. Washington, D. C.

Boyce, J. M., Jackson, M. M., Pugliese, G., Batt, M. D.,

Fleming, D., Garner, J. S., Hartstein, A. I., Kauffman, C. A., Simmons, M., Weinstein, R., Williams, C. O., and AHA Technical Panel on Infections Within Hospitals (1994). Methicillin-resistant staphylococcus aureus (MRSA): A briefing for acute care hospitals and nursing facilities. *Infection Control Hospital Epidemiology*, 15, 105–115.

Centers for Disease Control (1990). *Guidelines for preventing the transmission of tuberculosis in health-care settings, with special focus on HIV-related issues.* Morbidity and Mortality Weekly Report, Vol. 43, RR-13. Rockville, MD: author.

Egan, G. (1975). *The skilled helper: A model for systematic helping and interpersonal relating.* Monterey, CA: Brooks/Cole Publishing Co.

Eshleman, M. J. (1994). AIDS in the workplace: Implementing an AIDS policy. *Health Care Supervisor*, 13 (2), 51–57.

Federal Register (1987). Vol. 52., No. 163. *Hazard communication standard.*

Federal Register (1991). November 26, 1991. *Safe Medical Devices Act.*

Federal Register (1991). Vol. 56., No. 144. *Non-discrimination on the basis of disability in state and government services; Final rule.*

Federal Register (1991). Vol. 56., No. 235. *Occupational exposure to bloodborne pathogens standard.*

Federal Register (1991). Vol. 56., No. 187. *Omnibus budget reconciliation Act.*

Federal Register (1992). Vol. 57., No. 45. *Patient self-determination act.*

Garner, J. S., & Favero, M. S. (1985). *Guideline for handwashing and hospital environment control.* (PB85-923404) Springfield, VA: National Technical Information Service.

Goldsmith, S. B. (1994). *Essentials of long-term care administration.* Gaithersburg, MD: Aspen Publishers.

Halberg, K. J., & Waters, E. (1991). Functioning as a department head and supervisor: A new role for the activity coordinator. In P. M. Foster (Ed.), *Activities in action*, (p. 61–85). Binghamton, NY: The Haworth Press.

Heller, U. (1992). Surviving with the ADA: Hiring staff. *Nursing Homes*, August 1992.

Hunter, H. C. (1984). The activity director in a nursing care facility: How does she fit in? *Activities, Adaptation and Aging*, 4 (4), 13–43.

Jerris, L. A. (1993). *Effective employee orientation.* New York, NY: American Management Association.

Keller, M. J. (1984). Activity personnel as professional helpers. *Activities, Adaptation and Aging*, 4 (4), 51–60.

Maypole, D. E. (1985). Activity therapist continuing education needs assessment. *Activities, Adaptation and Aging*, Vol. 7 (2), 15–23.

Murphy, A. (1994). *Working with elderly people.* London, England: Souvenir Press.

Shank, J. (1985). Bioethical principles and the practice of therapeutic recreation in clinical settings. *Therapeutic Recreation Journal*, 4th quarter, 31–40.

Spindel, M. (1995). Agency pushes for ergonomics rule. *Provider*, July, 65–66.

United States Department of Justice, Immigration and Naturalization Service (1991). *Handbook for employers, instructions for completing form I–9* (Employment eligibility verification form). Washington, DC: author.

United States Department of Labor, Occupational Safety and Health Administration (1992). *Enforcement guidelines for occupational exposure to tuberculosis.* New York State Public Employee Safety/ OSHA National Office.

··· **F U R T H E R   R E A D I N G** ···

Hommel, P., & Wood, E. (1990). Guardianship: There are alternatives. *Aging*, No. 360, 6–12.

Iris, M. (1988). Guardianship and the elderly: A multi-perspective view of the decisionmaking process. *The Gerontologist*, Vol. 28, 39–45.

Jackson, V. R. (1994). The ethical value of a utilitarian approach to death and dying. *Activities, Adaptation and Aging*, Vol. 18, No. 3/4, 89–94.

Kimboko, P., & Jewell, E. (1994). A beginner's guide to ethical awareness in long-term care services. *Activities, Adaptation and Aging*, Vol. 18, No. 3/4, 5–26.

Kjervik, D., Miller, I., Jezek, K., & Weisensee, M. (1994). Decisions about guardianship for older persons: Incompetency criteria. *The American Journal of Alzheimer's Care and Related Disorders and Research*, July/Aug, 13–22.

Marinelli, R. (1994). Final life choices: Who decides? *Activities, Adaptation and Aging*, Vol. 18., No 3/4, 65–76.

Shavishinsky, J. (1991). *The ends of time: Life and work in a nursing home.* New York, NY: Bergin & Garvey.

Sylvester, C. (1982). Exploring confidentiality in therapeutic recreation practice: An ethical responsibility in need of response. *Therapeutic Recreation Journal*, 3rd qtr., 25–34.

Sylvester, C. D. (1985). An analysis of selected ethical issues in therapeutic recreation. *Therapeutic Recreational Journal*, 4th Quarter, 8–21.

United States Department of Justice (1991). *Nondiscrimination on the basis of disability in state and local government services: Final rule.* (Federal Register, Vol. 56, No. 144). Washington, DC: U. S. Government Printing Office.

United States Department of Justice (1994). *Enforcing the ADA: A status report update from the Department of Justice.* Washington, DC: author.

CHAPTER 3
Aging and the Physical/Psychosocial Needs of Residents

OBJECTIVES

After completing this chapter, you should:

- understand the aging process, including its physical, mental, and social aspects.
- know the systems of the body, disease processes, and medical terminology used in caring for the elderly.
- understand the psychosocial aspects of aging, and how medications effect residents.

INTRODUCTION

Delivering activity services to residents is a difficult task unless you first understand the medical needs of the residents you serve. Defining the aging process and clarifying the myths and stereotypes of aging will set the stage. A review of the body systems and disease processes offer a look at the situations that may be encountered during care. By considering the needs of specific age groups and medications used, a clearer picture of residents emerges.

The Aging Process

Studying the aging process will help you know the residents you will serve. **Aging**, defined by Atchley (1987), is ". . . a broad concept that includes phys-

ical changes that occur in our bodies over adult life, psychological changes in our mind and in our mental capacities, and social changes in how we are viewed, what we can expect and what is expected of us." He continues by stating that aging is not confined to one specific process, but has many "possible outcomes," both negative and positive. Another researcher, Krimsky (1969), offers this view of aging as ". . . a gradual progressive march toward greater maturity of mind and soul."

Aging Terminology

To comprehend the aging process, you should be familiar with the terminology used to describe each aspect. Hess and Markson (1980) trace the beginning of academic **gerontology** to the publication of three handbooks on the subject in the 1960s. Research continued, but interest in the field by politicians and decision-makers did not come until the passage of the **Older Americans Act**, adopted in 1965, and revised in 1973 and again in 1978. Gerontology is the study of old age, or the aging process, and according to Achenbaum and Levin (1989), seems to have no clear consensus of either definition or scope. A **gerontologist** is a person who studies or practices gerontology, but the position does not have clear cut boundaries in the medical field. A gerontologist may be a scientist, a sociologist, a researcher, or a medical person. **Geriatric medicine** is the study of illness and disability in the aged or elderly population. In a related area, Larue (1992) defines **geroethics** as ". . . consideration of ethical, moral and value issues as they pertain to elders."

Definitions that pertain to the indicators of age are also important to discuss. Atchley (1987) suggests that the three designations of age are **chronological age**, **functional capacity**, and **life stage**. Chronological age is the amount of years that a person has lived, according to birth records, and is not always a fair indication of the capabilities of a person. Classifications vary when chronological age is used as a determinant of job status or retirement eligibility. Functional capacity (i.e., mobility, appearance, and mental capacity) as an indicator of age may lead to incomplete conclusions and categorizations of people. Applying this theory as an indicator of age would classify many people as "old" because they have premature gray hair or mild confusion. Chronologically, they would be considered "young." Life stages as a view of aging (i.e., adolescence, young adulthood, middle age, and old age) relies on a combination of physical and social attributes to categorize individuals. Physical decline and social changes, such as retirement, begin during middle age and continue into old age. The stage of old age that Atchley discusses is marked by restricted activity, more cases of chronic ailments, and increased physical frailty. This stage is also the one where institutionalization takes place, if at all. Even though the life stage concept of aging allows for broader classifications of the aging process, no theory can accurately predict the true definition of old age.

Other terms that should be noted are **life span**, **life expectancy**, and **ageism**. Life span is the length of biological time that a human being can be expected to live. At this time, 120 years is thought to be the longest human life span. Life expectancy is the average amount of time that most people actually live. Rates of life expectancy through the next decade, are calculated as seventy-five years of age when men and women are considered together and are based on **mortality rates**. Ageism, a term coined by Butler (1974), refers to ". . . a process of systematic stereotyping of discrimination against people, because they are old-just as racism and sexism can accomplish this with skin color and gender."

Developmental Stages

Just as Atchley discussed life stages as indicators of age, there have been theorists who propose that certain development life stages generalize and explain the life cycle that includes aging. Through concept work first published in the 1950s and primarily used for educational settings, Havighurst (1969) looked to describe human development by defining developmental tasks for particular age groups in areas such as physical maturation, social and societal expectations and personal values. The tasks of old age that Havighurst discusses are thought to be a defensive strategy against aging that involve loss adjustment, learning and experiencing new concepts. Havighurst lists the primary tasks of old age as decreasing strength, beginning retirement and experiencing reduced income, adjustment to death of spouse, affiliation with age, civic obligations and changes in living arrangements. Another theory, offered by Erikson (1963), concludes that the life cycle is made up of a succession of psychosocial crises points that propel individuals in different directions according to their specific responses. During late adulthood or old age, Erickson proposes that the crises points faced by individuals are in fact critiques of their lives with resolutions toward peace and perspectives on past triumphs and shortfalls.

TASKS OF PERSONALITY DEVELOPMENT

Growing Stage	Task
Infancy	Learning to trust
Early childhood years	Recognizing identity as part of a family unit
School years	Skill development; constructive activities
Adolescent years	Developing identity as an individual
Young adulthood	Forming intimate relationships, raising a family
Middle years	Carrying out one's chosen work
Old age	Integrating life's experiences

Figure 3–1 Erikson's development tasks.

Stereotypes and Myths of Aging

Stereotypes are negative generalizations or prejudices against the aged, or old age in general. Any form of stereotyping is harmful because a label is given to something which can be negative and based on general feelings, rather than on specific individuals. The term ageism, discussed above, was developed in response to the discrimination and generalization of aging. Myths, on the other hand, are usually untrue facts that over time, have come to be accepted and believed as true. Myths about aging abound, and account for much of the stereotyping behavior that exists.

One of the biggest myths about aging is the concept reported by Butler (1974) which suggests the idea of chronological aging as a determinant of age. Since individuals have different rates of physiological and psychological changes, the use of chronological age can be quite misleading. Other myths include the idea that older people are nonproductive, inflexible, senile, or serene. Butler explains that when experiencing mild physical or mental changes, most individuals can still be actively involved in their lives, and make the adjustments and changes, if needed. Using a catch-all category such as senility (what we now call cognitive impairment) to describe older people is limiting and untrue. Many forms of confusion can be explained by depression, anxiety, medication, or symptoms of other physical ailments. Generalizing the majority of older people as "serene" is also without basis. Butler points out that the elderly often cope with many more stresses and life adjustments than other age groups. Epstein (1977) adds that myths and stereotyping that include ideas as "There is a pervasive hopelessness about old age . . ." do much to damage our ability to care for the aged appropriately.

Palmore (1977) and subsequent researchers have used the misconceptions about aging as a teaching tool to test the knowledge of health care workers in this critical area. By using an easy to follow true or false format, Palmore devised an aging facts questionnaire that provided a mechanism for assessing education about aging.

Theories of Aging

In an attempt to comprehend the aging process, many researchers have offered theories on how aging actually occurs. These theories can be classified as either biological or social. The following list contains a summary of some of the most prevalent aging theories.

Biological Theories of Aging. To answer the question "What causes aging?" biological theories of aging were proposed that were rooted in the medical or scientific analysis of changes that individuals experience as a result of living a normal life span.

The first four theories of aging have a genetic basis that are discussed by Schock (1977) and Zastrow and Kirst-Ashman (1994).

The **cellular genetic theory** proposes that DNA molecules are either damaged or changed over time, and results in misinformation about the production of body enzymes. The lack of ability of the cells to produce the crucial enzymes eventually destroys the cells, alters the chain of genetic information, and leads to cell death.

The **error theory** suggests that because of a build-up of errors in sending or receiving DNA information, the cells become overloaded, and cell destruction results.

The **program theory** asserts that a finite amount of DNA material exists in each cell in the body. DNA is removed as the cells age, and eventually the cells die.

Additional biological theories of aging have been postulated that have a cellular basis (involve discussion of human cells), but do not pertain to genetics.

The **wear and tear theory** assumes that similar to machinery or equipment, the cells of the human body "wear out" from stress through repeated use, and eventually cease to function. Some researchers suggest that this theory may not be valid because of all the built-in repair mechanisms that the body possesses to deal with wear and tear.

The **accumulation theory** suggests that dangerous or toxic materials collect in the cells of the body over time, and cause them to die.

The **free radical theory** asserts that certain chemicals, called free radicals, have high levels of oxygen, and react with other body processes to alter their structure, and eventually kill the cells.

The **cross-linkage theory** hypothesizes that alterations in the properties of molecules are caused by bonds, or cross-links, that form over time. Once the chemical properties of the molecules are altered, cells misfunction and die.

Some aging researchers explain the aging process through a series of **physiological theories** that address the breakdown of the control mechanisms in the body, or failure of particular organ systems to function. "Physiological" refers to the physical and chemical properties of living matter.

The **organ system theory** asserts that one system of the body, such as the cardiovascular system, deteriorates through a disease process, and subsequently leads to aging and death.

The **immunological theory** purports that an older person who has a weakened immune system that cannot produce antibodies to properly fend off disease experiences variations in cell structure. Cells invaded by foreign bodies are not able to mount a defense, which results in cell destruction.

The **stress theory** assumes that the stresses and strains of life deposit impaired material in the cell structure after each stressful episode. Over a lifetime, the harmful matter accumulates, and results in cell destruction and death.

Social Theories of Aging. The social theories of aging explain the aging process in terms of social adaptations and psychological factors.

The **disengagement theory**, formulated by Cumming and Henry (1961), suggests that as the aging client's role in society declines, higher levels of satisfaction with life emerge. The researchers postulate that aging members of society want to acknowledge they are no longer young, and "disengage" or withdraw from societal roles in order to begin the emotional process of preparing for death. This aging theory is controversial for many health care workers, especially activity professionals, who support a continued, active role for the elderly in society.

The **activity theory** theorizes that high amounts of social involvement in valued roles produce feelings of self-satisfaction and increased esteem. Although this theory more closely relates to the goals of activity professionals, critics find the theory limiting because it requires a person to be active in order to achieve happiness.

The **continuity theory** speculates that older adults make choices of adaptation to maintain their existing structure and role in society. They use "continuity," or techniques they are already familiar with to apply to all situations in life.

The **exchange theory** assumes that older adults will continue interactions as long as the benefits of the exchange outmeasure any negative aspects, and conversely, they will remove themselves from any exchange that does not have positive interactions.

Aging Research

Research in the last fifty years has provided professionals with new information about the aging population and the normal expectations of aging. Learning about the characteristics of normal aging, or "aging in the absence of disease" as defined by the National Institute on Aging (1993), helps us understand ways to avoid chronic diseases and disabilities so often associated with aging.

A landmark study that has provided much in the way of general information about expected aspects of aging is the Baltimore Longitudinal Study, conducted since 1958 at the National Institute on Aging in Baltimore, Maryland. The study that first began with men, then expanded to include women in 1978, seeks answers to questions about biological and behavioral aspects of aging, draws relationships between biologic and behavior aspects, and makes general conclusions about universal trends in aging. It is called a **longitudinal study** because it takes place over a length of time. Testing is conducted on the same participants every two years. Another way to study aging, not used here, is to perform a cross-sectional study at a point in time on a group of individuals. Data for the Baltimore study was collected in numerous areas, including immune function, cognition, personality attributes, dietary factors, heart, lung, and kidney function, and body composition.

Using the Baltimore Longitudinal Study data (1993), two themes emerge that have impacts against aging stereotypes. The first conclusion of the research is the fact that ". . . aging cannot be linked to a general or universal decline in all physical and mental functions." The second fact from the study is that "there is no single, simple, pattern to human aging." Another point drawn from the research is that the aging process is thought to have a great deal of variation, and is a very specific and individualized process.

On distinct issues, the study released some of their findings which are considered to be some of the aspects of normal aging. It is thought that the heart adapts as age increases, with output remaining almost the same as earlier years, but the incidence of coronary heart disease multiplies with age. If higher cholesterol levels exist in advanced years, it is considered a risk factor for heart disease. Lung capacity may decline approximately forty percent by age eighty. Mental skills are not thought to diminish as many propose. Personality factors usually remain constant over the entire span of life. Kidney and bladder function do decline over time, but incontinence can frequently be controlled by fitness and behavioral methods. Physical fitness is thought to decline up to ten percent every ten years. The pursuit of fitness is still encouraged, however, because there are links between moderate weight and living longer. Body fat does not decrease with age but redistributes itself in other areas (women in their hips and thighs, men in their abdomens). High frequency sounds may be harder to hear as one grows older, and men experience hearing decline more frequently than women. Vision declines with age, along with glare problems and difficulties in focusing in areas with low light.

The longitudinal nature of this work provides a continuing flow of important information on aging that will be read and studied in the years to come.

The Physical Aspects of Aging ....

When we think of aging, we most often think of the physical aspects, or outward signs, of decline that indicate aging is taking place. But there are actually three categories in which normal aging takes place: physical attributes, psychological factors, and the social arena. The physical area involves the health of an individual, and the proper operation of the systems of the body. The aging that takes place in the psychological part of an individual's being concerns the mind, feelings, and overall mental health. Social factors involve relationships, family, and the impacts on aging that come from issues such as satisfaction or isolation. By reviewing each body system, and understanding the diseases that may be present in the elderly, physical as well as mental and social problems that can occur, brings comprehension to the large task that activity professionals face in caring for the aging resident.

The Body Systems and Disease Processes

Defining physical components of the normal aging process begins with an overview of each of the key body systems. A body system is comprised of a series of organs and parts that coordinates and handles specific functions to maintain proper physical environment within the body. A brief review of the crucial factors in each body system is covered, along with a discussion of the physical changes that occur during aging.

To complement this body system review, some of the major diseases in each body system category associated with elderly residents is also mentioned. A disease is defined as a disruption of normal functioning within one or more systems or organs in the human body. Hegner and Caldwell (1994) report that conditions of disease

in the elderly can result from **trauma** (forceful injury to the body), congenital problems (those present at birth), chemical imbalances, blood supply problems, obstructions, abnormal cell growth, and infections. Other issues that may have a bearing on whether a particular disease develops include such "predisposing factors" as chronic conditions, genetic make-up, lifestyle, diet, sex, and, of course, age.

Diagnosing disease takes place by identifying **symptoms**, or the evidence of disease elements such as fever, pain, or vomiting.

Looking for clues about common disease factors in the elderly brings us to the results of the 1985 National Nursing Home Survey, United States Department of Health & Human Services (1989), which provides some clues to the prevalence of particular diseases in admitted residents. The survey shows that the leading category of disease on admission is heart disease. Other areas, such as mental disorders and diseases of the nervous system (Alzheimer's disease) are also highly represented in the survey. O'Morrow and Reynolds (1989) consider factors that cause healthy situations to occur versus disease-producing situations. They cite "enjoyable constructive recreation and use of leisure" along with "suitable exercise" and "love and belonging" as examples of factors that cause health-producing situations. Conversely, they mention "poor health factors," "stress," "sociocultural isolation and deprivation," and "excesses of deficiencies and deprivations" as determinants of disease-producing situations. Reactions to illness may also be different across cultures and varying developmental experiences.

It is assumed you will deal with disease in long-term care residents, but the situation may be complicated to manage for two reasons. First, a resident may be dealing with an **acute illness** phase of short duration, or a more **chronic** or extended pattern of illness of long duration. Second, as Saxon and Etten (1994) point out, residents may experience multiple health problems simultaneously that have conflicting drug and treatment regimens. Additionally, the symptoms of disease in elderly residents can be very different from the noticeable disease factors in other age groups, and often symptoms go undetected because of the reluctance of residents to report problems. To understand the variations in disease observation and reporting, many groups, such as the National Institute On Aging, Gastel (1994), have published clinician's guidelines that offer suggestions as to how to interact with elderly clients to gather clinical information. Disabilities, or conditions that restrict a person who is suffering from either an acute or chronic illness, are classified as major or minor. Atchley (1987) defines minor disabilities as those that cause limitations in areas other than employment, child care, or activities around the house. Major disabilities disturb the normal routine of primary activities such as employment, school, or child activities. Hess and Markson (1980) summarize by saying that ". . . health and illness are dynamic concepts that change with time, social circumstance, and values."

In long-term care settings, acute illness occurs, but with less frequency than chronic conditions. Most acute illnesses have an illness phase, followed by recovery. Chronic conditions, however, have gradually increasing medical requirements. Shivers and Fait (1985) point out that an individual suffering from an acute episode of an illness can often only focus on the illness and the people who are assisting with recovery. The narrow scope of the world to a person with an acute illness may appear to be a need only for physical comfort, nourishment, and rest. Kayser-Jones, Wiener, and Barbaccia (1989) mention the most common acute illnesses that cause residents of long-term care facilities to be hospitalized. These include symptoms of fever, cough, chest pain, changes in cognitive or emotional status, nausea, vomiting, and changes in cardiovascular status.

Chronic illnesses are very common among the elderly. Diseases such as arthritis, diabetes, hypertension, and hearing impairments are common chronic ailments noted by Lahey (1993). O'Morrow and Reynolds (1989) list illnesses in order of their most frequent appearance: heart condition, hypertension, chronic bronchitis, asthma, arthritis, diabetes, visual impairment, hearing impairment, and orthopedic impairment. Lahey mentions that a chronic illness does not often have a clear onset, and may begin with subtle changes that increase gradually over time. The Center for Corporate Health (1991) mentions that life skills such as remaining active, managing nutritional intake, maintaining social activity, and handling stress can assist in the prevention and management of chronic conditions. An individual's attitude toward chronic illness can have a great bearing on his or her behavior, according to Frye and Peters (1972). Influences such as family history, social class, ethnic background, educational status, occupation, religion, and recreational participation are all part of the development of an attitude to endure the length of a chronic illness. Burnside (1994) reminds us

that chronicity (possessing chronic conditions) may have implications for programming since multiple organ systems may be involved in the treatment of an illness.

The Integumentary System. The most visible system of the body is the one covering and containing all others. It is called the **integumentary system**.

Components of the integumentary system include the skin, oil and sweat glands of the skin, teeth, nails, and hair. The primary function of the integumentary system is to protect the rest of the body, maintain proper temperature, and act as a barrier and connection to the outside environment. The skin, thought to be the largest and most complex of the body systems, according to Saxon and Etten (1994), is comprised of a top layer called the epidermis, a second layer from the surface called the dermis, and the third or deepest layer called the subcutaneous tissue. See Figure 3–2 for a view of the components of the skin.

Aging factors related to the integumentary system, as reported by Hegner and Caldwell (1994) are:

- wrinkling of the skin caused by decreasing elasticity and fatty tissue
- loss of color from hair with the progression of from gray to white
- thickening of nails that cause brittleness and breakage
- weakening of blood vessels that cause spidery-looking hemorrhages in the epidermis
- slowing of production in the sweat glands

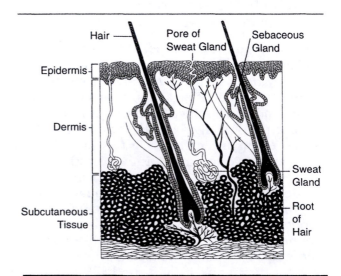

Figure 3–2 A view of the integumentary system.

- formation of moles, and other pigmentation changes
- missing teeth that require dentures or other dental work.

A chart highlighting the aging factors related to the integumentary system is shown in Figure 3–3.

■ *Integumentary*	Hair loses color and becomes thinner; skin dries, is less elastic, wrinkles develop, skin is fragile; fingernails and toenails thicken; sweat glands do not excrete perspiration as readily; oil glands do not secrete as much oil; increased sensitivity to cold.

Figure 3–3 A summary of the aging changes in the integumentary system.

Common diseases of the integumentary system that may be encountered by the elderly include:

- *cancer:* an abnormal growth of cells in one or more parts of the body.
- *decubitus ulcer:* a skin breakdown caused by pressure or friction and made worse by poor dietary intake.
- *infection:* bacterial or viral condition (i.e., a boil).

The Sensory System. Although not truly considered a body system, components of the sensory process as defined by Saxon and Etten (1994) are ". . . sight, hearing, taste, smell, touch, balance, and muscle sense." The purpose of the sensory organs is to aid a person in moving through the world by processing the information that comes in through the senses. All parts of the sensory process are important, but the two key components are the eye (necessary for vision) and the ear (necessary for hearing). A breakdown of the parts of the eye is shown in Figure 3–4, and the vital elements of the ear are illustrated in Figure 3–5.

Some of the aging factors related to the **sensory system** include a decrease in visual acuity and a decreased tolerance for glare. Saxon and Etten (1994) suggest that the vision changes cause increased risk for accidents. Verbal communication among the elderly may be at risk because of hearing loss or impairments. The work of Saxon and Etten report that more than half of all adults over age sixty-five may be experiencing hearing impairments of some sort that can, in turn, impact the quality of life of an individual. The sensitivity to taste may decrease with age, but researchers are not sure by how much. Olfactory ability (the ability to smell) also declines with age, and the elderly

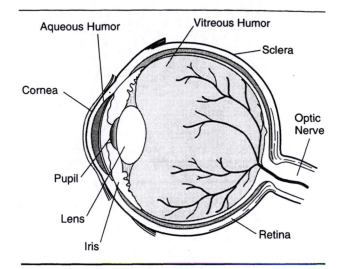

Figure 3–4 The key parts of the eye.

need stronger odors for recognition. Saxon and Etten point out that this is a safety factor in the prevention of accidents that are detected by odors. According to Saxon and Etten, there has been little research on the subject of touch. The sensation of touch is felt through the skin (integumentary system) and enables the body to react to hot, cold, or uncomfortable stimulation, and warns one of potentially dangerous situations. A greater increase in unsteadiness and imbalance is seen in the elderly because of changes that occur in the ear. Figure 3–6 shows some of the highlights of sensory changes that occur in aging.

The following is a list of some of the common diseases of the sensory system that can be seen in residents of a long-term care facility:

- *cataracts:* a murky or opaque film that forms over the eye because of protein changes in the majority of elderly, and causes impaired vision.
- *glaucoma:* a slow, progressive disease in which blindness results; because of a build-up of pressure in the eye.
- *tinnitus:* a common malady in older adults, especially those who have other hearing problems. This disorder is noted for the ringing or buzzing sounds that occur in the sufferer's ear.

The Cardiovascular System. The key elements of the **cardiovascular system** are the heart, arteries, veins, capillaries, and blood. The lymphatic and immune systems are also related to this system. The heart is a pumping muscle with four chambers that is responsible for the circulation of the blood through the arteries (largest passageways) to the veins, and finally into the capillaries (smallest passageways) and tissues and organs in the

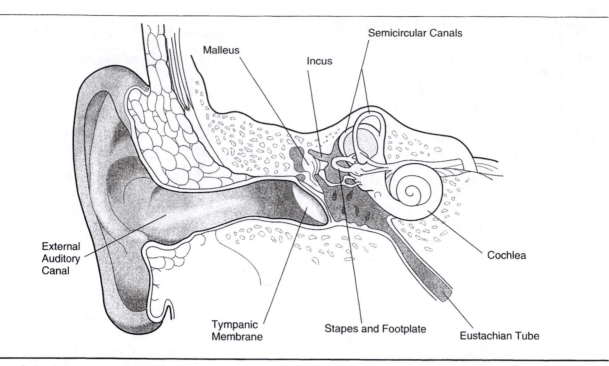

Figure 3–5   An overview of the ear.

- Degeneration of end organs
- Decreased sense of taste
- Decreased sense of touch
- Decreased sense of temperature
- Decreased sense of smell
- Decreased hearing ability
- Decreased sight

Figure 3–6   A summary of the aging changes in the sensory system.

body. The rhythm of the heart's pumping circulates the blood through the body. The blood, which comprises almost eight percent of an individual's body weight, according to Saxon and Etten (1994), contains red cells, white cells, platelets, and plasma. Red blood cells transport oxygen to different cells within the body. White cells are the body's protectors by preventing or interrupting attacks from bacteria and viruses. Plasma is the fluid that holds the other elements together. Platelets are necessary for blood clotting. The primary purpose of the cardiovascular system is to circulate the blood carrying oxygen and other key elements to vital tissues and organs. An overview of the circulatory system is shown in Figure 3–7.

As people age, the arteries often get clogged because of disease or lifestyle factors. The amount of blood that is pumped efficiently by the heart de-

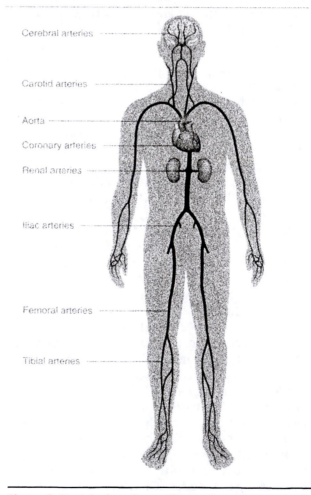

Figure 3–7   A look at the cardiovascular system.

clines over time and results in less oxygen reaching vital organs and other body tissues. Additionally, an aging heart may take longer to recover between beats. Figure 3–8 shows a summary of the aging changes that are anticipated in the cardiovascular system.

The following list contains some of the common diseases and conditions of the cardiovascular system (and immune system):

- *acquired immunodeficiency syndrome (AIDS):* a disease in which the immune system is damaged and the host is left vulnerable to many secondary infections that cannot be fought normally.
- *angina:* a term for the painful attacks that result when the heart does not receive the proper amount of oxygenated blood.
- *arteriosclerosis:* a disease in which the arteries harden, caused by diet, genetic history, obesity, smoking, and hypertension.
- *congestive heart failure (CHF):* a condition caused by the inability of the heart to pump adequate blood and oxygen to other areas of the body.
- *coronary artery disease:* a frequent disease among the elderly that occurs when the blood supply is blocked or slowed by clots or deposits in arteries surrounding the heart.
- *hypertension:* a condition evidenced by continuous or persistent elevated blood pressure that results in many other serious medical situations.
- *myocardial infarction:* heart attack; a situation that occurs when the heart rhythm stops or becomes erratic because the blood supply from the coronary arteries to the heart muscle is stopped or reduced.
- *phlebitis:* an inflammation of veins, most commonly found in the legs.
- *transient ischemic attack (TIA):* sometimes called "ministrokes," these attacks occur when the supply of blood and oxygen to the brain is suddenly stopped. A small number of brain cells may be effected.

- Fibrotic changes in vascular walls
- Narrowing of vascular lumen
- Increase in blood pressure
- Atrophy and fibrotic changes in myocardium
- Cardiac output decreased
- Less efficient chemical conversions

Figure 3–8 The aging changes present in the cardiovascular system.

The Respiratory System. The **respiratory system**, which some consider the most important system in the body, is comprised of the mouth, nose, sinuses, nasal cavities, throat (pharynx), voice box (larynx), windpipe (trachea), bronchi, and lungs. The main function of the respiratory system is to take oxygen into the lungs (inhalation) and exchange it for carbon dioxide, which is then expelled (exhalation). Other organs (i.e., the diaphragm) aid in the cycle. Hegner and Caldwell (1991) describe the first step in the process of respiration as "the air is warmed, moistened and filtered as it passes through the nasal cavities." The air continues through the throat, voice box, windpipe, and into the lungs. The exchange of gases (carbon dioxide and oxygen) takes place in the aveoli (the smallest air sacs) contained in the bronchia. Figure 3–9 illustrates the key organs and structures in the respiratory system.

The effects of aging related to the respiratory system are often seen as a decrease in overall lung capacity along with a change in the gas exchange process. Oxygen may not reach all tissues and organs at a proper rate. Additionally, sometimes the ability to cough is altered with age and a higher quantity of mucus accumulates in the lungs. This situation can be detrimental, and may lead to disease and even death. Figure 3–10 shows the aging changes that occur in the respiratory system.

The following list contains some representative examples of respiratory system diseases that could impact the elderly:

- *chronic obstructive pulmonary disease (COPD):* a chronic condition that may be the combination of obstructive bronchitis and emphysema, and results in restricted or obstructed breathing.

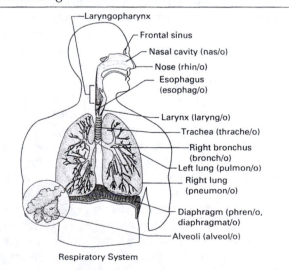

Laryngopharynx
Frontal sinus
Nasal cavity (nas/o)
Nose (rhin/o)
Esophagus (esophag/o)
Larynx (laryng/o)
Trachea (thrache/o)
Right bronchus (bronch/o)
Left lung (pulmon/o)
Right lung (pneumon/o)
Diaphragm (phren/o, diaphragmat/o)
Alveoli (alveol/o)

Respiratory System

Figure 3–9 The elements of the respiratory system.

- Decreased lung volume
- Reduced elasticity of lung tissue
- Diminished breathing capacity
- Enlarged alveoli
- Fibrotic changes in diaphragm and chest shape
- Diminished rate of gaseous exchange
- Changes in larynx
- Drier mucous membranes

Figure 3–10 A list of age-related changes in the respiratory system.

- *bronchitis:* an inflammation of the bronchi that causes a cough and mucus secretions. Chronic bronchitis may occur numerous times per year.
- *emphysema:* a chronic condition that results when the lungs are unable to expand and contract properly, resulting in destruction of cells in the lungs and retention of poor quality oxygen.
- *lung cancer:* cancer of the lungs that is normally caused by smoking or exposures to hazardous materials.
- *pneumonia:* this lung inflammation is usually caused by bacteria or viruses, and may be a result of other chronic conditions and can lead to death.

The Nervous System. Vital parts of the **nervous system,** such as the brain, spinal cord, and nerves are responsible for the key functions that coordinate and operate all body functions. The activities controlled by the nervous system include those of the central nervous system, the peripheral nervous system (which monitors voluntary functioning), and the autonomic nervous system, (responsible for involuntary body functions). The central nervous system is comprised of the brain, spinal cord, and surrounding membranes. The brain contains the cerebellum, responsible for muscle functionings. The cerebrum, the largest part of the brain, has control over thinking, reasoning, and movements that are voluntary. The brain stem contains pathways (neurons) that control involuntary processes in all the major organs of the body. Reflex movements are thought to be controlled by the spinal cord that leads from the bottom of the brain into the spinal column. The peripheral nervous system is comprised of cranial nerves that work to take messages of touch and feel to the brain. The autonomic nervous system contains nerves that relay involuntary messages about bodily and glandular functions. Figure 3–11 shows the structures of the nervous system.

The nervous system, like all the other major systems, is affected by the aging process. Some of the noted changes that occur with aging include slower functioning, movement, and response because the nervous system takes longer to handle changes. Additionally, changes may occur in sensory interpretation and in memory. A synopsis of the aging changes related to the nervous system are described in Figure 3–12.

Many of the diseases of the nervous system involve obvious changes in cognitive processes. Normal functioning in areas such as memory, comprehension, orientation, language, judgement, abstract thinking, and calculation change during a disease process. The following is a list of some of the more notable diseases and conditions involving the nervous system:

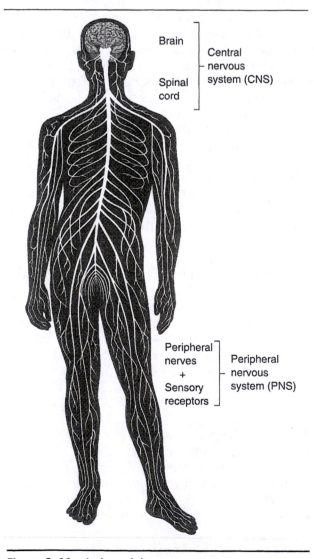

Figure 3–11 A view of the nervous system.

- Degeneration of end organs
- Loss of neurons
- Reaction time increased
- Decreased tactile sensitivity
- Decreased sensory perception
- Memory changes

Figure 3–12 Expected changes in the nervous system that accompany aging.

- *Alzheimer's disease:* a primary dementia in the elderly. The cause is unknown, and the disease is marked by a slow deterioration of cognitive functioning until death occurs.
- *cerebrovascular accident (CVA):* a condition in which the supply of blood to the brain is cut off, resulting in impairments in muscles, vision, speech, and memory.
- *multiple sclerosis (MS):* thought possibly to be caused by a change in enzymes or by a virus, this slow developing disease is marked by problems in the brain and spinal cord functioning that control motor and sensory skills.
- *multi-infarct dementia:* caused by strokes, this dementia results from a build-up of damage to the brain. Dementia symptoms are similar to those of Alzheimer's disease, but there is a relationship to a specific disease process which triggers the dementia, such as heart disease, hypertension, or other neurological problems.
- *Parkinson's disease:* a progressive disease in which shaking, rigidity of muscles, and very slow movement occurs because of an imbalance of certain chemicals in the brain responsible for transmitting information.

Functional disorders:

- *apraxia:* a deficit in gross or fine motor skills that results in an inability to perform previously learned functions regardless of desire or physical capability.
- *agnosia:* an abnormality in which an individual cannot perceive a visible object or person correctly.
- *amnesia:* a partial or total memory loss which may be temporary.

The Musculoskeletal System. Bones, muscles, cartilage, joints, ligaments, and tendons make up the **musculoskeletal system** that shapes and holds the body structure together, and allows the body to interact with the outside environment. The 206 bones and numerous joints allow for flexible movement, and the muscles, which number over 500, work with the skeletal system to provide pro-

tection for other body organs and parts and for voluntary and involuntary movement to occur. Figure 3–13 illustrates the skeletal form and Figure 3–14 shows the muscle system of the body.

There are many changes that occur in the musculoskeletal system as a result of aging. These include a decrease in calcium that leads to brittle bones and fractures. Hegner and Caldwell (1991) also mention a general loss of muscle tone, a decrease in stimuli response, and an increase in fat between the muscles. Figure 3–15 gives a summary of some of the aging changes in the musculoskeletal system.

The most frequently seen diseases or conditions of the musculoskeletal system include:

- *fracture:* a break in a bone caused by weakening because of disease (i.e., osteoporosis) or by accident or trauma (a fall in which a hip is broken).
- *rheumatoid arthritis:* a chronic situation in which an inflammation of connective tissues

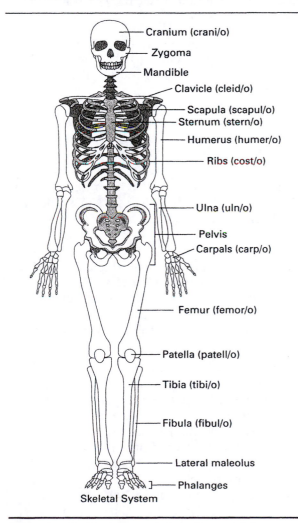

Cranium (crani/o)
Zygoma
Mandible
Clavicle (cleid/o)
Scapula (scapul/o)
Sternum (stern/o)
Humerus (humer/o)
Ribs (cost/o)
Ulna (uln/o)
Pelvis
Carpals (carp/o)
Femur (femor/o)
Patella (patell/o)
Tibia (tibi/o)
Fibula (fibul/o)
Lateral maleolus
Phalanges
Skeletal System

Figure 3–13 The human skeleton is part of the musculoskeletal system.

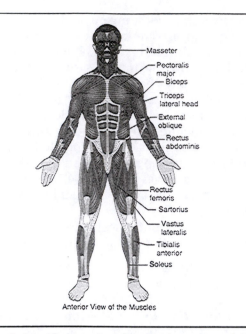

Figure 3–14 The muscles of the body are part of the muscoloskeletal system.

or membranes over the joints occurs because of an attack by antibodies in the connective tissues. Stiffness, joint pain, and joint irregularities occur.

■ *osteoarthritis:* also called degenerative joint disease (DJD), this disorder is another form of arthritis. Marked by a loss of cartilage, the bones become exposed to pain.

■ *osteoporosis:* a bone disease in which the bone tissue is absorbed at a higher rate than new bone can be formed. This results in a reduction of bone mass that can cause fractures and alignment problems.

The Digestive System. The **digestive system**, also called the gastrointestinal system, involves many organs and parts of the body to digest food from its starting point in the mouth through to disposal of waste from the anus. Some of the

■ Loss of muscle tone and strength
■ Increase in intramuscular fat
■ Glycogen (energy) storage diminished
■ Response to stimuli lessened
■ Smooth muscle walls of organs lose strength
■ Disks (pads) between vertebrae thin
■ Rib cage more rigid
■ Bones more porous and brittle

Figure 3–15 Musculoskeletal changes that are expected during the aging process.

body parts belong to other systems, such as the mouth and throat. Other organs, such as the esophagus, stomach, small intestine, large intestine, and rectum, are devoted entirely to digestion. Additionally, there are a number of secondary organs that work with the digestive process such as the teeth and salivary glands, the pancreas, the liver, and gallbladder. The purpose of the digestive system is to process food, turn it into fuel for the body, and distribute it accordingly. Waste products not needed by the body are disposed of on a routine basis. The digestive process begins when food is ingested, chewed by the teeth and mixed with saliva, and swallowed into the stomach. Once there, the food is further broken down and mixed with digestive juices. By the use of muscle action, it is expelled into the small intestine. Digestion is completed mainly in the small intestine where absorption of food and nutrients into the bloodstream occurs. The liver, pancreas, and gallbladder secrete fluids such as insulin (pancreas) and bile (from the liver into the gallbladder) to aid in the digestive process. Food (waste) not used in the digestive process is stored in the large intestine, and is eventually expelled through the rectum and anus. Figure 3–16 provides a look at the parts of the digestive system.

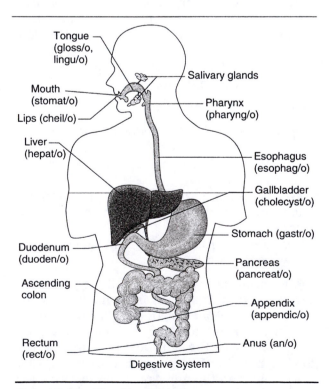

Figure 3–16 The digestive system.

Many organs are involved in the digestive system, and there are numerous changes that occur with aging that should be considered. As outlined by Hegner and Caldwell (1991), the beginning stages of the digestive process are impacted by the reduced sensitivity of the taste buds, along with fewer digestive enzymes available to process the food. Nutrient absorption is slower and the muscle action required during digestion may become weaker. Swallowing difficulties and dental issues also have a bearing on the aging digestive process, according to Saxon and Etten (1994). They also mention the self-image problems that occur because of loss of control over the rectal functions of the body. Figure 3–17 lists some of the expected impacts of aging on the digestive system.

The following is a partial list of some of the diseases and conditions of the digestive system that might be found in the elderly:

- *cirrhosis:* a disease in which deterioration and inflammation occurs in the liver, usually caused by alcoholism or nutritional problems.
- *diverticulosis:* a condition of the intestines in which a weakened wall allows sacs to protrude. When these pouches or sacs become infected, the condition is called diverticulitis.
- *hiatal hernia:* a painful condition in which a portion of the stomach is pushed through the diaphragm.
- *periodontal disease:* an inflammation or deterioration of the tissues surrounding the teeth. Problems can result in eating, chewing, and swallowing difficulties.
- *peptic ulcer:* a break in the lining of the stomach, esophagus, or duodenum from an excess of stomach acids.

The Urinary System. Comprising the **urinary system** are the kidneys, the urethra, the ureter,

and the bladder. The main function of the urinary system is to remove liquid waste from the body on a regular basis. The process begins with the kidneys, which act as a filter to remove waste products from the blood. The final product of this filtering process is called urine. Saxon and Etten mention that the kidneys are responsible for processing over forty-five gallons of fluid each day, although roughly one percent of that may actually be expelled as urine since most is recirculated and reused in the body. Figure 3–18 shows the basic structures of the urinary system of both women and men.

The alterations that the urinary system encounters during aging include a sharp decrease in kidney size over time, resulting in diminished capacity. The bladder becomes less efficient in holding and discharging urine. Blood flow changes also occur, and the entire filtration system is reduced in capacity. Figure 3–19 shows some of the expected age-related changes in the urinary system.

Some diseases and conditions that are frequently seen in the urinary system are listed below:

- *incontinence:* an inability to control bladder or bowel functions because of physical or cognitive changes.
- *renal failure:* either acute or chronic, renal failure is the inability of the primary function of the kidneys to occur.
- *urinary tract infection (UTI):* an infection of either the bladder, kidney, or other part of the urinary tract, caused by bacteria.

- Decreased number of taste buds
- Reduced digestive enzymes
- Thicker saliva
- More sensitive tongue
- Less efficient peristalsis
- Less effective gag reflex
- Poorer tolerance of some foods
- Slower absorption of nutrients
- Decreased chewing ability
- Ill-fitting dentures
- Weaker, less muscular walls

Figure 3–17 Aging changes in the digestive system.

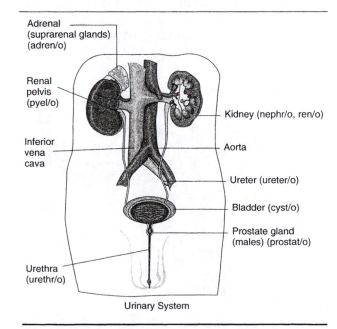

Urinary System

Figure 3–18 Structures of the urinary system.

- Kidneys decrease in size
- Scars replace renal cells
- Renal concentration is poorer with nocturia
- Bladder emptying becomes less efficient
- Filtration ability is reduced

Figure 3–19 Changes in the urinary system that may come as a result of aging.

The Reproductive System. The **reproductive system** is not one about which we would normally be concerned when talking about aging adaptations because the reproductive years were completed in middle age. Although there are two completely different organ systems for males and females, the function of the reproductive system in both remains the same: to produce the necessary cells to create a child and provide the hormones to maintain sex characteristics. The female reproductive organs are the vulva, mammary glands, the ovaries, uterus, cervix, and vagina. The male reproductive organs are the scrotum, penis, prostate gland, testes, and other glands that aid in the reproductive process. Figure 3–20 illustrates the female reproductive system and Figure 3–21 shows the male reproductive system.

Aging factors related to the reproductive system include a decrease in sexual response, weakening in the tissues and muscles, and a reduction in the level of the estrogen hormone (for women) and the testosterone hormone (for men). Figure 3–22 provides a summary of some of the anticipated changes that occur during the aging process in terms of the reproductive system.

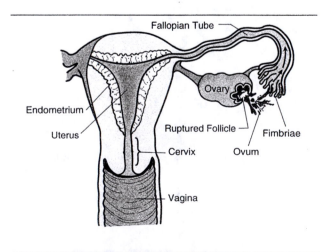

Figure 3–20 The female reproductive system.

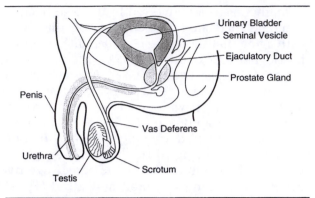

Figure 3–21 The male reproductive system.

In Males:
- Slower sexual response
- Delayed ejaculation
- Decrease in the number of sperm (but the number is still adequate for reproduction)
- Gradual decrease in testosterone levels

In Females:
- Decrease in estrogen levels
- Thinning of tissue of the vulva and vaginal walls, and a decrease in lubrication of the vagina. Elderly women are more prone to vaginal infections because of this.
- Weakening of breast tissues and muscles

Figure 3–22 Changes in the reproductive system that may come as a result of aging.

Although cancer and other problems can strike the reproductive system at any age, there are two forms of the disease that are very commonly seen in the elderly population:

- *cervical cancer:* a production of abnormal cancerous cells in the cervix. A pap smear test is usually done routinely on women to detect the presence of cervical cancer.
- *prostate cancer:* a frequent cause of cancer, especially in men of advanced age. The detection of abnormal cancer cells in the prostate results from a routine test that measures a specific protein called prostatic specific antigen (PSA).

The Endocrine System. The glands that comprise the **endocrine system** release hormones into the bloodstream on a specified basis to operate and control body functions. According to Hegner and Caldwell (1991), this is accomplished by hormone release from seven major glands. The seven glands are the pituitary, pineal body, adrenal glands, gonads, thyroid gland, the parathyroids, and the pancreas. The pituitary gland, located under the brain and sometimes referred to as "the master gland," works with the hypothalamus to control the growth process, the production of urine, and the work of many of the other glands. Researchers agree that the function of the pineal gland is not completely known. The adrenal glands release cortisone and adrenaline to control the water-to-salt balance in the body, as well as levels of other proteins. The adrenal glands are positioned on the top of each kidney. The gonads are the two testes in males and the two ovaries in women; each is responsible for releasing hormones that control sex characteristics. Body cell metabolism is regulated by the thyroid gland, and the parathyroid glands, also located in the neck area, regulate the utilization of minerals such as calcium. The pancreas, which we discussed earlier in relation to the digestive process, is in reality a gland that releases hormones to control the glucose level in the blood. Figure 3–23 illustrates the endocrine system.

Although aging factors related to the endocrine system appear to be more limited than the changes expected in some of the other systems, Saxon and Etten (1994) remark that overall hormone secretions decline with age. Some of the glands may become less active or may be reduced in size, causing the decline in production and release of hormones. Figure 3–24 provides a brief outline of the changes anticipated with aging in the endocrine system.

- Decrease in levels of estrogen and progesterone
- higher levels of parathormone and thyroid-stimulating hormone
- insulin production decreased

Figure 3–24   Changes in the endocrine system that may come as a result of aging.

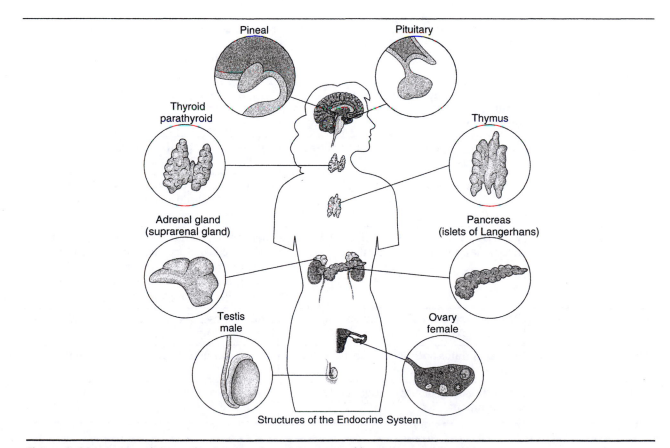

Structures of the Endocrine System

Figure 3–23   A view of the endocrine glands and the types of hormones produced.

The fluctuating changes in hormone production causes some common diseases and conditions in the endocrine system that include:

- *Addison's disease:* a disease marked by a deficiency of hormones produced by the adrenal cortex, resulting in weakness in muscles and fatigue.
- *Cushing's syndrome:* a condition in which an overabundance of adrenal cortex hormones are produced.
- *diabetes mellitus:* an inability of the body to produce the insulin necessary to control sugar levels. There are two primary types of diabetes: Type I is an insulin-dependent form that usu-

ally begins early in life, and Type II, or adult-onset, is a non-insulin dependent form and is most often seen later in life.

- *Grave's disease:* also called hyperthyroidism, this condition is caused by an increase in production of the thyroid hormone, and is evidenced by such symptoms as enlargement of the thyroid, fatigue, and weight loss.
- *hypothyroidism:* a lack of thyroid hormone is the chief cause of this disorder and results in such problems as depression, weakness, and fatigue.

An overview of each organ system and its function is illustrated in Figure 3–25.

SYSTEM	FUNCTION	ORGANS/BODY PARTS
Circulatory	Transports materials around the body: carries oxygen and nutrients to the cells, and carries waste products away	Heart, arteries, capillaries, veins, spleen, lymph nodes, lymphatic vessels, blood
Endocrine	Produces hormones that regulate body processes	Pituitary gland, thyroid gland, parathyroid glands, thymus gland, adrenal glands, testes, ovaries, pineal body, islets of Langerhans in pancreas
Gastrointestinal	Digests, transports food, absorbs nutrients, and eliminates wastes	Mouth, esophagus, pharynx, stomach, small intestine, large intestine, salivary glands, teeth, tongue, liver, gallbladder, pancreas
Integumentary	Protects the body against infection, regulates body temperature, eliminates some wastes	Skin, hair, nails, sweat, and oil glands
Musculoskeletal	Supports and protects body parts; allows the body to move	Muscles, bone, joints, ligaments, tendons
Nervous	Coordinates body functions	Brain, spinal cord, spinal nerves, cranial nerves, special sense organs such as eyes and ears
Reproductive	Reproduces the species, fulfills sexual needs, develops sexual identify	*Male:* Testes, epididymis, urethra, seminal vesicles, ejaculatory duct, prostate gland, bulbourethral glands, penis, spermatic cord *Female:* Breasts, ovaries, oviducts, uterus, vagina, Bartholin glands, vulva
Respiratory	Brings in oxygen and eliminates carbon dioxide	Sinuses, nose, pharynx, larynx, trachea, bronchi, lungs
Urinary	Manages fluids and electrolytes of body, eliminates liquid wastes	Kidneys, ureters, urinary bladder, urethra
Sensory	Helps the body detect changes in the environment	Eyes, ears, mouth, nose, skin

Figure 3–25 A summary of each body system listing the functions and associated organs/body parts.

Psychosocial Aspects of Aging ....

In addition to the physical changes that are a part of the aging process are the psychosocial impacts of growing older that must be examined for you to better understand your residents. The psychosocial aging process is made up of two categories: psychological changes and social changes.

Psychological Components

Atchley (1987) talks of psychological aging as a study of "mental dimensions" such as intelligence and perception while simultaneously considering human development. He mentions that certain processes of intelligence have links to physical aging such as perception, coordination, and reaction time. The higher mental processes (memory, creativity, problem solving, and thinking) fall into a psychological category since they are impacted by other factors.

Intellectual Changes. Atchley (1987) feels that research supports the claim that higher level functions that are more closely related to biological factors may be more impacted by the aging process, whereas functions based on learning or experience may not. Hess and Markson (1980) note changes in ability and intellect as part of the aging process that may become problematic. Some functions of intelligence such as the speed at which a response can be made, begin to decline early in life, and others such as verbal skills, remain at a constant level during the aging process. Hess and Markson also point out that cardiovascular disease may play a role in functional declines that often were attributed only to the aging process. All the researchers agree that measuring intelligence in any age group is difficult because agreement on a definition of intelligence has not been found.

Personality Changes. Studies have been conducted to look at personality adaptations in the aged populations, but contain few clear-cut results. A summary of the researchers' findings by Hess and Markson (1980) show that some of the studies support the stereotypes of aging (elderly with rigid, inflexible thinking). Hess and Markson feel that personality cannot be adequately studied in the aged population unless information from the earlier portions of an individual's life is included. Self-esteem, one of the factors related to personality, has great bearing on well-being and social conduct. Hess and Markson propose that self-esteem at the older adult level has been influenced ". . . not only by our childhood experiences but by social expec-

tations, roles and role changes." They also mention that older adults are more committed to the pattern of their lives and their roles and may feel a greater sense of self-esteem in that acceptance. Most researchers agree that even with acceptance, the aged population must endure many changes and losses that could impact self-image.

Social Components

At the same time that psychological factors are at work in the aging process, so too are the social aspects. External elements (cultural and environmental issues) cause changes in the elderly as well as internal causes (emotional adjustments and stress). Goldman (1971) speculates that during social aging, the greatest change the elderly person must deal with is the loss of choice over events. He suggests that choices are limited because of social or age discrimination, aging changes among friends, psychological limitations, loss of confidence, and an underuse of social skills. Atchley (1987) speculates that the roles a person "plays" in society, such as positions within an organization, along with experiences in the course of life, may all be influenced by age.

Maddox (1978) mentions that social aspects of aging involve how society views the "problem" of aging. As discussed earlier in the chapter, the myths and stereotypes set up and perpetuated by society at large may create some of the issues in social adjustments that occur later in life.

Loneliness. Loneliness is a reaction to many of the social losses and adjustments that the elderly must face. Burnside (1971) acknowledges that physical care has priority over emotional aspects, and often loneliness remains untreated. According to her, some of the common causes of loneliness are language and cultural barriers, geography, lifestyle, illness or pain, and approaching death. Burnside suggests that caregivers should determine the reasons for loneliness, and plan appropriate interventions to combat the problem.

Cultural Differences. Frye and Peters (1972) mention the impacts of family and group cultural traditions and how they relate to an individual's attitude toward the aging process and illness. Additionally, Gutmann (1977) feels that although the study of cultural aging impacts has been limited, it is safe to conclude that the ethnic elderly may have further burdens to adjust to socially because of their upbringing. He also found that socioeconomic status has a role in the life satisfaction of the aging population: those with higher socioeconomic status experienced greater levels of satisfaction with life. Cultural diversity is further discussed in Chapter 4.

Problem Areas in Psychosocial Adjustment

Dealing with change, loss, illness, and other alterations makes aging a stressful and emotional time. Hegner and Caldwell (1991) mention that the methods used by an individual to react to stress and change are often formed early in life.

Stress. Eisdorfer and Wilkie (1977) define a stressful situation as ". . . characterized by being novel, intense, rapidly changing, unexpected, as well as productive of fatigue, boredom, frustration or other similar state." When continually faced with upsetting situations and fears of loss or death, stress may occur as a reaction to the event. In a circumstance that induces stress, the body chooses either "fight or flight." Fight indicates that the body has decided to try to cope with the stress and adapt. Flight, however, indicates a retreat, a reaction, or perhaps physical or mental illness. Traditional life events such as marriage, divorce, or retirement can cause stress, especially when multiple events occur together. The impact of stress during life events was demonstrated by the Social Readjustment Scale, developed by Holmes and Rahe (1967).

Reactions to a build-up of stress may be handled through a series of coping devices called **defense mechanisms** which include **projection, denial, displacement, rationalization,** and **withdrawal.** Hamner (1984) defines projection as an attempt by one person to calm anxieties by "projecting" his or her feelings onto another person. Instead of expressing the feelings directly, the troubled individual attributes these feelings to another person, such as a caregiver. Denial, usually in the form of refusal to cooperate with caregivers or a particular situation, allows a person time to adjust to the numerous losses that are occurring. Displacement, as defined by Hamner, is the process of blaming another situation or person, as the source of a particular issue. She states that a typical example of displacement is negative comments from a resident of a long-term care facility, that have no specific basis. Rationalizing behavior, as discussed by Hegner and Caldwell, provides an explanation as to why something has or has not happened as a means of protecting an individual's true feelings. When stress becomes overwhelming and the traditional defense mecha-

nisms are not working, a resident may retreat and actually withdraw from the stressful situation.

Mental Illness. A key area that involves the social aspects of aging involves mental disturbances and mental illness. Shivers and Fait (1985) define a mental disturbance as ". . . any emotional response of sufficient severity to cause maladjustment or inability to function in a socially acceptable manner." There is a wide range of mental disturbance classifications developed by the American Psychiatric Association, many of which may explain the behavior of an elderly resident. It is thought that between fifteen and twenty-five percent of the elderly experience signs of mental illness. In addition, the American Psychiatric Association (1992) estimates that at least one-fourth of all elderly individuals who have dementia may have been misdiagnosed, and actually have a form of mental illness.The residents you work with may have a primary diagnosis of a medical problem, such as heart disease, but could also be undergoing treatment for an anxiety disorder or even have an undetected mental problem.

The residents who experience mental illness have to contend with misconceptions, fear, and stereotyping. By nature, most people are fearful of mental illness, and handle that fear through use of misinformation. Streamlining medical care has witnessed many more residents with true mental illness entering into long-term care facilities, thereby complicating service delivery. Hughes (1992) mentions that some of the behaviors and problems that may be a result of mental health issues include aggression, hostility, fear, anxiety, paranoia, and regression.

Depression. **Depression** is the most common psychiatric problem according to Billig (1987), and may be expressed either as a by-product of a mental disturbance or a disease. Depression "masquerades" as other physical problems such as headache, chest pains, and so forth, before a true diagnosis is made. The American Psychiatric Association (1995) estimates that depression effects at least twenty percent of individuals over age sixty-five. Common symptoms of depression include feelings of hopelessness, sadness, or loss of interest in normal activities for greater than two weeks. There also may be changes in appetite and level of fatigue or sleep. Suicidal thoughts or thinking about death may also occur, along with a variety of other physical symptoms. Kim and Rovner (1995) suggest that because of dementia and physical symptoms that can be attributed to other disorders, depression often remains untreated.

In addition to the problems of locating, diagnosing, and treating depression, Samuels and Katz (1995) mention other reasons for focusing on depression in the elderly. They suggest that research has shown that depression may be responsible for much of the weight loss seen in residents of long-term care facilities, and other negative responses to treatment by elderly patients. Samuels and Katz also propose that depression leads to increased medical needs, and can be related to higher mortality rates. Rovner et. al. (1991) first proposed the link between depression and mortality.

Depression is treatable through psychotherapy, and at times, drug therapy. The American Psychiatric Association (1992) notes that almost seventy percent of depressed patients (of any age) respond to one or more treatment methods.

Substance Abuse. To cope with life changes, losses, and other fears, some elderly people turn to substance abuse as a method of blocking painful situations. Drinking or drug abuse may start slowly, with little detection or awareness, but with increased physical problems or depression, substance abuse can get out of hand quickly.

Haugland (1989) relates that while drug and alcohol dependencies are the same, regardless of age, the number of elderly people who become chemically dependent continues to grow. Young (1988) speculates that the most common reasons for the elderly to abuse alcohol (that may eventually lead to an alcoholic condition) is because of adjustments to retirement, social isolation, bereavement, and illness or disability. He also found that abuse of legally prescribed drugs and over-the-counter medications was because of the same issues. Bernstein, Folkman, and Lazarus (1989) discovered that the elderly who misuse drugs often lack proper information about the drug's use.

Complications to substance abuse problems are the mental disturbances and other aging changes that occur, according to Lawson (1989). He postulates that often the elderly are not given treatment for substance abuse because their problems are not reported, or counselors may be reluctant to deal with elderly clients. Lawson suggests three methods of preventing substance abuse in the elderly: first, try to prevent those without problems from getting them; second, remove high-risk individuals from problem situations; and third, prevent problems that do exist from getting any worse.

Those individuals who have a chemical dependency and mental illness face even more coping difficulties than those dealing only with the normal stress of aging. Specialized training is required for staff members who assist with recovery and coping skills for these individuals.

Psychosocial Aspects of Activity Planning

How do the psychosocial aspects of aging relate to activity planning and participation? Frye and Peters (1972) summarize the important role that recreation plays in the social sphere by stating, "recreation activity may serve as a vehicle by which social contact is made . . . because of the very nature of much recreation activity, it can provide a natural climate or atmosphere for resocialization." They also suggest that a resident's ideas about his or her disability may have a bearing on his or her ability to participate in activity programs. Depression, as presented in the work of Iso-Ahola and Mobily (1982), is seen as an additional challenge to activity professionals because participation in programs was noted to be effected by its presence.

Death and Dying ....

The topic of death and dying plays an important part in long-term care. Saxon and Etten (1994) speculate that because approximately two-thirds of all deaths occur in either a hospital or nursing home setting, knowledge about death, dying, and grief is valuable to assist residents and their families.

Our view of the death and dying process is formed early in life and usually reflects the society and culture in which we live. Holmes (1978) describes key circumstances when there is the greatest cultural expectation in society for a death to occur: those who live dangerously, those living

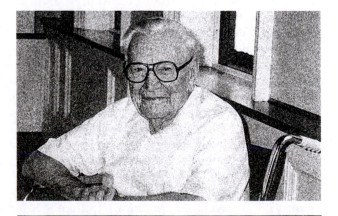

Figure 3–26 Aging is a process involving social, emotional, and physical factors, as seen here.

in times of crisis, those suffering from disease, and the very young, and the very old. The aging theories discussed earlier describe reasons for aging and offer explanations for the occurrence of death. Life expectancies are increasing, and the future holds the promise of a larger number of people who will experience old age. Kubler-Ross (1969) who wrote one of the classic books on death and dying, describes the overwhelming fear and discomfort that members of modern society have when accepting and dealing with death. Erikson (1967), when outlining his developmental theory discussed earlier in the chapter, speaks of the final life stage as a time to face the inevitability of death without fear.

According to Saxon and Etten (1994), death takes three forms. Physical death occurs when needed organs, such as the heart, no longer function. Social death is the level of isolation experienced by those who are dying. Psychological death is marked by withdrawal and detachment from society during the death process. Both Elder (1976) and Saxton and Etten (1994) discuss the work of Glaser and Strauss in developing the concept of the death trajectory. The course of death that individuals experience may be sudden, or lingering as in the case of a chronic illness. Whether or not the dying person is aware of his or her impending death also has a bearing on the level of communication between the dying individual and caregivers.

Hospice Care

Hospice care, which provides for the needs of a dying patient and his or her family by giving physical, mental, social, and spiritual support, is a relatively new phenomena. Buckingham (1983) suggests that the term "hospice" has its origins in the words "hospital" and "hospitality," both of which can be defined as "care and kindness to strangers." Becoming an increasingly popular option for patients in the later stages of a chronic or terminal illness, hospice care has been available in the United States since the late 1940s. Care is usually rendered in the home environment, which is preferred, but new hospice programs are being developed for use in long-term care facilities, hospitals, and specialized centers. Research presented by Elder (1976) and others indicates that individuals prefer to die at home rather than in institutions.

The philosophy of hospice care that Buckingham (1983) developed includes requirements for continuity of patient care, a symptom-free patient (when possible), maintenance of a patient's life-style, treatment of the patient as a person and with respect, resolution of problems of loneliness, isolation, and fear via caregivers, and provision of twenty-four hour a day care. Kubler-Ross (1969) has also remarked about the important aspect of listening and being present to hospice clients.

As part of the team who will provide care to the resident in the final months of life, you should be guided by all the normal programming principles as well as the fact that comfort and pain management may be an issue. In addition to the activity professional, the team may consist of a physician, nurse, hospice nurse, social worker, chaplain, nurses aides, dietician, and volunteer.

Williams (1992) suggests that activity professionals should focus on psychosocial issues in hospice such as receiving formal hospice training, and remembering the critical role that is played when listening to a patient, and acting as his or her confidant. The focus of your work as an activity professional is summarized by Nuland (1993) in his definitive book on the processes of dying in which he states "The greatest dignity to be found in death is the dignity of the life that proceeded it." If you have added to the quality of life of the person in the dying process, your contribution has been great.

Grieving

The **grieving process**, defined by Kneisl (1976) as "a response to loss," varies in length and intensity among individuals. Zastrow and Kirst-Ashman (1994) state that some ceremonies and rituals, such as funerals, are for the survivors and help ". . . initiate the grieving process so people can work through their grief." Two primary models exist for explaining the stages of the grieving process: the Kubler-Ross model and the Weisberg Model. The Kubler-Ross Model (1969) has been widely documented and outlines five key stages of grief: denial, anger, bargaining, depression, and acceptance. A summary of the stages of the Kubler-Ross Model is shown in Figure 3–27. The Westburg Model, outlined by Zastrow and Kirst-Ashman (1994), was originally developed in 1962, and contains more steps than the Kubler-Ross model: shock/denial, emotions erupt, anger, illness, panic, guilt, depression/loneliness, re-entry difficulties, hope, and affirming reality. Both Kubler-Ross and Westburg feel that grief sufferers may go back and forth between stages and some may never fully achieve the final grief stages.

Techniques for staff and residents to handle fears about death and grieving for the resident

STAGES OF GRIEF	
Denial	Resident refuses to accept the truth
Anger	Resident may act out feelings, directing anger at caregivers and family
Bargaining	Resident attempts to "make deals" for more livable time
Depression	Resident comes to full realization that situation cannot change and feels saddened about things that will be left unfinished
Acceptance	Resident recognizes that death is part of the natural progression of life

Figure 3–27 The Kubler-Ross stages of grief.

losses they experience routinely by working in a long-term care facility, need to be formulated. Recent changes in the availability and use of advance directives has added to the moral and ethical issues with which staff have to deal. Researchers have found that staff anxiety about the death process may be a function of the age of the caregiver (older caregivers are less anxious), and whether or not death education was available. Franklin (1994) found in her study that many facilities formed an ethics committee, and used in-services and counseling for staff to improve knowledge and coping skills concerning the death process. Families and residents often were offered counseling and staff support to assist them with their grief.

Zastrow and Kirst-Ashman (1994) offer these general tips on how to assist others with the grieving process: use crying and talking to express the loss, refrain from self-doubt and questioning, accept that some people may be uncomfortable with death, and recognize that guilt is expected.

Understanding Medications ....

An estimated thirty percent of all prescription drugs are consumed by the elderly, according to Sheahan, Hendricks, and Coons (1989). Therefore, the potential for problems in functioning and programming are increased. A medication is a drug or other agent, prescribed by a physician, dispensed by a nurse, and taken to relieve symptoms or disease process. Residents in assisted living, residential, or personal-care homes have more freedom in the use of medication, and in many states, residents in these settings take their own medications with available help and supervision.

Treating and providing comfort for the large list of possible physical and mental conditions described above account for many of the reasons for the high prescription drug use that is encountered in the long-term care facility. Shimp and Ascione (1988) feel that appropriate drug therapy can add to the quality of life for many elderly, but some serious risks exist, such as residents who are on numerous medications. Cooper (1988) adds that some common drug-related problems in nursing homes occur because of unnecessary drugs that were ordered or drugs that had adverse reactions with each other.

Pharmacokinetics, which MacLennan and Singleton (1984) define as ". . . the changes which occur in the body's ability to handle medications," involves functions such as absorption, distribution, metabolism, and excretion. In general, Lamy (1988) found that the elderly have more negative impacts with the use of drugs because their bodies are less able to absorb, process, and dispose of the drug appropriately. Saxon and Etten (1994) comment that the effectiveness of drug use in the elderly is impacted by their special responses to drugs and their higher than normal misuse of drugs. Because of the changes in various body systems from aging, drug efficiency may be seriously altered.

Drugs are prescribed for the elderly for many purposes, which range from treating illness and symptoms to alleviating anxiety and depression. Medications can be in different forms such as capsules, tablets, creams, patches, injections, or suppositories, and may be administered orally (by mouth), rectally (through the anus), topically (to an external part of the body), or injected.

Drugs may be **generic** or have a brand name from a particular company. A generic drug is one that contains the same active ingredients as the brand name. An example is Tylenol (brand name): its generic name is acetaminophen. Drugs can be prescribed by a physician or bought **over-**

the-counter (OTC) with no physician prescription required.

Drugs are classified into various categories based on their action or function within the body systems. Figure 3–28 shows a list of some typical drug classifications, along with their functions and examples. Additionally, Saxon and Etten describe some of the commonly used drugs for treatments of diseases and conditions in certain organ systems. They remark that it is common for digitalis or nitroglycerin to be prescribed for disorders of the cardiovascular system. Digitalis adds strength to the beating heart and nitroglycerin helps shrink blood vessel size. Arthritic conditions often are helped by using anti-inflammatory drugs such as aspirin, and osteoporosis may be aided by taking calcitonin.

Psychotropic drugs, those drugs designated for use in psychiatric drug therapy, will probably be used in your facility. Some of the subclassifications in the psychotropic category are anti-anxiety drugs, anti-depressant drugs, and anti-psychotic drugs (see Figure 3–28). It is vital that you be familiar with these drugs for several reasons. First, a portion of your resident population may be taking psychotropic drugs at one time or another. Second, these drugs must be carefully monitored for both the reason why a resident was placed on the drug, and the behavior of the patient that is noted while he or she is taking the drug. These drugs can be considered **chemical restraints**. A chemical restraint is a medication that causes a resident to be restricted in movement or behavior. The rationale for the use of these drugs must be documented by the medical staff, and any other interventions that have been used prior (and subsequent) to the administration of the drug. Third, you should know about psychotropic drugs because of the impact they have on the residents who are taking them. Pakes and Pakes (1982) recommend that recreation personnel become aware of not only the effects of medication on their residents, but also expected side effects. Side effects include restlessness, pacing, unsteady gait, lethargy and decreased speech. A permanent side effect to prolonged usage of anti-psychotic drugs is called **tardive dyskinesia**, in which involuntary movements are present.

Understanding the different classifications of medications that you will encounter as you review the medical records of your residents, will help you see the impacts the drug regimen has on participation in programming. MacLennan and Singleton (1984) propose that activity participation has a side benefit of helping to reduce or eliminate certain unnecessary drugs that residents are taking. They also mention the successful work of other researchers in using the "drug holiday" concept, which proposes a drug-free day for all residents who can participate. Research has shown that benefits of the drug holidays include increased alertness that enhances socialization and activity participation, closer contact between staff and residents, and could pave the way for a decreased need for some medications in some cases.

DRUG TYPE	DRUG ACTION	EXAMPLES
Analgesic	Relieves pain	Aspirin, Acetaminophen
Anti-anxiety	Reduces fear and anxiety	Valium, Librium, Xanax, Ativan
Antibiotic	Combats infection	Penicillin, Cipro, Amoxicillin
Anti-depressant	Mood enhancement	Zoloft, Prozac, Paxil, Elavil
Anti-hypertensive	Lowers blood pressure	Lopressor, Tenormin, Monopril, Lozol
Anti-inflammatory	Reduces inflammation	NSAID, Ibuprofen, Naprosyn
Antipsychotic	Lessens psychotic symptoms	Thorizine, Haldol
Diuretic	Promotes urine output	Lasix, Hydrochlorothiazide
Hypnotic	Induces sleep	Dalmane, Restoril, Halcion
Laxative	Promotes bowel elimination	Milk of Magnesia, Dulcolax, Doxidan
Diabetic	Alters blood sugar	Glucotrol, Insulin, Micronase
Steroid	Decreases inflammation	Prednisone, Hydrocortisone

Figure 3–28 Common drug classifications used to treat the elderly.

Medical Terminology ....

After reading and absorbing all the information in this chapter, you will be tested on your knowledge about your residents by reading resident medical records and other documentation. To complete the medical picture, you should understand the specialized medical terminology with which you will be working. The information presented here will also be useful when you tackle documentation and medical records in Chapter 12.

Medical terminology is defined as the abbreviations, symbols, and words that assist health team professionals render care. Two categories of medical terminology are addressed: medical language and common abbreviations.

Medical language is a form of communication, both written and spoken, that relies on combining word "roots" with prefixes and suffixes. **Word roots** are the building blocks, or elements of the word, and usually are names for a body part or medical condition. An example of a word root is "cardio," which means "heart." A **prefix** is a word part that is placed before a word root to add meaning. An example of a prefix is "peri," which means "around." If we combine "peri" and "cardio," we have the word pericardio, which means "around the heart." A **suffix** is a word part that is positioned at the end of a root word to change or add meaning. An example of a suffix is "ia" which means "a disease" or "condition of." By combining the prefix, root word, and suffix, we get pericardia, which means "a disease or condition of the outside of the heart." Most of the common diseases and many medical procedures can be broken into a word root with a prefix, a suffix, or both. At times an additional combining vowel may be necessary to make the word connection work. Figure 3–29 gives some examples of word roots, prefixes, suffixes, and combinations.

Common abbreviations in the medical world are designed for two reasons. The first reason is to make documentation quick and easy; the second has to do with conformity by having a universally accepted system for expressing care issues, diagnoses, and medication administration. Common abbreviations exist for time (such as in medication administration times), and for weights and measures. Phrases that are used in physicians orders ("discontinue") can be shortened to "dc." Some frequently seen diagnoses have abbreviated forms such as "A.D." for Alzheimer's disease. Review the summarized list of more frequently seen abbreviations shown in Figure 3–29 and check with your medical records or nursing director for any specialized medical terminology in your facility.

SUMMARY

A basic understanding of the aging changes that residents encounter is vital in formulating a significant program to address residents' needs. Aging theories, along with gerontological studies, create a structure for viewing the aspects of aging. Physical concerns of residents as related to the

MEDICAL LANGUAGE

Prefixes
a—from, without. *Example:* anemia, without adequate blood
ante—before. *Example:* antemortem, before death
contra—against, opposed. *Example:* contraindicated, against the usual treatment
dys—difficulty. *Example:* dysuria, difficulty urinating (also used to describe painful urination)
hyper—above, in excess of. *Example:* hypertension, high blood pressure
hypo—under, a deficiency of. *Example:* hypotension, low blood pressure
pneum—lung. *Example:* pneumonia, a condition involving the lungs

Word Roots or Combining Forms
arthr(o)—joint
cardi(o)—heart
dermat(o)—skin
gastro(o)—stomach
hem(o)—blood
neur(o)—nerve
pneum(o)—lung, air
thorac(o)—chest

Suffixes
algia—pain. *Example:* neuralgia, pain in nerves
asis or *osis*—state, condition, or process. *Example:* arteriosclerosis, hardening of the arteries
ectomy—removal of. *Example:* laryngectomy, removal of the larynx or voice box
emia—blood. *Example:* glycemia, sugar in the blood
itis—inflammation. *Example:* gastritis, inflammation of the stomach
oma—tumor. *Example:* lipoma, fatty tumor
ostomy—creation of an opening. *Example:* colostomy, surgical opening into the large bowel (colon)

COMMON ABBREVIATIONS

Diagnosis
AD—Alzheimer's disease
ASHD—arteriosclerotic heart disease
CHF—congestive heart failure
COPD—chronic obstructive pulmonary disease
CVA—cerebral vascular accident (stroke)
DM—diabetes mellitus
HOH—hard of hearing
MI—myocardial infarction (heart attack)
MS—multiple sclerosis
PVD—peripheral vascular disease
TIA—transient ischemic attack (mini-stroke)
URI—upper respiratory infection
UTI—urinary tract infection

Figure 3–29 A summary of commonly used medical abbreviations and terminology (*continued on next page*).

Weight/Height
in. or *"*—inch
kg.—kilogram
lb.—pound
wt.—weight
ht.—height

Time
a.c.—before meals
p.c.—after meals
a.m.—morning
p.m.—evening or afternoon
h.s.—hours of sleep (bedtime)
hr.—hour
b.i.d.—twice a day
t.i.d.—three times a day
q.i.d—four times a day
q.2h—every two hours

Measurements and Volume
cc—centimeter
l.—liter
ml.—milliliter
oz.—ounce
pt.—pint
qt.—quart

Resident Orders
ADL—activities of daily living
ad lib—as desired
bm—bowel movement
c̄—with
C—Celsius
dc—discontinue
Dr.—physician or doctor
Dx—diagnosis
F—Fahrenheit
noct—at night
npo—nothing by mouth
O₂—oxygen
per—by
po—by mouth
prn—whenever necessary
qs—sufficient quantity
Rx—treatment (take)
s̄—without
spec—specimen
stat—at once, immediately
tinct—tincture
ung or *oint*—ointment

Figure 3–29 A summary of commonly used medical abbreviations and terminology (*continued*).

disease processes in the body systems are important to comprehend. Psychosocial components of aging are also key factors in the adjustment of residents in the facility. The areas of death and dying, medication impacts, and medical terminology are also necessary for a full appreciation of the many changes that take place during the aging process.

R E V I E W   Q U E S T I O N S

1. Explain the differences between chronological age, functional capacity, and life stage.
2. What is the crisis to be solved in Erikson's old age stage of development?
3. Name two expected aging changes that occur in the sensory system, and two common diseases or conditions.
4. In which body system are dementia conditions classified? How do Alzheimer's disease and multi-infarct dementia differ?
5. What causes diabetes mellitus? What are the two types?
6. What is another name for "aging in the absence of disease?"
7. What is the most commonly treated psychiatric problem, and how treatable is it?
8. What are the five stages of grief in the Kubler-Ross Model?
9. Define pharmacokinetics, and explain why it is important in the treatment regimen of the elderly?
10. What is a psychotropic drug?

O N   Y O U R   O W N

1. Use medical record information or assistance from your Director of Nursing to determine the top three diagnoses in your facility. Work with those diseases or conditions, gather information, and design two new programs to respond to your findings that will assist residents.
2. Using each of body system classifications, list one or two aging changes and diseases that occur in each category.
3. Compare and contrast the disengagement theory, activity theory, continuity theory, and exchange theory. Which one has the most application for use in an activity department and why?
4. Using Figure 3–29, make up five words using word roots, prefixes, and suffixes.

R E F E R E N C E S

Achenbaum, W.A., & Levin, J. (1989). What does gerontology mean? *The Gerontological Society of America*, Vol. 29, No. 3, 393–400.

American Psychiatric Association (1992). *Mental illness: There are a lot of troubled people*. Washington, DC: author.

American Psychiatric Association (1994). *Facts about: Mental health of the elderly*. Washington, DC: author.

American Psychiatric Association (1995). *Psychiatric medications*. Washington, DC: author.

Atchley, R. (1987). *Aging: Continuity and Change, 2nd edition*. Belmont, CA: Wadsworth Publishing Co.

Atchley, R. (1989). A continuity theory of normal aging. *The Gerontological Society of America*, Vol. 29, No. 2, 183–190.

Bernstein, L. R., Folkman S., & Lazarus, R. S. (1989). Characterization of the use and misuse of medications by an elderly, ambulatory population. *Medical Care*, 27 (6), 654–663.

Billig, N. (1987). *To be old and sad. Understanding depression in the elderly*. New York, NY: Lexington Books.

Buckingham, R. (1983). *The complete hospice guide*. New York, NY: Harper & Row.

Burnside, I. M. (1971). Loneliness in old age. *Mental Hygiene*, Vol 55, No. 3, 391–397.

Burnside, I. M. (1994). Education and preparation for group work. In I. Burnside & M. G. Schmidt (Eds). Working with older adults: Group process and techniques, 3rd ed. (65–74) Boston, MA: Jones and Bartlett.

Butler, R. N. (1974). Successful aging. *Mental Hygiene*, Vol. 58., No. 3, 6–12.

The Center for Corporate Health (1991). *Taking care of today and tomorrow: A resource guide for health, aging and long-term care*. Reston, VA: author.

Cooper, J. W. (1988). Medication misuse in nursing homes. *Generations*, Summer, 56–57.

Cumming, E., & Henry, W. (1961). *Growing old*. New York, NY: Basic Books.

Eisdorfer, C., & Wilkie, F. (1977). Stress, disease, aging and behavior. In J. Birren and K. Schaie (Eds.) *Handbook of the Psychology of Aging*. (251–269) New York, NY: Van Nostrand Reinhold Company.

Elder, R. G. (1976). Dying and society. In R.E. Caughill (Ed). *The dying patient: A supportive approach*. (1–29). Boston, MA: Little Brown & Co.

Epstein, C. (1977). *Learning to care for the aged*. Reston, VA: Reston Publishing Co.

Erickson, E. (1963). *Childhood and Society, 2nd edition*. New York, NY: Norton.

Franklin, M. (1994). Death and dying fears overcome by progressive strategies. *The Journal of Long-Term Care Administration*, Winter, 4–9.

Frye, V., & Peters, M. (1972). *Therapeutic recreation: Its theory, philosophy, and practice*. Harrisburg, PA: Stackpole Books.

Gastel, B. (1994). *Working with your older patient: A clinician's handbook*. Bethesda, MD: National Institute on Aging, National Institutes of Health.

Goldman, S. (1971). Social aging, disorganization and loss of choice. *The Gerontologist*, Summer, 158–162.

Gutmann, D. (1977). The cross-cultural perspective: Notes toward a comparative psychology of aging. In J. Birren & K. Schaie (Eds.). *Handbook of the Psychology of Aging*. (302–339). New York, NY: Van Nostrand Reinhold Company.

Hamner, M. L. (1984). Insight, reminiscence, denial and projection: Coping mechanisms of the aged. *Journal of Gerontological Nursing*, Vol. 10. No. 2, 66–81.

Haugland. S. (1989). Alcohol and other drug dependencies. *Primary Care*, 16 (20), 411–429.

Havighurst, R.J. (1969). Adulthood and old age. In R. Ebel (Ed.), *Encyclopedia of educational research*. New York, NY: Macmillan Publishing Co.

Hegner, B., & Caldwell, E. (1991). *Geriatrics: A study of maturity, 5th edition*. Albany, NY: Delmar Publishers Inc.

Hegner, B., & Caldwell, E. (1994). *Assisting in long-term care, 2nd edition*. Albany, NY; Delmar Publishers Inc.

Hess, B., & Markson, E. (1980). *Aging and old age: An introduction to social gerontology*. New Yok, NY: Macmillan Publishing Co. Inc.

Holmes, T. (1978). Death and dying. In G. Usdin & C. Hofling (Eds.) *Aging: The process and the people*. (47–95). New York, NY: Brunnel/Mazel publishers.

Holmes, T. H., & Rahe, R. H. (1967). The social readjustment rating scale. *Journal of Psychosomatic Research*, Vol 11, 213–218.

Hughes, M. (1992). *Mental health problems and the nursing home resident.* LaGrange, TX: M&H Publishing Co.

Iso-Ahola, S. E., & Mobily, K. E. (1982). Depression and recreation involvement. *Therapeutic Recreation Journal,* 3rd quarter, 48–53.

Kayser-Jones, J. S., Wiener, C. L., & Barbaccia, J. C. (1989). Factors contributing to the hospitalization of nursing home residents. *The Gerontologist,* Vol. 29, No. 4, 502–510.

Kim, E., & Rovner, B. (1995). Epidemiology of psychiatric disturbances in nursing homes. *Psychiatric Annals,* 25: 7, 409–412.

Kneisl, C. R. (1976). Grieving: A response to loss. In R. E. Caughill (Ed). *The dying patient: A supportive approach.* (31–46) Boston, MA: Little, Brown & Co.

Krimsky, J. (1969). Prescription for successful aging: An essay. *The Ohio State Medical Journal,* February, 154–158.

Kubler-Ross, E. (1969). *On death and dying.* New York, NY: Macmillan.

Lahey, M. (1993). Acute care vs. chronic care models of service to the elderly: Implications for therapeutic recreation. In M. Lahey et. al. (Eds.) *Recreation, leisure and chronic illness: Therapeutic rehabilitation as intervention in health care.* Binghamton, NY: Haworth Press.

Lamy, P. (1988). Actions of alcohol & drugs in older people. *Alcohol & Drugs Generations,* Summer, 9–13.

Larue, G. (1992). Geroethics. In G. Larue & R. Bayly (Eds). *Long-term care in an aging society: Choices and challenges for the 90's.* (147–167) Buffalo, NY: Prometheus Books.

Lawson, A. W. (1989). Substance abuse problems of the elderly: Considerations for treatment and prevention. In G. W. Lawson & A. W. Lawson, (Eds.) *Alcoholism and substance abuse in special populations,* (p. 95 –113), Rockville, MD: Aspen Publishers.

MacLennan, B., & Singleton, J. (1984). Drugs, activities and the elderly: Implications for service delivery. *Activities, Adaptation & Aging,* Vol.4(4), 75–82.

Maddox, G. (1978). The social and cultural context of aging. In G. Usdin & C. Hofling (Eds.). *Aging: The process and the people.* (20–46), New York, NY: Brunnel/Mazel publishers.

National Institute On Aging (1993). *In search of the secrets of aging.* (NIH publication 93-2756), Washington, DC: Public Health Service, author.

Nuland, S. (1993). *How we die: Reflections on life's final chapter.* New York, NY: Vintage Books.

O'Morrow, G., & Reynolds, R. (1989). *Therapeutic recreation: A helping profession. (3rd edition).* Englewood Cliffs, NJ: Prentice Hall.

Palmore, E. (1977). Facts on aging: A short quiz. *The Gerontologist,* Vol. 17, No. 4, 315–320.

Pakes, D. L., & Pakes, G. E. (1982). Anti-psychotic drug side effects and therapeutic recreation program considerations. *Therapeutic Recreation Journal,* 1st quarter, 12–19.

Rovner, B., German, P., Brant, L., Clark, R., Burton, L., & Folstein, M. (1991). Depression and mortality in nursing homes. *Journal of The American Medical Association,* Vol. 265, No. 8, 993–996.

Samuels, S., & Katz, I. (1995). Depression in the nursing home. *Psychiatric Annals,* 25:7, 419–424.

Saxton, S., & Etten, M. (1994). *Physical change & aging: A guide for the helping professions, 3rd edition.* New York, NY: The Tiresias Press Inc.

Sheahan, S. L., Hendricks, J., & Coons, S. J. (1989). Drug misuse among the elderly: Covert problem. *Health Values,* 13 (3), 22–29.

Shimp, L. A., & Ascione, F.J. (1988). Causes of medication misuse and error. *Generations,* Summer, 17–21.

Shivers, J., & Fait, H. (1985). *Special recreational services: Therapeutic and adapted.* Philadelphia, PA: Lea & Febiger.

Shock, N. (1977). Biological theories of aging. In J. Birren and K. Schaie (Eds.) *Handbook of the Psychology of Aging.* (103–113) New York, NY: Van Nostrand Reinhold Company.

U.S. Department of Health & Human Services (1989). *The national nursing home survey: 1985 summary for the United States* (DHHS Publications No. PHS 89–1758). Hyattsville, MD: author.

U. S. Department of Health & Human Services (1993). *With the passage of time: The Baltimore longitudinal study of aging.* (NIH publication No. 93–3685). Washington, DC: National Institutes of Health.

Williams, J. (1992). Transition of the hospice patient to the nursing home. *Activities, Adaptation & Aging,* Vol. 16(3), 41–49.

Young, T. J. (1988). Alcohol use and abuse among the elderly. *Journal of Behavior Technology Methods and Therapy,* 23 (2), 1–5.

Zastrow, C., & Kirst-Ashman, K. (1994). *Understanding human behavior and the social environment.* Chicago, IL: Nelson-Hall Publishers.

F U R T H E R R E A D I N G

Berkovw, R., & Fletcher, A. (1992). *The Merck manual of diagnosis and therapy. 16th edition,* Rahway, NJ: Merck Research Laboratories.

Berndt, D., & Ray, R. (1979). Leisure and the process of aging: Reference points for professional development. *Therapeutic Recreation Journal,* 1st quarter, 50–63.

Bollinger, R. (1974). Geriatric speech pathology. *The Gerontologist,* June, 217–219.

Burger, S. (1982). Three approaches to patients care: Hospice, nursing homes and hospitals. In M. Hamilton & H. Reid (Eds.). *A Hospice handbook: A new way to care for the dying.* Grand Rapids, MI: Eerdmans.

Caughill, R. (1976). *The dying patient: A supportive approach.* Boston, MA: Little, Brown & Co.

Cousins, N. (1983). *Anatomy of an illness as perceived by the patient.* New York, NY: Bantam Books.

Daley, D., & Campbell, F. (1989). *Coping with dual disorders: Chemical dependency and mental illness.* Center City, MN: Hazelden.

Epstein, C. (1977). *Learning to care for the aged.* Reston, VA: Reston Publishing Co.

Elias, M., & Ellas, P. (1977). Motivation and activity. In J. Birren & K. Schaie (Eds.). *Handbook of the psychology of aging.* (357–383). New York, NY: Van Nostrand Reinhold Company.

Fonrose, H. (1978). Medical care in the geriatric population. In M. Mitchel (Ed.) *A practical guide to long term care and health services administration.* Green Vale, NY: Panel Publishers.

Foster, P. (1983). Activities: A necessity for total health care of the long-term care resident. *Activities, Adaptation & Aging,* Vol. 3(3), 17–23.

Friedan, B. (1993). My quest for the fountain of age. *Time,* Sept. 6, 61–64.

Gilford, H D. (1988). *The aging population in the twenty-first century: Statistics for health policy.* Washington, DC: National Academy Press.

Goldsmith, S. B. (1994). *Essentials of long-term care administration.* Gaithersburg, MD: Aspen Publishers.

Grigorian, H. M. (1970). Aging and depression: The involutional and geriatric patient. In A. Enclow (Ed.). *Depression in medical practice.* West Point, PA: Merck, Sharp & Dohme.

Hilton, J. (1988). *Strategies for identifying blind and visually impaired nursing home residents.* New York, NY: American Foundation for the Blind & The Delta Gamma Foundation.

Indiana State Board of Health (1991). *Nursing home activity directors course.* Indianapolis, IN: author.

Kiernat, J. M. (1983). The effect of hearing loss on the activities of older persons. *Activities, Adaptation & Aging,* Vol. 4(1), 39–47.

Lawton M. (1977). The impact of the environment on aging and behavior. In J. Birren and K. Schaie (Eds.) *Handbook of the psychology of aging.* (276–301) New York, NY: Van Nostrand Reinhold Company.

Leitner, M., & Leitner, S. (1985). *Leisure in later life: A sourcebook for the provision of recreational services for elders.* Binghamton, NY: Haworth Press.

Linn, M., Linn, B., & Gurel, L. (1972). Patterns of illness in persons who lived to extreme old age. *Geriatrics,* Vol. 27, 67–70.

Lipton, M., & Nemeroff, C. (1978). The biology of aging and its role in depression. In G. Usdin & C. Hofling (Eds.) *Aging: The process and the people.* (47–95) New York, NY: Brunnel/Mazel publishers.

MacNeil, R., & Pringnitz, T. (1982). The role of therapeutic recreation in stroke rehabilitation. *Therapeutic Recreation Journal,* 4th quarter, 26–33.

McDowell, C. F. (1986). Wellness and therapeutic recreation: Challenges for services. *Therapeutic Recreation Journal,* 2nd Quarter, 27–38.

Merriam, S., & Mullins, L. (1981). Havighurst's adult development tasks: A factor analysis. *Activities, Adaptation & Aging,* Vol. 1(3), 9–22.

Murphy, A. (1994). *Working with elderly people.* London, England: Souvenir Press.

Portnoy, E. (1981). Aging sensory losses and communication behavior. *Activities, Adaptation & Aging,* Vol. 2(1), 59–66.

Rancourt, A. (1991). Programming quality services for older adults in long-term care facilities. *Activities, Adaptation & Aging,* Vol. 15(3), 1–11.

Schmidt, M. G., & Burnside, I. (1994). Demographic and psychosocial aspects of aging. In I. Burnside & M. G. Schmidt (Eds.). *Working with older adults: Group process and techniques,* 3rd edition, 8–23, Boston, MA: Jones and Bartlett Publishers.

Stein, S., Linn, M., & Stein, E. (1986). Patients' perceptions of nursing home stress related to quality of care. *The Gerontological Society of America,* Vol. 26, No.4, 424–430.

Sternberg, J., Spector, W., Drugovich, M., Fretwell, M., & Jackson, M. (1990). Use of psychoactive drugs in nursing homes: Prevalence and residents' characteristics. *Journal of Geriatric Drug Therapy,* Vol. 4(3), 47–60.

Stinson, F. S., Dufour, M. C., & Bertolucci, D. (1989). Alcohol related morbidity in the aging population. *Alcohol Health and Research World,* 13(1), 80–87.

Teaff, J. (1985). *Leisure services with the elderly.* St. Louis, MI: Times Mirror.

Tedrick, T. (1991). Aging, developmental disabilities and leisure: Policy and service delivery issues. In J. Keller (Ed.) *Activities with developmentally disabled elderly adults and older adults.* Binghamton, NY: Haworth Press.

Thomas, B. (1988). Self-esteem and life satisfaction. *Journal of Gerontological Nursing,* Vol. 14, No. 12, 25–30.

U.S. Senate Special Committee on Aging in conjunction with The American Association of Retired Persons (1984). *Aging America: Trends and Projections 2nd printing.* Washington, DC: author.

Williams, M. (1984). Alcohol and elderly: An overview. *Alcohol Health and Research World,* Spring, 3–9.

C H A P T E R   4
Getting to Know Residents, Staff, and Families

KEY TERMS......................................

activity assessment
resident status form
daily census form
Minimum Data Set
    (MDS)
activity assessment data
    collection form
medical record
transfer sheet
face sheet
responsible party
progress notes
attending physician
physician's orders
medication orders
standing orders
clothing and
    possessions inventory
advance directive

power of attorney
release forms
activity photo release
    form
activity trip release form
resident council
resident satisfaction
life satisfaction
quality
quality assurance
resident concern form
sandwich generation
activities of daily
    living (ADLs)
family council
reminiscence
practitioner behavior
    or conduct

OBJECTIVES..

After completing this chapter, you should:

■ understand and use the stages of the initial activity assessment process as you meet your new residents.

■ have gained knowledge about the reactions and needs of family members during the resident's stay in the facility.

■ meet your co-workers in a suitable manner and apply the principles of professional conduct you have acquired.

INTRODUCTION

Serving the needs of your residents requires a full knowledge of their medical and leisure status. Learning about the resident through contact with family members brings additional useful information to assist in planning. The family has a unique set of concerns that should be addressed as you build your program. Knowledge about your conduct as a professional on the job and learning about your co-workers are two other valuable strengths you will need to succeed in your position.

Learning About Your Residents ....

Your residents and their needs are the reasons you and the rest of the health care team are employed. Too often, adequate time is not spent by team members on identifying key sources of information about residents in order to provide quality care.

In addition to understanding the physical and psychological aspects of aging, and the common disease processes in geriatrics that were covered in the last chapter, it is important for the activity professional to take opportunities to interact with residents, family members, other relatives, and staff to build a foundation of information about each resident to determine and meet their activities needs. The **activity assessment**, social history, and other information can be gleaned from your formal and informal encounters with these individuals.

Your Role in the Admission Process

The easiest way to begin the process of information gathering is by means of the pre-admission process. Depending on the size of your facility, you may be part of the daily admissions committee, which reviews potential admission applications. It may also be the policy of your facility for family members to meet or tour with department heads rather than the admissions director. In this case, a great opportunity to learn about a new resident and his or her family in an informal setting is provided. It also gives you time to market your program to the potential new resident and the family. Although the meetings are held for the purpose of admission, and are technically considered to be "formal," much extra information critical to your activity history and initial assessment efforts may come up at this time. Many facilities opt to take the admission process to a more detailed level by performing site visits, either in the home or hospital, to assess potential admissions. This step provides more of a glimpse into an applicant's life, particularly during home visits. Staff members such as the social service director, the administrator, director of nursing, and, of course, the activity professional, can expect the added benefit of increased rapport once the individual has entered the facility because some of the initial clinical assessment and fact-finding has taken place in the comfortable, familiar territory of the individual's own home. The opportunity to see someone in his or her own environment allows an easier translation of their needs once they enter the facility. An activity professional can gain much knowledge by participating fully in the pre-admission process.

If your facility does not allow you to take part in the pre-admission process, it probably has communication mechanisms in place so you can be apprised of any upcoming admissions, discharges, or room changes. Normally, this information is handled through the use of a **resident status form**, completed by the director of social services or director of admissions, and forwarded to each department so they are aware of the change. The resident status form, whenever possible, is drawn up a day or two before the anticipated change to allow adequate facility preparation. Another form most facilities use to communicate changes in resident status is the **daily census form**. The responsibility for completion and distribution of this form is usually left to the social service or admission director, and a copy of the daily census form is sent to all departments. An example of the resident status change form is shown in Figure 4–1.

Initial Resident Meetings

Notification of resident admission by means of the resident status form and the daily census form prepares you to make contact with your new resident shortly after he or she is admitted. Some facilities have successful, formal admission procedures that involve specific contact time with the new resident by each department on the first day of admission. For example, the activity department might visit the new admission within the first hour of admission and greet the resident

with a balloon or plant. If your facility does not have a definite admission welcoming procedure, you may wish to develop one that will avoid visits by all departments at the same time, or duplication of effort.

As you meet each new resident for the first time, you will be given the opportunity to reassure and acclimate the resident to the facility and begin your activity assessment process for their activity programming needs. As you will learn in Chapters 8 and 12, part of the planning and documentation process for activities is based on a detailed activity assessment. An activity assessment is a process of collecting key pieces of information about an individual resident to assist in activity planning and documentation. Figure 4–2 shows the stages of the assessment process. It is the critical first step in the activity planning process, and includes such resident information as physical and mental limitations, identified recreational interests (past and present), religion, occupation, and previous work history. Other health care team members such as the charge nurse, the social worker, and the dietician will conduct their own resident assessments based on information they need for health care planning in their areas. The activity assessment is done formally, along with those of the other health care team members, by compiling the **Minimum Data Set (MDS)** after the first fourteen days of admission. The preparation stages of gathering information for use in the activity assessment, however, starts with your first contact with the new resident. Use of the **activity assessment data collection form**, shown in Figure 4–3, guides you in accumulating the data you need for thorough assessment documentation requirements and program planning. When reviewing this form, be aware of the kind of things you should be looking for as you meet the new resident. Remember, the assessment phase of each discipline begins with the first meeting.

Depending on the health and mental status of the resident, you may be able to pick up some information in introductions and initial conversations you have with the resident. In addition to possible conversation (or a monologue, if the resident is unable to converse), an activity professional should be casually looking around the room for clues about the resident's hobbies, interests, and past. Items like pictures, momentos, diplomas, style of clothing, and prized possessions are powerful indicators of areas that can be pursued to guide you in activity planning. The family or friends who accompanied the resident

---

Resident Status Form

Date form completed: _____ Form completed by: _____
Resident Name: _____
Sex: ___Male ___Female

TYPE OF STATUS CHANGE:
Admission

    Date of admission: _____
    Time (if known): _____
    Admitted from: _____
    Admitted to room: _____
    Payment source: _____
    Laundry done by: Family/Facility   (circle one)
    Comments: _____

    _____

Discharge

    Date of discharge: _____
    Discharged to: _____

Room Change

    From room _____ to room _____
    Effective date of room change: _____

Payment Source Change

    From: To:
    ___Private ___Private
    ___Medicare ___Medicare
    ___Medicaid ___Medicaid
    ___Other ___Other

Figure 4–1 A resident status form is a communication tool for keeping departments informed.

Tasks in the Assessment Process

Resident Conversations

Resident Observations

Family/Friends/Significant Other
Conversations

Review of Medical Record

Meetings with Co-workers/
Health Care Team Members

Completion of Assessment
Preparation Form

MDS Initial Assessment

Figure 4–2 The assessment process.

on this first day can also be crucial in helping you learn. You should introduce yourself, and ask to schedule a meeting with, or make a telephone call to, appropriate family for further assessment information. If the new resident is unable to provide you with much information because of medical or mental status, input from family and friends becomes vital in preparing an accurate activity assessment.

After your brief initial conversation with the new resident and his or her family, set up a time with the resident when you can stop back to talk further, or have the resident join an activity, if appropriate. This is also your opportunity to check with the resident and family member to see if they need anything, or if everything is in order. If there is a special request for something (i.e., use of a telephone by family), handle the request personally.

Understanding Ethnicity and Cultural Diversity

Sensitivity and understanding of **ethnicity** and cultural diversity issues are crucial as you meet your residents and begin to plan for their needs. Barresi and Stull (1993) define ethnicity as ". . . a large group whose members internalize and share a heritage of, and a commitment to, unique social

---

ACTIVITY ASSESSMENT DATA COLLECTION FORM

A. Personal Data

    Resident name: _____
    Prefers to be called: _____
    Date of admission: _____
    Date of birth: _____
    Marital status: _____
    Religious preference: _____
    Cultural heritage/background: _____

    Siblings:

       Name   Relation   Address/phone
    Children:

       Name   Address/Phone
    Grandchildren

       Name   Address/Phone

B. Medical Information

    Diagnosis   Medication

    Diet: _____
    Medical limitations/precautions: _____
    _____
    Allergies: _____
    Mobility/ambulation: _____
    Mental status/orientation: _____
    Mood/behavior: _____
    Vision/hearing/speech: _____
    ADL skills: _____
    Adaptive equipment: _____
    Bowel/bladder continency: _____
    Eating skills: _____

C. Activity Pursuits/Interest and Need Review

    Past occupation(s): _____

    Hobbies/interests (current): _____

    Hobbies/interests (past): _____

Needs Assessment:

Needs Area	Capabilities	Restrictions	Recommendations
Social			
Physical			
Creative			
Educational			
Spiritual			
Awareness			
Integration			

Figure 4–3 A data collection form helps you gather information.

---

characteristics, cultural symbols, and behavior patterns that are not fully understood or shared by outsiders." Cultural diversity, a similar sounding term, relates to the different cultural experiences that ethnicity may dictate.

Ethnic minorities exist within twenty percent of the general population, and account for eleven percent of the elderly population, according to Barresi and Stull. The elderly minority groups (called "minority" because it is thought that minority is a factor in most ethnic groups), are one of the fastest growing segments of the elderly population, and are expected to grow to fifteen percent of the population by the year 2025. The most frequently mentioned ethnic groups were thought to be (in order of frequency) German, Afro-American, English, Irish, Spanish, Italian, and Mexican. Barresi and Stull commented that because only six percent of those surveyed were identified as Americans, it pointed out the highly diverse ethnic backgrounds that exist.

Why is the study of the cultural diversity of the ethnic elderly so important? One reason is that in our goal to provide individual services to our residents, the diverse background and cultural factors are critical to understand. Another consideration is the fact that those residents who are viewed as elderly and part of a minority group have been said to be in "double jeopardy," or as Thomas (1988) states, they may face ". . . the dual discrimination of ageism and racism."

A resident who is an immigrant and part of a minority group may encounter further communication problems as the activity professional tries to meet his or her needs. In Morrison and Zabusky's work (1980), the immigrant experience is described in this way: "In moving, people create cultural and linguistic gaps. Their own habits and phrases are the products of one place; arriving in another they confront habits and phrases no more comprehensible to them than theirs are to the strangers about them." When defining the immigrant experience in terms of the aged population, Norman (1985) has coined the term "triple jeopardy," to mean, ". . . at risk because they are old, because of the physical conditions and hostility under which they have to live, and because services are not accessible to them."

To combat these potentially damaging threats to understanding their care needs, Yeo (1993) suggests that consideration of these culturally sensitive factors can assist in their care. One of the elements that she feels is important is the use of an ethnically sensitive activity program. Yeo suggests using ethnic volunteers to donate leadership and continuity, making special celebrations for traditional cultural holidays, and providing calendars and other marketing materials in more than one language. Other vital care factors that assist in maintaining a cultural balance include use of native language for communication, traditional foods, and the provision of religious services. These suggestions, and your own ideas, should motivate you to consider all aspects of a person's background as you plan a personalized program.

Reading the Chart and Other Documentation

Before your initial meeting with the resident and his or her family, you should stop at the nurses' station to review the new chart, or **medical record**. Medical records in your facility, or care documentation by contributing departments, are usually kept in a chart system (a spring loaded method for holding and protecting documents) or a binder system. Both systems use tabs to separate different areas of the medical record to allow quick and easy access to specific areas of interest. At this early stage in the admission process, many of the other departments may not yet have contributed information to the medical record. You will find such data as the **transfer sheet** (if the resident was admitted from a hospital or other facility) that outlines the person's medical information and personal data at the time of transfer. The first sheet of the medical chart, also called the **face sheet**, is specific to the guidelines of your facility, and includes basic information about the resident (the diagnosis, date of birth, last address, social security number, medical insurance numbers, **responsible party**, next of kin, funeral home designation, and so forth). There may also be an initial entry by the charge nurse and possibly some **progress notes** from the nursing staff and other departments that briefly outline their findings as they met and examined the resident. The **attending physician**, who has agreed to care for the resident while he or she is in the facility, may have been contacted for **physician's orders**, a list of care directives that the physician makes on behalf of the resident. The initial physician's orders might include:

- **medication orders**, related to a specific medical diagnosis
- a request for a professional consultation for the resident (i.e., speech therapist)
- other guidelines such as the amount of physical activity recommended for the resident.

The physician's orders help you understand the needs and limitations of the resident as you begin your activity planning.

Your facility may also have a policy for **standing orders**, or physician's orders that are effective under certain circumstances. For example, your facility may have a standing order policy that states certain laboratory work be performed upon admission for every resident. The attending physician is aware of the facility's standing order policies (hopefully he or she assisted in forming the policies), but can override the policy if it is medically unsuitable for a particular resident.

You may also find completed forms such as **clothing and possessions inventory** (a detailed list of all clothing and possessions that the resident brought to the facility), **advance directive**

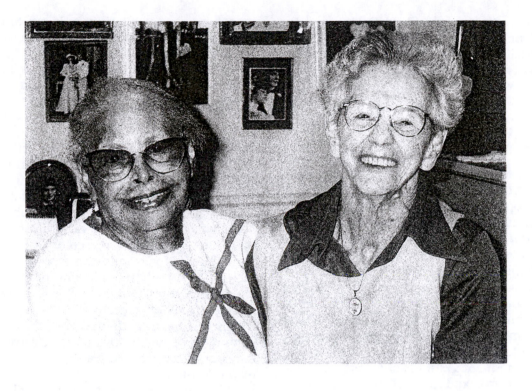

Figure 4–4 Acknowledge and celebrate cultural diversity when setting up an activity program for your residents.

declaration, **power of attorney** designation (granting financial management authority to a particular person under certain circumstances), and **release forms** for such items as facility photographs (for use in activities, publicity, and on the medication cart for identification by nursing), and resident attendance on facility outings. These forms are completed by the incoming resident or a family member at the time of admission. A sample of the **activity photo release form** and **activ-**

ity trip release form are shown in Figure 4–5. It should be noted that only the resident may complete and sign an advance directive declaration, based on the guidelines in your state.

As you review the medical record, use this opportunity to reacquaint yourself with the medical terminology, diagnoses, disease names, drugs, and other notations you find. If you do not understand something, ask the charge nurse. You can also use the standard reference materials such as the

ACTIVITY PHOTO RELEASE FORM

I,_____, give my permission for the publication, reproduction, use, or reuse of any photograph of _____.
I understand that photographs are used in the facility for identification, publicity such as the newsletter or press releases, and in displays in facility areas.

Resident Signature	*Date*
Responsible Party	*Date*
Witness	*Date*

ACTIVITY TRIP RELEASE FORM

I, _____, do/do not wish to attend trips outside the facility. I understand that medical concerns or limitations should be discussed with my physician prior to any trip.

Resident Signature	*Date*
Responsible Party	*Date*
Witness	*Date*

Figure 4–5 Examples of activity photo release and activity trip release form.

Physicians Desk Reference (*PDR*) (1995), and the *Merck Manual*, Berkow & Fletcher (1992) to research specific drugs or diseases. These and many other books are published annually, and should be available at the nurses' station or nursing office.

Resident Interests Dictate Program Planning

As you meet and learn about your residents, either through individual new admissions or a whole resident population as a new employee, a central theme should be forming in your mind: *The interests and individual needs of your residents should dictate your activity program planning!* It seems simple, but many activity professionals ignore this crucial point, and base their program planning on their own "agenda." Continue the information-gathering process on both a formal and informal basis with residents to determine their needs. The goal is to collect as much data about each resident's past history, lifestyle, and interests as possible, and to couple that with medical needs and restrictions in order to arrive at a plan for meeting activity needs. The informal methods of learning about residents come through a series of casual conversations with the residents, their families, and friends. Additionally, your review of the medical record, resident observations, and conversations with other department heads or consultants add further knowledge. Norris, Hawes, Murphy, Nonemaker, Phillips, Fries, and Mor (1991) mention in their MDS training manual that speaking with nursing assistants and nonlicensed staff members can often yield much direct resident information that will be valuable in the assessment process.

Formally, you can converse with your residents individually about their activity interests, and meet as a group through resident's council to air the residents' desires for programming. In the course of this text, we expand on this idea as we discuss activity program planning in Chapters 8, 9, and 10, and when we cover documentation and medical records in Chapter 12.

Resident Council

A formal arena for learning about resident activity interests is through participation in the **resident council**, an organized setting for residents to meet on a regular basis to vent concerns and express needs. Initially organized by either the activity director, social worker, or both, the resident council is open to all facility residents to meet independently and participate in facility decisions and planning.

Meetings may be held monthly or more frequently, with resident officers such as president, vice-president, secretary, and treasurer managing the meeting. Participation from administration may be requested, and department heads may or may not be invited to attend the meetings to respond to specific departmental concerns. Silverstone (1977), in her work on resident councils, talks about the purpose of a successful resident council, and states, "There are some jobs in every home which residents can carry out better than staff, such as selecting the color of furnishings, the choice of foods, and the type of activities." Merrill (1979) advises that one of the primary functions of a resident council is to actively promote the activity program within the facility. As we discussed earlier, the residents are always the guiding force for the planning of activities and the council format is just another area for information gathering.

Although her study focused primarily on resident councils in residential facilities, Silverstone suggests a number of ways to increase resident participation in meetings that have implications for long-term care facilities. First, support and publicity for the council, in the form of posters, announcements, and newsletter articles are crucial to communicating the importance of the meeting and soliciting membership. Regularly scheduled meetings with good group dynamics, possibly led by a staff member, if requested, are also vital. All participants should have an opportunity to speak and the meeting itself should be open to all residents. It should remain private from nonresidents, unless staff or others are specifically invited by the residents to attend.

Meetings should have a format, and minutes kept and read at the following meeting to check on progress. If department heads or administrative staff are invited to the meeting, and remark that a specific follow-up is to be performed, this should be noted in the minutes of the meeting. Getzel (1983) offers the comment that adjunct committees can be formed to allow more active residents to work on projects with department heads or as directed by the council.

Silverstone (1977) also notes that there may be impediments faced by activity professionals in forming a resident council, such as having uninvolved administrators or staff present, lack of resident interest, or a minority of residents regularly running the show.

The above issues are manageable when you consider the biggest problem that activity directors face in assisting resident councils is the changing abilities of the long-term care resident over the past few decades. The **continuum of care**, discussed in Chapter 1, shifted in the last decade or so, and changed the type of residents who are now typical in a long-term care facility. Because of the more fragile nature of the resident, both physically and mentally, there may be fewer residents in your facility who are able to participate in a full resident council session. This creates a dilemma of balancing on the one side the rights of residents to participate in their own decision-making through enrollment in the resident council, against the realities of their conditions and abilities on the other. As the long-term care client continues to advance in frailty, the resident council participation issue becomes more pronounced.

Resident Satisfaction and Life Satisfaction

During the dialogue of the resident council, issues are brought to the activity professional concerning **resident satisfaction** and **life satisfaction**. Resident satisfaction is defined as the level of **quality**, or measure of excellence, that residents perceive the delivery of care in the facility to be. Zinn, Lavizzo-Mourey, & Taylor (1993) suggest that resident satisfaction can be a primary indicator of care quality. The Nursing Home Resident Satisfaction Scale (NHRSS) used as the basis for their study, proposes questions to residents to test satisfaction, including: "Do you like the daily schedule? . . . How would you rate the daily schedule? . . ." Their study showed that the NHRSS was accurate in measuring resident satisfaction, although there were no significant findings related to resident satisfaction as a factor of age, specific facility, gender, or cognitive functioning.

As it relates to activity planning, resident satisfaction is defined by how pleased residents are with the number, type, and frequency of programs offered, and to what extent the programs adequately address their needs. The residents' ability to participate in the planning of programs is necessary and critical. Byrd (1983) studied the effects of control and choice in institutional life and concluded that ". . . when these individuals are forced to assume some measure of control over the activities programs at their respective institutions, there is a subsequent increase in satisfaction with both the quality of the institution and the quality of their own lives."

Your definition of quality for the activity department that you monitor on a regular basis (**quality assurance**), discussed in Chapter 14, should include both resident concerns of satisfaction and programming/documentation issues.

When predictors or indicators of quality are used in general studies of resident satisfaction, Linn (1974) found that obvious factors such as a comfortable, pre-planned facility that included specific use areas such as ". . . a recreational area . . . ," influenced ultimate resident satisfaction. Portnoy (1985) studied elderly needs and found that effective communication between staff and residents could be seen as a very significant factor in measuring a person's satisfaction and adjustment to an institutional setting. Additionally, Brown, Nelson, Bronkesh, & Wood (1993) discuss how residents utilize ". . . surrogates of quality . . . " to view their pleasure or displeasure with their entire care experience. By applying "surrogates" in terms of activities, a surrogate is seen as someone who smiles, shows a special interest in resident concerns, or brightens a significant day. Each of these are representations of the larger quality of service that the entire organization has to offer.

Some facilities measure resident satisfaction more formally by designating a staff member to collect issues from residents, staff, or family, and distribute these issues to the appropriate department to ensure proper resolution. Lanza, Lawyrk, and Piegari (1983) successfully utilized a patient representative model for resolving concerns that were not receiving attention in normal channels. By using a staff member charged with traditional patient representative duties based on a hospital model, requests and concerns were monitored in each department and residents were satisfied and assured that their needs were being met. Other facilities have devised a **resident concern form** (see Figure 4–6) to keep track of resident complaints or problems. The overall responsibility for monitoring this form may be left with the administrator, social worker, or the activity professional. The forms have two parts to allow the department which is reporting the complaint to retain a copy until the problem is actually resolved.

Life satisfaction is a general term, and applies to residents' overall feelings of adequacy in various aspects of their lives. The hypothesis has been that as individuals become more involved in active pursuits, and basic needs are met, the sense of satisfaction with life is higher. Not only is the activity department challenged with the task of

---

Resident Concern Form

A. REPORT OF CONCERN

    Resident name: _____

    Room number: _____

    Nature of concern: _____

    _____

    Reported to: _____

    Date issue occurred: _____

B. REVIEW AND FORWARDING OF CONCERN

    Reviewed by: _____

    Date: _____

    Forwarded to: (Name): _____

               (Department) _____

C. RESOLUTION AND FOLLOW UP OF CONCERN

    Description of how issue was resolved: _____

    _____

    _____

    _____

    Is any further follow up required? _____

    _____

    Signature of person handling resolution: _____

Figure 4–6 Handling residents' issues can be done with a resident concern form.

meeting needs through innovative programs, but also has the additional responsibility of contributing to the increase of life satisfaction with effective program planning.

In linking life satisfaction more directly to participation in activity programs, Larson (1978) reviewed thirty years of literature on life satisfaction and older adults, and concluded that individuals who fostered high interaction with their social environment and generally maintained an active lifestyle had a higher degree of life satisfaction than those who did not. Agostino, Gash, and Martinsen (1981) expanded on Larson's conclusions and discovered that life satisfaction is more highly correlated with residents' participation in activities that are classified as active (either in a group or individually), rather than passive. Passive participation in programs did not show the same life satisfaction impact.

Meeting Family and Friends of Your Residents ....

Your first visit with your new resident may give you the opportunity to meet and speak to the extended family. Learning as much as you can about the family will give you a clearer picture of the sources of information you need to follow up on your resident.

As discussed earlier, contacting family, friends, and neighbors for assistance in learning about your new resident is part of your assessment process. Family members may be out of the area physically, or even if in the area, out of touch socially. A family can be a subjective term, and may mean that friends and neighbors are actually considered family to a particular resident, even though grown children may live nearby. You may encounter feuding families, disinterested or disgusted relatives, or family members who appear hostile to you. All of these reactions are expressions of the involvement that family members play in the caregiving team.

Understanding the Needs of Family Members

Before you can gain the trust of families, and solicit their support for information about your new resident, you must first understand them. Looking at families as part of the "unit of service" that health care professionals must deal with when a resident is admitted, is suggested by Helphand and Porter (1982). They feel that meeting resident needs is enhanced by forging an early partnership with the family.

The family members, who accompany your resident, may be part of a growing segment of nonprofessional caregivers who have been caring for their loved one at home. The caregiving that they performed was most likely done without any formal training, usually with limited resources, and conducted while juggling numerous other responsibilities. Schwartz (1979) may have coined the term **sandwich generation** whereas Soloman (1983) uses the term "intergenerational crunch" to describe the generation of adults who range in age from forty to sixty as the middle-aged children who have responsibilities as a spouse, parent, or grandparent, and who have elderly relatives who rely on them for care. More recently, Stone and Kemper (1989) narrowed the "sandwich generation" definition to describe those individuals raising at least one child under the age of fifteen and simultaneously caring for an elderly or disabled parent. Their work estimates that the "sandwich generation" accounts for ". . . 1 out of every 13 persons with children under the age of 15."

Of the many family members who were in this predicament, and others who faced different caregiving challenges, most faced some form of the burdens of caregiving as researched by Cafferata and Stone (1989). The researchers report that the general effects of caring for a disabled person may result in loss of time from employment, decreased time spent in personal pursuits, increased anxiety and concern, and dwindling financial resources because of health care costs. Additionally, Cafferata and Stone discuss the difference between objective and subjective caregiving burdens. Objective burdens are routine tasks (such as assisting with **activities of daily living [ADLs]**) skills whereas subjective burdens are viewed as part of either "role conflict" or "role strain." Role conflict develops between the caregiver and the expectations of the person receiving the care. For example, a disabled person may expect a higher level of care when being taken care of by his or her own child. Role strain occurs when the caregiver attempts to care for her relative and assume other demanding roles such as mother, grandmother, and spouse.

Role reversal and a shift in dependency needs are other stress factors with which many families have to cope. Hirschfield and Dennis (1979) discussed the guilt that caregivers feel in relation to what they perceive as their responsibilities. Their study suggested that caregiver feelings of loneliness, depression, and resentment were also common. Additionally, the caregiver may be looking ahead to his or her own inevitable aging process and become anxious.

Once the resident has entered your facility, you may notice that some families cope with their feelings by becoming distant, others by getting involved, and others by simply watching everything from the sidelines. Horowitz and Lanes (1992) document the phenomenon of family and friends who become "witnesses" to caregiving. They may casually observe, or they may take on a more active role of thinking and speaking for the resident with a mix of sympathy and resentment. Fox (1986) reports that other families may assume an assertive role by being "vigilant" and "vocalizing" and involve themselves actively with all aspects of the caregiving.

Armed with that information, you as the activity professional must be prepared for the complex situations you may face as you approach the new resident. Along with the resident comes a complicated family dynamic that now will be a challenging part of your day.

Involving Family Members in the Activity Program

Entering the facility with this emotional baggage, the families need the understanding and support of the whole team. As the activity professional, you will have many opportunities to involve the family in constructive outlets that will benefit not only the residents and family members, but your program as well.

When you first meet the family, do not be discouraged by a lack of interest, or too much interest, in your program. As discussed earlier, these reactions are understandable. In the early stages of a resident's admission, you should try to gain a rapport with the resident and his or her family, and seek vital information about the resident to assist in your assessment. As you speak with families about their relatives, take the time to get to know them, too. They have to feel comfortable with you before they will give you the information you need. Do not get so focused on questions about the resident that you ignore obvious questions about them. And, while you are conversing, look for areas or skills they may have that may help with future programs.

Whenever possible, arrange to talk with families privately, instead of on-the-run, or in corridors. Allow enough time for them to express their feelings. If families need assistance for issues that are out of your area of expertise, make referrals for them, then follow up to see that the issue was handled. Give families a status report on the progress on the resident, and try to include positive information whenever possible. Family members should be personally invited to be part of programs when feasible but posters, flyers, and a newsletter are also great ways to inform them about the program. Families may wish to be direct participants by attending programs as motivators for the resident, volunteer to help with specific programs, or help with behind-the-scenes work. Any involvement from families benefits you and your program.

Family Council

Many facilities include a **family council** as part of activity and social service programming options to allow families to participate in facility operations in a controlled and productive manner. A family council can be a formal meeting of family members on a scheduled basis to discuss specific topics, such as advance directives, or it may operate as an informal gathering of family members who meet to talk about their own coping issues. Staff members may act as facilitators to open the discussion or may not be involved at all, except to schedule space in the facility for the meeting to be held. Helphand and Porter (1982) suggest that some of the objectives for family groups may be to form an association between the family and the staff, to educate families about expected facility policies and issues related to aging, and to create an arena to air concerns. Formation of a family council may provide an outlet for the adjustment issues that families are often faced with as they place a family member in a long-term care facility. Having an opportunity to express feelings such as resentment and guilt in a safe setting that includes other families dealing with similar issues can be comforting. In addition, the educational information that is included in family council meetings such as speakers, films, and literature, assist in reducing anxiety and building better communication with staff and administration.

In order to coordinate the formation of a family council (if one does not already exist), begin by speaking to your administrator and your co-workers in social services to gain some history on how a family council has worked in your facility in the past. Do not be discouraged if you find that a family council has not been a steady part of the activity calendar. It is often difficult to maintain interest in such a group when many of the members have different situations and residents come and go from the facility for many reasons. In her work on understanding family adjustments to institutionalization, Soloman (1983) mentions that family members have different needs as they experience the various institu-

tional "crises" of a resident's admission. A family member's need for support or education may vary based on the stage in which the resident is involved. For example, at the early stages of admission, a family member may benefit more from education and reassurance whereas in the later stages of a resident's illness, when the patient is closer to death, a family member may welcome the support of other families to help them begin the grieving and understanding process.

A technique that can be offered through the activity department to family members and residents to help them at any stage of adjustment is the **reminiscence** process. This will be discussed further in Chapter 10. Reminiscing, or recalling past, long-term memories, is part of a life review process that has therapeutic value for residents and family members. Weiss, Blake, and Koscianski (1991), in their study of family council members, suggest that using reminiscing between family and resident can have positive effects such as establishing credibility and reminding each of past successes as well as increasing self-esteem and decreasing depression. They further illustrate that family council members who receive training in reminiscence techniques feel more confident by having the skills to relate to their resident.

No matter what shape your family council structure has taken before, you will find it to be an important collaborative effort with social services to re-establish and motivate your family group for added programming benefits.

Merging With the Facility and Your Co-workers

As a new employee, fitting into the facility and meeting your co-workers means a positive start for you on the job. Each facility handles the new employee start-up process differently, so you may spend more or less time meeting your co-workers than is suggested here.

Introductions to Staff

Meetings with co-workers are usually set up within the first week or so of employment. Establishing professional relationships with co-workers up front helps you as you progress in your career in the organization. Determine in your first few meetings things such as areas of overlap between your departments, immediate concerns, and specific policies that you should be aware of in order to interact with other departments. If you sense any problems, request a second meeting to resolve issues, or see your administrator. Problems handled in the early stages are easier to solve than issues that have grown larger through avoidance or frustration.

You may be introduced to the general staff at a large meeting or maybe your facility has a policy of assigning you a "buddy" to introduce you around the building. You will meet many people in a short span of time, and you will not remember all the names, but make a point over the next few weeks to try to really meet and remember a few new staff members each time you are out on the resident floors.

Meeting Attendance

As an activity professional, you will be required to attend a number of meetings held throughout the facility on a regular basis. Chapter 2 discussed the type of meetings in which you may be involved. You need to find out what level of participation is required from you at certain meetings (this information usually comes from your administrator). For example, are your department head meetings held weekly with a very formal agenda and very little chatting by attendees, or do you have a daily, informal meeting with your administrator and fellow department heads? Are you expected to review charts and have specific recommendations ready before you come to the interdisciplinary care plan meetings, or does your group spend time at the meeting reviewing the chart together and having lengthy discussions about each resident? As a safety committee member, are you expected to do rounds and complete a safety checklist audit before a meeting, or are you part of a group that reviews incident reports and prepares a meeting agenda before the committee meets?

As you can see, there is more to attending a meeting than taking up chair space. You are a professional member of the team, and should come prepared and ready to participate in any meeting you attend. Meetings are meant to further ideas and make progress on resident issues. If you are unclear about your role, or sense that many of the meetings you attend are not productive, speak to your administrator or the committee chairperson well in advance of the meeting for clarification.

Practitioner Behavior and Standards of Practice ....

As a professional activity person, you have probably joined the field with some experience or training in the field of recreation or activity planning and implementation. If you are completely new to the industry, you should focus on gaining the proper credentials that meet your career objectives.

Long gone are the days when some people considered the activity profession a frivolous one. Today, professional activity and recreation organizations exist (which will be discussed in Chapter 19) which mandate a certain level of competency and job performance expectations called **practitioner behavior** or **conduct**. As an activity professional, you have a code of ethics to adhere to, as does the registered nurse, the administrator, and the registered dietician. Your certifying body—national, state or local organization—may already have set ethical standards for your conduct. Being certified by an outside organization is different than meeting the qualifications for your position. If you are not yet affiliated with a professional organization, bear in mind these general guidelines for acceptable behavior as an activity professional:

1. Act as a highly ethical role model for all team staff.
2. Uphold resident rights in all interactions and programs.
3. Show empathy and concern for resident illness and discomfort.
4. Explore the unique qualities of each resident and provide programs to reflect these qualities.
5. Seek continuous education to refine and improve your skills.

Joining an organization of activity or related professionals can be an enlightening experience. Not only will you feel validated as you see that many other professionals are facing the same challenges as you, but you will gain access into ideas and resources to stimulate your programs.

SUMMARY

Meeting and learning as much as you can about your residents, families, and staff puts you at an advantage as a team member. You work more efficiently and effectively if you know details about the people with whom you serve and work. The learning process is not a static one; rather as needs of residents change, and as some of your co-workers move on, you must continue the gathering of information to provide the best care to your residents.

R E V I E W   Q U E S T I O N S

1. What are the methods for collecting resident information during the activity assessment process?
2. How does resident satisfaction relate to quality assurance and quality indicators?
3. Name three of the issues that family members may be coping with as their relative is admit-ted to a long-term care facility.
4. Why is a resident status form or similar document important?
5. What are some of the suggestions made by Yeo to help make a program more ethnically sensitive?

O N   Y O U R   O W N

1. What other ways can you think of in order to increase your knowledge about new admissions when residents cannot assist you, and family members may be unavailable?
2. Devise a method to measure resident satisfaction that involves all departments.
3. Using the needs of family members as a guide, develop a presentation to a first family council for a facility.
4. In a paragraph, write your own code of ethics for your department.

R E F E R E N C E S

Agostino, J. N., Gash, T., & Martinsen, J. (1981). The relationship between recreational activity programs and life satisfaction of residents in Thunder Bay homes for the aged. *Activities, Adaptation and Aging,* 1 (4), 5–15.

Barresi, C., & Stull, D. (1993). Ethnicity and long-term care: An overview. In C. Barresi & D. Stull (Eds.) *Ethnic elderly and long-term care.* (p. 2–30), New York, NY: Springer Publishing Co.

Berkow, R., & Fletcher, A. (1992). *The Merck Manual of Diagnosis and Therapy.* 16th edition, Rahway, NJ: Merck Research Laboratories.

Brown, S. W., Nelson, N., Bronkesh, S. J., & Wood, S. D. (1993). *Patient satisfaction pays: Quality service for practice success.* Gaithersburg, MD: Aspen Publishers.

Byrd, M. (1983). Letting the inmates run the asylum: The effects of control and choice on the institutional lives of older adults. *Activities, Adaptation and Aging,* Vol. 3 (3), 3–11.

Cafferata, G. L., & Stone, R. (1989). The caregiving role: Dimensions of burden and benefits. *Comprehensive Gerontological Supplemental Issue, A+B,* 3: 57–64.

Fox, N. (1986). *You, your parent and the nursing home.* Buffalo, NY: Prometheus Books.

Getzel, J. (1983). Resident councils and social action. In G. S. Getzel & M. J. Mellor (Eds.), *Gerontological social work practice in long term care,* (p. 179–185). Binghamton, NY: The Haworth Press.

Helphand, M., & Porter, C. M. (1982). The family group within the nursing home: Maintaining family ties of long-term care residents. *Journal of Gerontological Social Work,* Vol. 4 (1), 51–62.

Hirschfield, I. S., & Dennis, H. (1979). Perspectives. In P. K. Ragan (Ed.) , *Aging parents,* (p. 2–10).

[Monograph]. University of Southern California Press.

Horowitz, K. E., & Lanes, D. M. (1992). *Witness to illness: Strategies for caregiving and coping.* Reading, MA: Addison-Wesley Publishing Co.

Lanza, S. E., Lawyrk, S. C., & Piegari, R. M. (1986). Establishing a patient representative program. *Contemporary Long Term Care,* February 1986, 36–39.

Larson, R. (1978). Thirty years of research on the subjective well-being of older americans. *Journal of Gerontology,* 33(1), 109–125.

Linn, M. (1974). Predicting quality of patient care in nursing homes. *The Gerontologist,* Vol. 14 (3), 225–227.

Merrill, T. (1979). *Activities for the aged and infirm.* Springfield, IL: Charles C. Thomas Publisher.

Morrison, J., & Zabusky, C. (1980). *American mosaic: The immigrant experience in the words of those who lived it.* New York, NY: E. P. Dutton.

Norman, A. (1985). *Triple jeopardy: Growing old in a second homeland.* London, England: Centre for Policy on Ageing.

Norris, J. N., Hawes, C., Murphy, K., Nonemaker, S., Phillips, C., Fries, B. E., & Mor, V. (1991). *Resident assessment instrument training manual and resource manual.* Natick, MA: Eliot Press.

Physician's Desk Reference (1995). Montvale, NJ: Medical Economics Data Production Company.

Portnoy, E. J. (1985). Communication and the elderly patient. *Activities, Adaptation & Aging,* Vol. 7 (2), 25–29.

Schwartz, A. N. (1979). Psychological dependency: An emphasis on the later years. In P. Kagan (Ed.), *Aging parents.* (p. 117–125). [Monograph]. University of Southern California Press.

Silverstone, B. M. (1977). *Establishing resident councils: Guidelines for residents and administrators desiring to organize or strengthen resident councils in residential facilities for the elderly.* New York, NY: Federation Of Protestant Welfare Agencies.

Soloman, R. (1983). Serving families of the institutionalized aged: The four crises. *Journal of Gerontological Social Work*, Vol, 5, (1/2), 83–96.

Stone, R. I., & Kemper, P. (1989). Spouses and children of disabled elders: How large a constituency for long-term care reform? *The Milbank Quarterly*, Vol. 67, Nos. 3–4

Thomas, B. (1988). Self-esteem and life satisfaction. *Journal of Gerontological Nursing*, Vol. 14, No. 12, 25–30.

Weiss, C., Blake, D., & Koscianski, V. (1991). Enhancing family council members' ability to relate to and reminisce with older disoriented residents: Replication and extension. *Topics in Geriatric Rehabilitation*, Vol. 7 (2), 45–59.

Yeo, G. (1993). Ethnicity and nursing homes: Factors affecting use and successful components for culturally sensitive care. In C. Barresi & D. Stull (Eds.) *Ethnic elderly and long-term care*, (p. 161–177). New York, NY: Springer Publishing Co.

Zinn, J., Lavizzo-Mourey, R., & Taylor, L. (1993). Measuring satisfaction with care in the nursing home setting: The nursing home resident satisfaction scale. *The Journal Of Applied Gerontology*, Vol. 12, No. 4, 452–465.

F U R T H E R   R E A D I N G

Barresi, C. M., & Stull, D. E. (1993). *Ethnic elderly and long-term care.* New York, NY: Springer Publishing Co.

Barrett, L. (1994). Supporting end of life decision making. *Activities, Adaptation and Aging*, Vol. 18, No. 3/4, 77–88.

Bartlett, M. (1944) Married widows: The wives of men in long-term care. Journal of Women and Aging, Vol. 6 (1/2) 91–106.

Curry, T., & Ratliff, B. (1973). The effects of nursing home size on resident isolation and life satisfaction. *The Gerontologist*, Autumn, 295–298.

Fain, S. (1985).The art of teaching professional ethics. *Therapeutic Recreation Journal*, 4th Quarter, 69–74.

Heim, P., & Piegari, R. (1987). Visitation program lifts spirits of hospitalized nursing home residents. *D.O.N.*, December, 38.

Pieper, H. (1989). *The nursing home primer: A comprehensive guide to nursing homes and other long-term care operations.* Whitehall, VA. Betterway Publications, Inc.

Schlessinger, B. (1989). The 'sandwich generation': Middle-aged families under stress. *Canada's Mental Health*, 37, September, 11–14.

Schwartz, A. N., & Vogel, M. (1990). Nursing home staff and residents families role expectations. *The Gerontological Society of America*, Vol. 30, No. 1.

Spence, D. A., & Wiener, J. M. (1990). Nursing home length of stay patterns: Results from the 1985 national nursing home survey. *The Gerontological Society of America*, Vol. 30, No. 1, 16–20.

Weiss, C., Bieber, J., Peterson, C., & Wold, L. (1983). Danger: T.R. at work. *Therapeutic Recreation Journal*, 1st Quarter, 12–17.

C H A P T E R 5
• • • • • • • • • • • • • • • • • • • •
Supervising Your Staff Through Effective Management Techniques

KEY TERMS..

management
leadership
probationary period
performance appraisal
anniversary date
disciplinary action

warning notice
termination
communication
delegating
consultant
intern

OBJECTIVES...

After completing this chapter, you should:

- Know the traditional tasks that will be required of you as a supervisor.
- Understand the way messages and communication are handled throughout the facility.
- Begin the process of forming your own management style through a review of various management issues.

• •

INTRODUCTION

With both your staff and/or volunteers, you will have numerous opportunities to practice the management skills you need to control and direct your department. Familiarizing yourself with your staff and gently guiding them to satisfactory performance is one of your management initiatives. By learning to handle the core aspects of management (hiring, orienting, and job counseling), you will be able to forward your department's objectives. Issues in the areas of communication and management also need to be addressed carefully.

Accomplishing tasks through other people is the easiest definition of **management**. Regardless of whether you are coming to your position as a seasoned manager or discovering management issues for the first time, your knowledge base of this critical subject area will serve you well as you navigate the complicated waters ahead.

You are already considered a professional in your field because of your training, and now by employment in your area of expertise. You are beginning the transition from professional to manager, which Lombardi (1993) and many other experts consider a critical growth stage in your employment. In his book on health care management, Lombardi mentions some of the adjustments a new manager makes include switching his or her orientation from a self-directed, clearly established situation as a professional to a less defined, fluctuating circumstance as a manager. Easing into the transition becomes easier if you understand some of the key elements and responsibilities of your new role.

Adding to the stress of making this new transition from professional to manager may be lingering feelings of nonacceptance by your peers or your administrator. Halberg and Waters (1991) discuss the phenomenon of activity professionals who do not accept themselves as department head managers because of a lack of professional competence, or a suspicion that staff members view them as wanting to have fun with residents instead of being serious-minded professionals. Even more disturbing, Halberg and Waters discovered that many activity professionals do not feel they are department heads, and are uncomfortable with that role. With such a large portion of time needed for managing people (Lombardi's [1993] estimates over sixty-five percent of a manager's time), the need to find a comfort zone as a manager is extremely important.

Assessing Your Staff ....

You have staff and/or volunteers working for you. Congratulations! Your administrator obviously feels that you are up to the challenge of managing people. After you have had a chance for brief conversation with each of your new employees, it is time to begin learning what you can about them and their past work patterns.

An easy way to start the process is to review your staffing time schedule and peruse your employees' personnel folders. You will get an indication of the length of service of each employee, any disciplinary notices, absenteeism records, and from time records, the best time to schedule a departmental welcome meeting.

Before you have the departmental meeting, plan at least a fifteen- to thirty-minute private meeting with each employee. This enables you to get to know them and their issues better. Sometimes these meetings yield trivia, and others give you a sense of the tone of the department and where problems lie that need attention. Your role in these meetings should be to say very little, and allow your employee a chance to talk without interruptions.

At your formal first meeting, you should come prepared with an agenda that includes any comments on the private meetings you had with others (i.e., any departmental issues which resulted from the meetings), and a brief outline of your background and approach to the department. Establishing yourself as a leader with specific expectations is important, but indicating or mentioning radical changes will not endear you to your new employees. Even though your individual and group meetings may have given you clues to areas you want to change within your department, you would be wise to say "Many of you have mentioned that you would like to expand our sensory program so we will be looking at that over the next few weeks," instead of "There are big problems with our sensory program which will be changed by the end of the month." Observing and studying your department during the first few weeks and months helps you clearly judge what changes may need to be made. Impulsive moves only result in double work (you have to make another change to correct the first one), and you may lose the respect of your ability as a leader from your staff.

Handling Traditional Supervisory Tasks ....

Job situations vary with the size of the building, the type of administrative structure, and the number of employees. Perhaps you have only one employee who has been with the organization for ten years but requires attention, or you may have five employees who work on different floors of a large building and who are used to being independent. The American Health Care Association (1988) lists three areas of responsibilities for supervisors that should guide their management of employees:

- quality of work activities (ways to help employees gain more from a job)
- industry competence (technical guidance and support)

- control (assuring that facility and department policies are followed).

We will discuss areas of supervisory practice and illustrate key elements of a manager's knowledge that will assist in getting a satisfactory performance from all the employees under your jurisdiction.

Leadership

Acting as a leader and setting standards for your staff in a **leadership** role is the first step in establishing a successful work environment. Lombardi (1993) defines leadership as ". . . the catalyst of all action in any group," and suggests that effective leadership takes on an even more important role in health care settings because of the crisis-oriented nature of health care delivery. Residents have medical situations which occur at any time, and a cool-headed leader knows how to lead the staff and bring the event to a successful conclusion.

What are the qualities of an effective leader? Making decisions and sticking to them, taking charge in difficult situations, and setting clear job and role responsibilities are some aspects of good leadership. In discussing patient satisfaction, Brown, Nelson, Bronkesh, and Wood (1993) talk about leaders "modeling quality," and cite additional leadership traits as listening to others, having vision, and seeing value in the people and their work. Zenger (1985) adds that leaders use good communication skills when speaking of an organization's values, and in turn, develop loyal followers.

Being a leader and being a supervisor or manager go hand in hand. As a manager, it helps your supervisory style if you have natural or learned leadership skills. All managers, no matter what their abilities, face similar supervisory tasks that shape their department's effectiveness.

Recruitment

Your staff may be stable at the moment, but at one time or another, most managers face the prospect of replacing a staff member. The opening may result from resignation, or an employee may have been terminated by you for poor performance or other issues. If a staff member resigns, request the resignation be put in writing according to your facility policies (i. e., the amount of notice required for individuals who resign may be equal to the amount of vacation time they accrue annually). This resignation period gives you a chance to find a suitable replacement (and possibly have the new person trained) before your current employee leaves. When an employee resigns, you should meet with the individual to determine the cause of the resignation. The written resignation letter may not hold all the facts, and you should know of any problems, if they exist. When a job opening becomes available because of a planned termination you initiated, you should make some coverage arrangements before the termination takes place. No matter how a staff opening occurs, you are responsible, as supervisor, to ensure your residents' activity needs do not suffer during this transition stage.

An employee opening creates an opportunity, although when you are faced with the prospect of filling a position, the situation appears to be less of an opportunity than a headache. When someone leaves, you have the chance to rethink the position and make adjustments that may better suit your residents' needs. You may want to include more responsibilities in your assistant's job description, or perhaps make a change in the job title that would sound more attractive. Redoing the job description and clearly addressing the salary, hours, benefits, and union membership (if applicable) are important before you begin to recruit new employees.

Your recruitment process should start internally, preferably within your own department. Are there staff members who are qualified, and who could be promoted or moved from part-time to full-time? Some facilities require the posting of internal job openings for a specified number of days before external recruitment begins, or working with a personnel department to screen applicants. If no one from your in-house staff is interested or qualified, place a newspaper advertisement (if budget permits), or contact local activity organizations or schools with an appropriate major that suits your program. Establishing contact with other activity professionals in the area helps at times of staff replacement because they often know of interested and qualified individuals. If you place a newspaper advertisement, be sure to include a brief description of the position, if it is full- or part-time, if weekends or evenings are involved, hours, and rate of pay (optional). Be sure that the ad is clear, and to whom you wish applicants to respond, either by telephone, coming to the facility to complete application materials, or by sending a resume. Include the facility name, address, telephone number, and a contact name in the advertisement. Placing advertisements is usually approved by your administrator, be sure to check your facility policy.

Interviewing

A good advertisement or helpful activity contact may have elicited some responses. If you speak to applicants by telephone before setting up interviews, try to get a sense if they are suitable for the opening. You can learn much about your candidates from the interview scheduling telephone call. Are they brisk and shrill in voice, or do they have difficulty taking down the directions to the facility? If you are reviewing resumes or applications, look beyond the qualifications and experience that you require. Neatness, grammar usage, and completeness count, and give you a good indication of the person you are going to meet during the interview.

Interviews should be scheduled allowing adequate time (at least twenty to thirty minutes) to review the position requirements, question the applicant, and conduct a tour. After you become experienced at handling interviews, you will be able to assess a candidate in the first few minutes, and give an abbreviated interview if you know for a fact they are unsuitable for the position. The interview itself should start on time and be held privately. You may form opinions about an applicant who comes late to an interview, but the applicant may also look less favorably on your facility if you kept him or her waiting twenty minutes for no explained reason. Once the candidate is seated and some "small talk" has taken place, take control of the interview by asking the candidate your prepared questions. If the answers to your questions take you off course, be sure to remember your focus. You will want to ask about past experience, reasons for wanting to work in a long-term care setting, commuting time, and accomplishments. Be prepared for "canned," or insincere, answers that some candidates offer; you may have to dig below the surface to get the answers you want. Have a copy of the job description available to review in detail with the candidate.

In the next segment of the interview, you should outline the goals of your department, responsibilities of the position, and describe the type of person you are seeking. Discuss the specifics of the position, and include hours, weekend coverage, and benefits. If the salary is not predetermined by administration, it may or may not be brought up by the candidate. Some applicants feel uncomfortable, but be prepared to disclose either your set salary figure or the salary range for the position, based on the experience of the applicant. If the applicant does not bring up the issue of salary, ask what range or amount they are currently making and the amount they are seeking. This can be tricky because some candidates are not always honest, or their answers may effectively eliminate them as a candidate.

In the last area of the interview process, allow the candidate to question you about any information you have already covered, or bring up any new issues. Again, the tone and type of information they deem important may be enlightening. For instance, if they often ask about the condition of your parking lot in snowy weather, you may predict attendance issues on bad weather days. If the candidate questions you about the specific aspects of your program, and shares enthusiastic accomplishments of his or her own, the person may be a good match for your department. Be careful of what people do not ask about. When candidates do not follow up on basic information they should know about the job, let that be a warning sign.

Following the question phase, conduct the facility tour. By asking selected residents and staff in advance, introduce your candidate to targeted colleagues and residents, and get their feedback afterward. Observing your applicant in resident situations (which are often unpredictable, even on tours) will give you further information on his or her viability as an employee. Does the applicant appear comfortable? Outgoing or reserved? Does he or she ask questions about what he or she sees, or does he or she want the tour to end? What kind of resident or staff interactions were made? Your opinions may change as you walk a candidate through the building. The outgoing, perfect activity assistant in the office may be transformed into a nervous, mousy type during the tour.

If you have not discussed references, obtain permission in writing from the candidate to check some business and personal references. The business references hold the most clout since former bosses can comment on work performance whereas personal references are often from friends or long-time associates, and can be biased in favor of the applicant. Close the interview by giving the candidate a clear indication of your timetable for filling the position, and when your next contact with him or her will be made.

The Hiring Process

Consideration of hiring a person to fill your position is based on the application that lists experience, the interview in which you received personal impressions and personality indications, and from a reference check. When a candidate meets your parameters in these areas, and you can offer a salary that is suitable for you both, you are ready to make your top candidate a job offer. Gather your notes of all the conditions of the position (hours, salary, and so forth) as well as any special items that you discussed (i.e., pre-employment agreements about an unpaid vacation after the third month of employment), and call the candidate and review the list. Employees may be paid as salaried, hourly, on-call or as temporary employees, depending on your facility policies. Give the applicant a brief time (if needed) to decide if the terms are acceptable, and to get back in touch with you. Some hirings are "negotiated" with issues like vacations or salary reviewed back and forth between the employer and the applicant. You may find that negotiations are more a part of the hiring process for department head positions.

If the applicant accepts your offer of hire, secure a firm starting date for the position. An overlap of time between the outgoing activity staff member and the new employee is preferable, but if that is impossible, ask if the new person can come in for a day, or even a few hours, to spend with your current employee.

Put all the information that you and your candidate agreed on in writing, and mail a copy to him or her prior to the starting date. This reaffirms your interest in your new employee and gives an opportunity to cover any misunderstood items well in advance of the starting date. Include in the mailing any personnel information to be completed and instructions on scheduling a pre-employment physical.

Orientation and Training

Now that the starting date is scheduled, begin preparing for the new employee's first day. Nothing is worse for a new person than to not feel welcome or to lack structure in the first few days and weeks. An absence of planning on your part may mean that your new employee is placed in situations where he or she is not prepared to handle certain issues, or may get erroneous information from someone else who is trying to help. The habits formed in the first few days are critical, and you are in charge of seeing that your new person gets off to the right start.

Initially, explain to the new employee how long the orientation lasts, who conducts it, and how time is to be spent in the first week or so. When you personally answer questions, rather than sending the person here or there, it helps in bonding. Watch for any problem areas during the orientation session. Small issues can grow to unmanageable size quickly without your intervention. Feedback from other staff, co-workers, and residents is also helpful.

After the orientation checklist has been completed by the employee, meet with the new person to determine if there are any issues that need to be addressed. In many instances, you may have noted minor problems during orientation that need to be mentioned to the employee, about which he or she may be completely unaware. Also, situations may arise with some new employees where extending the orientation period becomes necessary. If you need to add more orientation time (with permission from your administrator), there should be a clear limit and purpose for the extension.

Scheduling

Developing a written schedule for all employees in your department brings order to the delivery of your program. At the time of hire, an employee's hours and work days were discussed and agreed upon mutually. Your job as manager is to write a work schedule for all your employees based on two factors. One item is the time period during each day that your department is "open," (i.e., 9:00 a.m.–8:00 p.m.). These are the hours when staff is available. With the demands of addressing needs for the cognitively impaired residents increasing, more activity departments are expanding their view of their traditional day. The second consideration in scheduling is the availability and working agreements of your staff. If you have arranged for your two staff members to rotate and work every other weekend, give them days off during the week to compensate. Consider your staffing budget, and the number of hours staff are slated to work each day. What about breaks, lunch, and dinner? Are meals paid or unpaid time? Are meal breaks one-half hour or one hour

in length? Is it your facility policy to encourage staff to remain on premises during lunch?

An easy way to create a work schedule is to list the full name of each employee in the left-hand column and use the horizontal space to write out the dates of the schedule period you are covering (i.e., fourteen days or one month). Start your draft schedule by roughing in the dates you know people are working, such as weekend rotation time. Then fill in the rest of the schedule, using your program calendar as a guide. Remember to stagger time to cover evening programs, be sure to allow full staff for days when key meetings are held, and take into account your department's special needs. Your schedule should be posted in a visible area in your activity office or other accessible spot. Employees should know when you plan to post a new schedule which should be at least one week prior to the end of the old schedule. Set up a clear departmental procedure for your employees so they understand how far in advance they must request time off in writing. An example of a work schedule is shown in Figure 5–1.

Supervision

Ensuring that your employees are doing their job in support of your whole department is part of your responsibility as a manager. The length of service for your employees has some bearing on the amount of supervision they may require, but all of your employees need attention, observation, and follow-up on their projects on a regular basis.

You can accomplish supervision through either direct or indirect methods. Handling supervision directly means physically observing your staff in different situations (running a program, interacting with a resident, or speaking to a family member). The spontaneity involved in observing staff under varied conditions at different times gives you a clearer picture of their conduct. Direct supervision can also be accomplished by doing side-

Activity Department Work Schedule														
Time Period: _____ Prepared by: _____														
Employee Name/Title/Status	Jan 17S	18M	19T	20W	21T	22F	23S	24S	25M	26T	27W	28T	29F	30S
Caglianone, M., Director FT	9–5	12–8	—	8–4	9–5	10–6	—	—	9–5	8–4	9–5	—	10–6	10–6
Martinez, E., Asst. FT	—	9–5	12–8	—	8–4	12–8	10–6	9–5	12–8	—	10–6	12–8	9–5	—
Zarski, J., Asst. PT	—	—	8–4	4–8	4–8	—	4–8	—	—	4–8	—	8–4	4–8	—

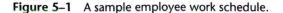

Figure 5–1 A sample employee work schedule.

by-side programs along with your assistant, and making casual observations. When you establish a team atmosphere with your staff, supervisory visits feel comfortable and nonthreatening. If you come around infrequently, you and the staff may feel out of place. The best way to gain the most information about your staff and their programs is to make frequent casual, nonpurposeful "drop-in" visits to all sites where staff and residents are found. If you stop by and ask what new project they are working on instead of questioning them about the lack of attendance at yesterday's program, you will certainly receive a warm welcome, and begin to learn more about your employee. The ideal characteristics of a management and supervisory style was viewed by Halberg and Waters (1991). They found that the most impactful supervision counts on the activity professional looking at tasks of subordinates equally with the maintenance of morale. Save the negative issues for an office visit in private unless you see something of a serious nature (i.e., a safety infraction). Some supervisory issues have to be handled on the spot, but in a private location and with tact.

Some indirect ways you learn about your employee and supervise them are through verbal and written communication in the facility. Your co-workers, families, and residents, whether asked or not, will provide you with feedback on your employees. You should not use their comments as your only guide; your personal observations are the real gauge of performance. Are your employees interpreting your written work schedule correctly and showing up for work on time and on the correct days? Are they completing request slips for time off that they need?

Written communication, in medical records, memos, and so forth, is another representation of

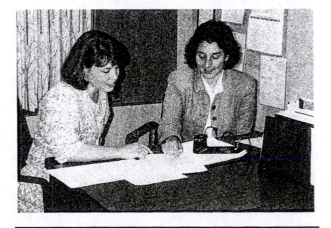

Figure 5–2 Holding regular meetings with employees helps you communicate and avoid conflict.

your department by your employee. Through these forms of communication, you may be able to see indirect aspects of your employee's performance that you can evaluate along with your direct observations.

Your reason for supervising, either directly or indirectly, is to measure your employee's performance against their job description for the position. Look for opportunities for praise, ways that you can help the employee succeed, and indications of any further training that may be needed. Most facilities have a **probationary period** of employment, lasting from thirty to ninety days, on average. Your close observation of the employee, along with help and guidance, assists the employee in completing his or her probationary period, and becoming a permanent member of the staff.

Another part of your task as supervisor is to provide your employees with recognition and praise as positive motivation for continued success. Some theorists postulate that as a manager, you should look for as many positive items to comment on to employees about their performance to keep their interest up, and reserve the negative observations for rare occasions. Recognition, in small daily doses, helps in bonding your staff to you, and helps them realize their worth. Formal praise, such as yearly bonuses, rewards, or honoring them during National Activity Professionals Week, goes a long way toward increasing their positive work and hopefully, their work performance.

The role of supervisor may feel uncomfortable to you at first, but after some experience, and with any luck, a good mentor for guidance, you will gain the confidence you need to face any situation. Most seasoned managers have made many mistakes and had their share of good decisions and questionable ones. Some of the most critical tips that the majority of managers agree on includes pitching in to help employees, being available, having a positive attitude, handling employee discussions in private, and being clear about expectations in the first place.

Employee Evaluation

After you new employee has spent his or her probationary period of employment under your direction and guidance, a **performance appraisal** should be prepared by you and presented to the employee in a private conference. Not all facilities require this, but many find that having a written summary of the employee's overall performance during the probationary period accomplishes two objectives: first, the employee is made aware of the strengths and weaknesses in his or her performance, with suggestions for areas in which to improve; and second, the employer is forced to seriously evaluate an employee and decide if continued employment is suitable. If it is recommended to continue employing the individual, then the employer spells out clear objectives for future performance. Halberg and Waters (1991) additionally illustrate that factors such as motivation of performance and identification of training needs are other purposes of the appraisal process.

The performance appraisal session should take place privately, with enough time allotted to cover the material without continued interruptions. Your facility probably uses a standardized form that has a rating score and a space for comments under a few key categories such as absenteeism, quality of work, quantity of work, and rapport with residents and staff. You may have the opportunity to devise your own form in which case you can make the rating criteria very specific for the job you are evaluating. There should be a space (and time) set aside to listen to any comments the employee may have and an opportunity should be given to him or her to write personal comments down on the form, if desired. Before you close the meeting, alert the employee to the next scheduled performance review. According to your facility policy, reviews may be done annually on the **anniversary date** of employment, or may be required every six months or on some alternative schedule. An original copy of the performance appraisal form should be placed in the employee's personnel folder, and if your policy permits, the employee may request a copy of the completed form as well.

Employee Counseling and Discipline

During the course of your supervision, you may encounter clear indications that some areas of your employee's performance require your intervention. If you notice something minor for the first time, you may opt to make a mental note of it but not bring it up to the employee. If you begin to see patterns of noncompliance with facility policies (i.e., repeated absences or lateness) or trends that involve safety concerns (i.e., leaving potentially dangerous work materials in the Alzheimer's unit), gather your thoughts and speak to the employee about these issues. Educate him or her on the seriousness of the issues, and request a return to compliance with the policies. Once you have spoken formally with an employee about performance issues and document your meeting, you have taken **disciplinary ac-**

tion. Depending on your facility's guidelines, you should start a discussion with a verbal counseling session. During a verbal session, have a written summary of the points you wish to cover that will be reviewed with the employee, and document it in his or her personnel record. In many facilities, a verbal counseling is written on an employee disciplinary form, but the employee may not be required to sign it. The reason the session is called verbal counseling, although a written copy is kept, is to ensure that a record of the session is retained for future use in the employee's folder. Some employee incidents never get further than the verbal warning stage, which is really the desired result. The intent of the verbal counseling session is to alert an employee about areas of concern so that he or she can take steps to make improvements before the issue escalates.

Should there be further instances of noncompliance on a particular matter, a written **warning notice** is issued. This step is more serious, because your facility, like many others, probably has a formal disciplinary procedure. These include verbal warnings as the first step, followed by first, second, and third written warnings that lead to suspension and termination, if required. The written warnings are documented on the employee's disciplinary form which includes space for reasons for disciplinary action, date of infraction, date of last warning (if applicable), remedial measures expected, signatures of both employee and supervisor, and space for any employee comments. When a written warning is given to an employee, it is often the facility policy that the session be witnessed by another management employee. In the case of a unionized facility, the entire disciplinary process may be spelled out in the union contract, and special circumstances may apply. The employee is asked to write his or her comments on the form, if desired, and sign that he or she has received the warning (even if he or she does not agree with it). There are occasions where an employee refuses to sign the document. In this circumstance, a witness to the warning session becomes useful. Your witness signs as management verification that the employee refused to sign the warning slip, and that the third party witnessed the conference.

If after repeated attempts to help an employee comply with the policies of the home, and the employee does not accomplish this, further warning notices may be written. In each case, the warnings should include a statement that gives an indication of the expected next step in the disciplinary process if compliance is not achieved.

For example, at the time a third warning notice is issued for absenteeism, a notation should be placed on the warning notice that states, "A further incident of absenteeism over the next ____ days will result in a suspension from the facility." The employee is then aware of the consequences for further noncompliance.

Before your employee attends a verbal counseling session, inform your administrator of your plans. The administrator will review the facility steps, and give you some guidance as to how to handle the situation. By the time you have reached the stage of suspension or termination (a situation that many never face), you should be in close contact with your administrator about the steps you are taking, including showing the administrator a rough draft of your disciplinary forms at each stage for his or her comments. If you do suspend an employee for a period of time, be sure your administrator agrees as to the length of time. A one-day suspension may be adequate for simple noncompliance issues like continued absentism, but additional days may be required for more serious issues. You should clearly state on the warning slip the number of days of suspension, including the return to work date. These days are, of course, unpaid.

Termination

One of the most trying situations you can face as a manager is the need to terminate an employee. By the time an employee situation escalates to this point, there usually have been numerous counseling sessions concerning the issues under discussion. It should be mentioned that most facilities have a list of items (i.e., stealing or defacing facility property), that are causes for immediate **termination**, with the proceeding steps. Should you face the termination of an employee, be sure that all efforts have been made (and documented) to attempt to correct the behavior before this step is taken. If the disciplinary process stages are followed, you should feel secure that you have carefully given the employee every opportunity to improve without success. If your administrator approves, proceed with the termination in private, but with another department head (or your administrator) as a witness. Your notes on the reasons for termination should be clearly written on the termination slip, along with the dates of all past warning sessions. The employee should be offered the opportunity to give verbal and written comments as well as sign the document. Surrendering of facility equipment and keys occurs at this time, and often, it is helpful to have another

department head escort the terminated employee to his or her work area to gather personal things to minimize the shock to the rest of the facility. Once the terminated employee has left the facility, you should notify key staff and your other departmental employees of the departure. It is not professional behavior to discuss the specific details with other staff, only that the termination occurred.

You may be thinking, "I could never do that!" Well, you can and you may have to some day, if you have an employee who is not suitable for the delivery of activity services to your residents. Your job as a manager is to give a carefully screened and oriented employee every chance to do a super job. But when serious issues cloud a performance, and begin to take a disastrous toll on the operations of your department, you have no choice but to take action. If your attempts to bring the employee back to a good and reliable performance do not work, termination may be a necessary option. You should know that terminations are very unpleasant, even for managers with years of experience. A self-assuring thought you should have at this time is that you did everything in your power to help the employee achieve a good performance. You spoke to, worked with, counselled, and documented the areas of concern with him or her. If all that was done, and potential employees still are unable or unwilling to accept the responsibilities of the position, then you did not fire them; they fired themselves! If you think of the situation that way, you will feel better. And if you have to do it again, you will be strengthened by your experience.

On the flip side, most facilities have a formal procedure for handling grievances. This is for employees who have an issue that they feel cannot be resolved through the normal channels of bringing it to you for solution. Your employee may come to you with an unresolved issue that may have nothing to do directly with job performance (i.e., feels that the last raise should have been more, or unhappy that he or she has to work the next holiday). With an internal grievance procedure in place in your facility, your employee has the option of pursuing the issue further within the guidelines, if desired. Keep all notes of any conversations you have with employees concerning their conferences with you on the issues because they may become necessary if the grievance procedure is used.

Managing Issues Between Departments ....

As the main advocate for your department, you will be rewarded with good interdepartmental relationships and a harmonious activity department team for your efforts in communicating effectively and constructively at every opportunity.

Communication Skills

Each day you have numerous occasions to inform, alert, listen, discuss, seek opinions, and teach employees, co-workers, families, and the administrator. In the American Health Care Association (1988) training materials for managers, they report that ". . . communication requires an exchange of information that assures mutual understanding." The **communication** opportunities that you have available to you should not be taken lightly because they are your means of getting things accomplished.

The types of communication you have available to you are written, verbal, and body language. In outlining the differences in communication formats, The American Health Care Association (1988) ranks face-to-face verbal communication as the most effective form of exchange of ideas because there is the most chance of the message being understood with time for eye contact and other feedback. Verbal communication is used in meetings, conferences, resident interactions, and the telephone.

Written communication (i.e., memos, letters, newsletters, and reports) has permanence, and the opportunity to provide a more detailed message. There is, however, little feedback from the receiver when this method is used.

Body language, which The American Health Care Association calls "non-verbal communication," is a more subtle form of communication that gives clues into the real message that a communicator intends to make. For example, if you participate in a meeting where the speaker is trying (verbally) to be enthusiastic about a project but keeps yawning, what message do you take away from that meeting?

In your department you will have many ways of applying all forms of communication. You will have verbal, face-to-face communications with your staff, supervisor, and resident and family interactions. Memos to your staff, letters to families, budget reports to the administrator, your activity calendar, and your activity work schedule are all important forms of written communication that you must handle regularly. With a positive attitude, your body language will support your feelings. Use your knowledge about nonverbal communication to help unravel unclear messages from other co-workers and residents.

Talking to Your Administrator

As we mentioned earlier, keep your administrator informed of the status of your departmental issues. It is important to gain direction and support from your administrator on supervisory issues that could be inflammatory. Resignations, employee conflicts, recruitment efforts, warning notices, and possible grievance situations comprise the information the administrator needs from you to understand the workings of your department. If your administrator is unavailable, be sure to document your information and leave it for review. Keep a photocopy of your memo for your records.

Holding Meetings and Facility Functions

Previous discussions focused on your role as a meeting attendee, but how should you prepare if you host a meeting or other facility function? First, know your target audience. If you are having an activity department meeting, prepare differently for that gathering than for a planning meeting you are chairing on the new chapel with the board of directors. Have an agenda in place before the meeting. For some meetings, it is useful to circulate the agenda to all participants before the meeting to prepare them for the upcoming discussion. Make sure the meeting spot accommodates all the meeting attendees, and that there are enough materials (hand-outs, agendas, and so forth) for each participant. Assert yourself as the person in charge of the meeting by starting it on time, managing the flow of discussion, and including as many participants as you can in the discussion process. End the meeting on time with a recap of the key points and items. All of us, as health care managers, have spent hours of unnecessary time at meetings at the mercy of ill-prepared hosts who did not follow some of the key points in meeting etiquette. As a result, less of the objectives of the facility were met. As an activity professional, use every chance to hone your leadership skills and forward the image of the activity professional as a key member of the management team.

Establishing Your Own Management Style ....

The practice of good management techniques is ongoing, and fits each new manager and situation differently. You may work in a facility where formality is the common practice, so your style should adjust to that tone. On the other hand, your facility might be casual, and you can have a more relaxed manner. In most cases, the management style of the administrator or administrative team (owners, board of directors) often sets the tempo for the rest of the building. For instance, if your administrator is very precise in his approach to handling problems (i.e., written documentation done for every meeting, however brief), some of that will no doubt rub off on you because he or she expects you to manage issues in a similar way. Do not be discouraged if your manner appears to be unique; there are many examples of individuals with completely different management approaches coexisting happily in the same organization.

In a report from Halberg and Waters (1991), determining a particular supervisory method for an activity professional can be accomplished according to the personality and internal values of the supervisor and subordinate along with the unique characteristics of the facility.

Another way that a style is formed evolves from the handling of the daily onslaught of conversations, writing, conferences, and other issues that Lombardi (1993) calls "administrivia." Some issues help your style, others hinder it, but all have an impact on creating the successful manager in you.

Attitude and Assertiveness

Developing a positive mindset and learning to assert yourself as a person are two steps in the process of forming a management style. Hitting the highs and lows of managing people and running a demanding program can cause the most spirited person to lose sight of goals from time to time. Cultivating an overall positive approach to deal with people and problem solving will make your whole outlook (and results) seem brighter. Kranz and Frauen (1986) talk about using "attitude maintenance" by always allowing yourself time to prepare for anything, going over your successes to motivate future performances, and using mental imagery to see the results you desire in a planning stage. Handling failures on a large or small level is helped by a positive attitude.

Establishing assertive techniques in your dealings with people, regardless of whether they are staff or residents, should help you express more of your needs to those around you. In all of your business dealings, you and your department have rights or entitlements to certain expectations of performance. When these expectations are not met, or are not handled in the manner in which you had hoped, you should use assertive measures to let your opinions be known concerning the situation. Assertiveness, the confident and persuasive method of allowing your feelings to be expressed, is not the same as aggression. An aggressive approach to problem solving might be complete control of the situation whereas an assertive view might be the simple expression of feelings on the subject. Feeling more comfortable in your role as manager allows you to test more assertive techniques, and allowing yourself to try more assertive techniques will increase your level of comfort as a manager.

Issues in Management

There are a number of areas that should be addressed in the area of management that can help you be your best as an activity professional supervisor.

Listening. Being a good listener is such a simple idea one would not think it necessary to mention. Many managers, however, forget that lending an ear at times can be very helpful to co-workers, families, and residents. Listening is a skill that can be developed for more effective use through some guidelines formulated by Franz and Frauen (1986). They suggest that listening habits can be improved by not giving into the many distractions that cloud our work day (resisting second-guessing of the ideas of the speaker and not offering advice unless asked).

Active listening, which involves a process in which the listener accepts responsibility for interpreting the message that is being spoken, requires the listener to look for clues about feelings through body language and reserve opinions while trying to understand the view of the speaker. Being an active listener means that any barriers to receiving a clear message, such as making assumptions or disinterested listening, must be eliminated.

Developing good listening skills will help in all facility interactions and relationships. One of the most difficult times to be a good listener is during a situation of duress where a resident may be angry or an employee unhappy with a decision. Sharp listening skills, coupled with calm intervention, are important tools when seeking solutions.

Conflict Resolution. A hidden danger in all work groups and departments is the potential for conflict at any time. Even conflict that appears to have roots in only one department will have effects on the rest of the facility, if not properly resolved. Some issues of conflict seem to appear out of nowhere, but most have been forming for a while unnoticed. With practice, Lombardi (1993) suggests that you can look for warning signs of conflict to come (i.e., criticism, changes in performance, avoidance of others, and excuse-making) in order to head off potential conflicts. Resolving conflicts effectively involves time to collect the information about the issue and an attempt to mediate a fair conclusion that satisfies both parties. Your goal is to be sure that the policies of the facility that govern the services to the residents are upheld.

Time Management. With the shrinking resources available in health care, the activity professional has to view time as a valuable commodity and use it wisely. Some of the suggestions for managing time more effectively range from the suggestions of Cunninghis (1984) to set clear job priorities, delegate any duties, and remove time wasters, to the ideas of Lombardi (1993) that include planning a priority, developing better telephone management skills, and shortening meetings. Franz and Frauen (1986) feel that being a good listener automatically helps save time because messages do not need to be repeated. Certainly, general organization, daily "to do" lists, and goal setting will also be effective.

Stress and Burnout Control. Stress is an unavoidable fact of daily work in a long-term care facility and may be more acute in a fast-paced activity department. The stress itself may not change, but your ability to handle it can be al-

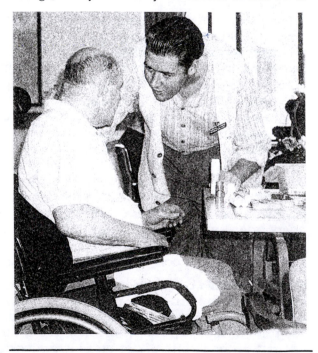

Figure 5–3 Active listening is an important communication skill.

tered. Cunninghis (1984) gives a fair overview of the suspected reasons why an activity professional could have stress, ". . . the very qualities that lead people to choose a helping profession . . . are quite possibly the same ones that make them more vulnerable to high levels of stress. These people often are sensitive with high ideals, great enthusiasm, and a desire to be useful and needed." She also discusses stress factors, such as small departments with no staff, that can lead to isolated feelings, the general view of the activity profession, and demanding job expectations. Some of the daily rigors of the job of a health care manager (information overload and being overwhelmed by numerous requests) are described by Lombardi (1993) as a negative influence over productivity.

Most experts who talk about stress management suggest taking time for yourself each day to recharge, leaving the job behind at the end of the day, learning to relax, and not being so hard on yourself.

Delegating Authority. **Delegating** is a great way to manage time and, coincidently, relieve stress. You, as the manager, are in charge of the overall work load for your department. It is your responsibility to look at the tasks at hand and the resources you have (staff and otherwise), and find ways to effectively assign some work functions to other staff members and still get the job done. Delegating work should not be a dumping of all the unpleasant tasks, but instead a match of duties with skills and abilities. Any assigned work has to have specific instructions and the due date for completion. Your responsibility does not end by delegating work to someone on your staff and waiting for the work to come back complete. You must monitor and follow up on any assigned work to be sure the directions have been understood, the quality is present, and the requested due date is met.

Dealing With Consultants. Having **consultants**, either as part of your larger parent company or as outside agents, is becoming a common place occurrence for many activity professionals. Learning to work effectively with consultants without losing sight of your departmental objectives is crucial. A consultant is usually someone with a background that includes field experience in long-term care as well as certification and/or a degree in activities or recreation leadership. The person may also be a regional corporate representative from your facility headquarters who does not have a direct background in activities, but instead has training in nursing or a related field.

The reasons for employing consultants varies from facility to facility. In one facility, it may be the practice of the corporate quality assurance staff to do monthly programming audits, and in another, an outside consultant may be brought in to work with new staff or help launch a new project. Because the reasons are different, so are the services that a consultant provides to a facility. A consultant can do everything from statistical reports to staff evaluations and program observations, normally functions independently instead of as a direct member of the care team, and usually does not actively participate in the implementation of programs. Cunninghis (1984) suggests that the consultants who are most effective include the activity staff in their planning, give a full report to the activity personnel that they serve, and are aware that proposing major changes would seriously impact the morale of the staff.

A recommended plan for working with consultants is to first secure direction from your administrator about the scope of the consultant's responsibility. After meeting the consultant, give an overview of your department and projects, and ask for a summary of his or her role. If there are any discrepancies in the two versions of consultant responsibility, check with your administrator for clarification. After your role is defined, ask the consultant to provide you with an exit conference meeting or a report before he or she leaves the facility each time. You may be able to include your administrator in these meetings. There is a reason your department requires a consultant at this time. You can derive many benefits from a consultant's stay if you approach the issue openly and cooperatively.

Handling Interns.   With proper organization and planning, providing opportunities for new students in the field of recreation or activity direction should be a welcome addition to your department. The advantages of having student **interns** in your program are that they are usually enthusiastic helpers and a new link to the community for your residents. A disadvantage is that interns may be a drain on your program if you are sent students by professors or instructors who expect you to design the scope of an internship for them and the student. No student should be accepted as an intern without first going through a series of procedures that protect the residents as well as the student. First, the prospective student or instructor should make formal contact with you or your administrator, by telephone or by letter. Second, the student should contact you directly to arrange for an interview. Schedule only a limited number of interns at any one time. Once you have interviewed the student and assessed the scope of his or her internship process along with the role of your department, make a determination as to whether you are able to accommodate the student or not. Unfortunately, a disservice has frequently occurred with interns when they are not properly represented in the initial stages of an internship request. Without a courteous application and a clear expectation of the program, activity professional department heads should be reluctant to accept interns.

When conditions are met and an intern starts, be sure to use the same orientation procedures that you would use for a new activity staff member. This is another neglected area that leads to trouble if not handled properly. If the intern does not provide an accountability sheet for hours, set one up. Also, be aware of reporting responsibilities of both the intern and the person who is monitoring him or her. Check ahead of time on the amount of staff time the intern may need for interviews, and verify whether or not the intern is expected to photocopy large quantities of facility policies or documents as part of classwork. Some facilities request that interns who do not have instructors to provide this required material bring in their own copy paper, and do their copying of permitted facility documents on off hours.

Despite all the potential start-up hassles, interns can be a delight for your residents and your staff. They will be busy working on their class projects and many of your residents will be happy to help. Do not, however, rely on them to fill in for your normal staff, or just handle "boring" jobs like filing. That is unfair to them, and they would not get a well-rounded picture of the profession.

SUMMARY

Taking the time to firmly establish yourself as a full-fledged manager is worth the effort when you feel confident to lead your employees and volunteers through a successful job performance. Gaining practice and a measure of comfort with assessing your staff, conducting various supervisory tasks, handling communication issues among departments, and developing your own management style are critical to your success as an activity professional.

R E V I E W   Q U E S T I O N S

1. What are the three areas of responsibility rated by The American Health Care Association for supervisors to guide their management of employees?
2. What are the components of the interview process?
3. Under what circumstances should a warning notice be given?
4. Why is a performance appraisal important?
5. What type of communication is also called nonverbal communication?

O N   Y O U R   O W N

1. Using your facility as an example, name five ways to improve your time management on the job.
2. If routine methods of communication do not seem to be motivating staff to work on a special resident project, what other methods can you think of to get results?
3. How would you handle explaining a difficult termination of a very popular employee to residents, staff, and volunteers.?

R E F E R E N C E S

American Health Care Association (1988). *Effective supervisory skills: A guide to leadership development in long term care facilities.* Cranford, NJ: Didactic Systems.

Brown, S., Nelson, A., Bronkesh, S., and Wood, S. (1993). *Patient satisfaction pays: Quality service for practice success.* Gaithersburg, MD: Aspen Publications.

Cunninghis, R. (1984). *A professional guide for activity coordinators.* Willingboro, NJ: Geriatric Educational Consultants.

Halberg, K., & Waters, E. (1991). Functioning as a department head and supervisor: A new role for the activity coordinator. In P.M. Foster (Ed.) , *Activities in action* (p. 61–85), Binghamton, NY: The Haworth Press.

Kranz, J., & Frauen, J. (1986). *Professional resource development.* Englewood Cliffs, NJ: Prentice Hall.

Lombardi, D. N. (1993). *Handbook for the new health care manager: Practical strategies for challenging times.* Chicago, IL: American Hospital Publishing.

Zenger, J. H. (1985). Leadership: Management's better half. *Training,* December, 44–52.

F U R T H E R   R E A D I N G

Bader, G. (1991). Good guys finish last: Understanding organizational politics. *Health Care Supervisor, 10(1),* 23–26.

Bassett, L. (1992). How motivation defines productivity. *Topics in Health Information Management,* Vol.13, (2), 65–72.

The Bowman Gray School of Medicine of Wake Forest University (1984). *Scheduling staff can be a challenge.* (Respite report, Winter, 3–7) Winston–Salem, NC: author.

Conway, M. (1985). Performance appraisal system for therapeutic recreation. *Therapeutic Recreation Journal,* 1st Quarter, 44–49.

Davidhizar, R. (1989). The two-minute manager. *Health Care Supervisor,* 7(3), 25–29.

D'Antonio-Nocera, A., DeBolt, N., and Touhey, N. *The Professional activity manager and consultant.* Ravendale, WA: Idyll Arbor, Inc.

Eigen, B. (1990). *How to think like a boss and get ahead at work.* New York, NY: Carol Publishing Co.

Eptig, L.A., Glover, S., & Boyd, S. (1994). Managing diversity. *Health Care Supervisor,* 12(4), 73–83.

Howe, C. (1981). Select concepts in management for therapeutic recreation specialists. *Therapeutic Recreation Journal,* 1st Quarter, 11–17.

Keller, M.J. (1985). Creating a positive work environment for therapeutic recreation personnel. *Therapeutic Recreation Journal,* 1st Quarter, 36–43.

Ogborn, S. (1994). Running effective meetings, running effective groups. *Health Care Supervisor,* 13(2), 69–77.

Schillinger, K. (1988). Professionalism vs. unionism: A dual loyalty dilemma. *Therapeutic Recreation Journal,* 3rd Quarter, 15–30.

C H A P T E R 6

Creating and Maintaining Environmental Areas

OBJECTIVES..................................

After completing this chapter, you should:

- be able to organize your office to execute effective programs
- know how to use the environment to assist in programming efforts
- be able to manage your work and storage areas to accommodate your resident's needs and your facility layout
- start to develop a working rapport with other department staff to expedite your time and enhance your space

INTRODUCTION

This chapter focuses on establishing a methodical and accessible system for utilizing your office space and the program areas that you and your staff serve. The use of various environmental modifications will help to make your programs more acceptable to residents. Additionally, you will gain insight into the benefits of good staff relationships as a critical resource for program building.

Setting up your office and program areas in a organized manner is a key step to establish successful practices and gain professional acceptance in the job. Your office is your base of operations, and should incorporate all the necessary items to run your department. Program areas, used by your staff and set up primarily for use in assisting residents, need to be arranged in an efficient way that allows materials to be accessible but uncluttered. Storage spaces should be organized so that seasonal equipment and supplies are easy to reach, and a regular supply inventory can be conducted quickly.

Your Office ....

If you are like most activity professionals, you work with minimal office space and experience many distractions. You may be one of the growing number of activity professionals to have your own office, or you might be using part of your ac-

tivity room. Most facilities that have available space recognize the need for privacy, and provide an office for the activity department head and/or staff. Other facilities, because of a lack of space, funding, or awareness, do not allot an adequate office area to the activity professionals on staff. An office is a place to do work quietly, and can be a plush expanse with designer furniture or a simple niche carved out of an old housekeeping closet. If you spend the majority of your time with residents, time in your office is limited. Regardless of the shape or size of your office area, work with what you've been given, and set up the space to make it work for you.

Elements of a Successful Office

If you are given an office, there are a few factors you should consider as you begin to set it up. With what size space are you working? Do you have a bowling-alley shape, a standard-type office, or the converted closet style that was mentioned earlier? The size will determine your ultimate use of the office. For example, the renovated closet may allow you to use the area only for your own documentation needs, such as preparing the monthly calendar, whereas a standard size office will permit you to use the office for your planning, departmental meetings, and visits by other staff members or residents. If you are worried about the size you have to work with, remember the activity professionals who do not have a private work space!

The next area to consider in organizing your office is the furniture and equipment you have been given. At the very least, you need a desk or work table with a chair. Access to a telephone is vital to any activity professional and it should be close at hand. A locking file cabinet, bookcases, and shelves are necessary for storing books and files, and for locking up valuable items such as a petty cash box.

Another fundamental item is a storage closet for supplies. Ideally, at least one small storage closet or area should be located in, or very near, your office, or perhaps one could be located adjacent to, or in, your main activity room.

Two often overlooked elements when setting up a workable office space are proper temperature and lighting. Although consideration of these factors may appear unnecessary, your productivity will be directly effected by extremes in either temperature or lighting. You cannot maximize the efficiency of your office if you cannot see your desk or you have to wear a heavy coat year round!

Setting Up Your Resource, Filing, and Storage Systems

Making your office work for you means having an organized system for filing and retrieving information and supplies.

Resource Information. Your desk should have two resources that you will establish and continually develop over the life of your position. The first is a detailed telephone and address directory of contacts, entertainers, volunteers, local groups, and other key people connected to your program. A rotary file with alphabetized tabs is an easy way to access information quickly. The best way to organize your cards is either to separate them into key groups by tab (i.e., entertainers) or to color code the cards for groups (i.e., a purple dot on the right hand corner to designate the person as a volunteer). With such a system in place to identify particular groups, you can use your files to obtain a contact or mailing list quickly. Another tip to make your telephone and address file more useful is to keep brief but current notes on the back of the card of pertinent details concerning a volunteer or entertainer. For example, you may wish to note that a certain performer, although loved by your residents, is always ten minutes late to every booking. This information will be important to your staff the next time they use the file to schedule a program. You may want to use the back of your directory cards to record the last time a particular performer came to your facility, or include a list or a volunteer's upcoming vacation schedule to help when planning.

The second resource you should have on your desk is the **community resource file**. This file contains all the organizational support programs in your local community, county and state, as well as national groups that your residents or their families need to satisfy their activity or adjustment needs. A file box that holds a 4-inch x 6-inch size card or larger works best to manage this information since it will be updated continually if the file is used properly. Each card should contain the name, address, telephone number, and contact person for organizations and groups that have pertinent information, programs, or support for your residents, families, and staff. A brief description of the service provided is also helpful. Some examples of community resource contacts may include Alzheimer's disease support groups, hospice information, bereavement seminars, senior centers, restaurants that cater to elderly clients, and government publications, just to name a few. File these organizations alphabetically, or by larger categories, such as "support groups." When maintained properly, this file is invaluable when referring either your residents, families, or staff to alternate assistance that exists outside your facility, or to add new information to your own programs. Notations on referrals or other changes in data should be made right on the card so the file is always updated for use by anyone on your staff.

If you have inherited old files for either your telephone directory or your community resource file, review all entries with your staff and check on any questionable listings before you use or share the information in your program planning.

Filing Systems. Setting up your office files properly is one of the most critical things you do to help your staff (and yourself!) succeed. There are at least three ways that you can organize your files; in folders in a cabinet, in binders, and in "hot files" for high visibility.

Determine if files exist in your office in the following areas, and if they are not available, establish them:

1. Activity calendars for the last three months.
2. Attendance/interest/participation files for programs.
3. Budget/petty cash information.
4. Census forms.
5. Confidential files (used infrequently to record information too sensitive for inclusion in the

medical record (i.e., documentation of abusive remarks made to a staff member by a resident's family).

6. Contracts for services such as retired senior volunteer program (RSVP), or internship agreements.
7. Employee information.
   a. Application forms
   b. Personnel information
   c. Training materials
8. Entertainer information.
9. Idea files for future programs.
10. Information from other facilities.
11. Mailing lists.
12. **Material Safety Data Sheets.** An Occupational Safety and Hazard Act (**OSHA**)-required sheet describing hazardous substances (glue, paint) with which your staff or residents may have contact. Sheets must be available for all substances, and staff must receive in-service training on each.
13. Monthly/quarterly reports to administration, if required.
14. Newsletter.
15. Organization information (brochures, flyers).
16. Purchase orders (if applicable).
17. Resident roster and room lists.
18. Seminar information.
19. Survey information.
20. Vendor/catalog information.
21. Volunteer services.

There are some items that are easier to store in separate three-ring binders, and kept on a nearby shelf for reference by all activity staff members. The first and most utilized binder should be your departmental **policy and procedure manual**. In this volume, keep an alphabetical collection of your departmental policies, the written steps required to perform any task or function within your department. Have available procedures on everything from how to run a current events group to the detailed responsibilities of the activity department during a facility disaster. Update the information in this binder frequently. Specific guidance on how to write policies and procedures is included in Chapter 12.

Another binder that many activity professionals find beneficial is one that contains a compilation of vital medical record information for each resident. You may wish to keep copies of the **face sheet** (first page of the medical chart) filed in the binder for quick reference to specific data (i.e., the name of the responsible party, medical billing numbers, original admission date, **diagnosis**, and

other vital statistics. In some facilities, the admission director maintains a face sheet book to which you can refer. In addition to considering the advantages of keeping copies of resident face sheets, establish a system for maintaining awareness and accountability for the documentation requirements that your facility must follow for each resident. Have a form, or file, for collecting data on documentation requirements such as the name of the resident, date of original admission, date of last Minimum Data Set completed, goals, and progress note schedules (if required in your state). Along with the resident information, schedule, in written format, a monthly or quarterly list of documentation that is coming due for completion along with a list of the responsible staff members from your department. This schedule along, with your collected medical information on each resident, serves two purposes: first, it is a method to ensure that all documentation work is being delegated to the appropriate staff members, and second, it is a tool to prepare quality assurance audits.

Two other categories of information that you may find useful in a binder format are the federal and state regulations for activities and your **in-service education** data. Having a copy of your state and federal (if required) regulations handy on a shelf makes referral easy for staff. In-service education is defined as the ongoing staff training necessary for a particular job title during the course of employment. Your in-service binder should hold educational materials for general staff programs including activities, programs for the activity department staff, any special resident or family training events, attendance sheets, and a current planning calendar for your upcoming education courses. Housing the staff in-service materials in a binder is beneficial because of the frequency of your programs, and the ease of having all your forms related to in-service in one location. There will be more information on the subject of in-service education in Chapter 18.

Some office materials, such as the items on the list below, should be kept in a "hot" file on your desk or in another special spot such as a bulletin board, so they can be found quickly:

1. Last survey report.
2. Facility provider numbers (if applicable), facility employment identification number (EIN), facility tax exempt number (if applicable).
3. Current resident room list.
4. Employee/volunteer blank applications.
5. Copies of current activity calendars/newsletters.

6. Frequently called telephone numbers.
7. Project lists.

Storage Closets. In an adjacent storage closet or a locked area of your office, keep a stock of consumable program items such as construction paper, glue, pens, pencils, tape, scissors, markers, paint and brushes, "instant" projects for drop-in volunteers, and so forth. You may also wish to keep items of value such as sing-along books, musical equipment, and photographic materials where they can be monitored.

Office Problems

Regardless of whether you have your own office or share with someone else, you will no doubt have to contend with distractions that can effect your success. Depending on your location, you may have to cope with frequent drop-in visitors who interrupt your work. Be assertive in handling other staff members or even residents who constantly demand your time on a repetitive basis. Your goal, of course, is to be available and work cooperatively with staff, and certainly with residents, but you should put some restrictions on individuals who require an excess of your attention. The simplest way to handle this type of problem is to anticipate the attention that these individuals may require in advance, and schedule meetings at a mutually convenient time. If you know that one of your residents appears at your door every Thursday at 1:30 p.m. to read her latest letter to you, and the planning for your 2:15 p.m. activity is usually disrupted, speak to the resident earlier in the day, and schedule a visit at 4:00 p.m. when you will be free. The same principle applies to drop-in staff members, family members, and volunteers who drain your time resources. Using your time in your office wisely is an important management skill.

Physical office problems such as noise, lighting, or temperature issues should be addressed with the maintenance director and your administrator. At times, a simple change can make a great difference in your ability to use your office.

Sharing your office with another staff member or having an office that is part of a larger room can be challenging, but many activity professionals deal with this every day with success. If you share your space with another staff member, establish some time that each of you can use the office without interruptions. You may also wish to devise a method to inform each other that privacy is required at a particular moment (i.e., an impromptu conference with a distraught family member). If your office is within a larger space, such as your activity room, try to use the room for quiet times at off hours, or attempt to establish an "office hour" that staff recognize as your private time.

Your Program Areas

Program areas are those spaces in your facility that hold small and large activities, as well as individual conferences. Any of the following areas may be available: a large formal activity room, a series of wing day rooms, a lobby, a wide area in front of the nurses station, or an alcove that you find empty. In addition to the number and kind of spaces you have around you, the number of floors in your building should be taken into consideration. Your method of program planning for large group programs will be impacted directly by the layout and size of your facility.

In a large facility with numerous floors, you may opt to set up a **decentralized system** for delivering larger group activities. In the decentralized system, you regularly use a series of rooms in the facility to host programs, some of which occur simultaneously. Cohen and Day (1994) refer to this method as the "dispersed" model of activity environmental planning. In facilities with many levels, residents can benefit from this approach by having many of their programs in the day room or alcove right on their floor. Noise control and excessive stimulation, however, during programs, may be a problem. The decentralized or dispersed model offers more flexible scheduling options, but can be difficult to monitor when programs in progress are in more than one area. In smaller sized facilities, (ones with fewer staff members or facilities with an accommodating activity room), a **centralized system** may be more sensible. This method allows the bulk of group events to be held in one designated area. With a centralized activity "headquarters" for most programs, you may find better staff cooperation and easier orientation and recognition for residents. Cohen and Day (1994) refer to centralized programs as "unified" activity scheduling, and cite accessibility to all residents and easy surveillance of the areas as key positive factors. The downside of the centralized or unified model is the "institutional feel" of a large activity room that may not work well for intimate group settings.

For smaller group programs, you may use a dining area in off hours, lobby, alcoves, or any other available space that is safe and free from too many distractions.

Individual programs are normally conducted in semiprivate facility spaces or at the bedside. As Olson (1994) notes in her book, the trend toward specialized care required for the frail elderly is rapidly growing. The frail group of the geriatric long-term care segment requires more programming attention in formats such as bedside or in-room programming. The activity professional has to address the issues of reaching more clients by way of individual bedside programs versus the larger traditional group dynamics.

Outdoor areas in the front or back of the facility, and enclosed patio spaces are excellent, but many times overlooked, spots for all types of programming.

Environmental Modifications in Programs

Space availability in your facility, although a major consideration, should be weighed against the impact that a particular environment has on engaging positive interactions and increasing participation in programs. McClannahan (1973) discovered that certain functional aspects of room design, such as the use of pedestal-type tables and short-seated chairs with arms and high backs, actually increases an individual's level of interaction and movement in the environment. With greater individual mobility and higher activity functioning, body processes work more effectively and ". . . retard the degenerative processes associated with aging." In describing architectural considerations in long-term care design, Skaggs and Hawkins (1994) comment that attention should be given to allow ". . . exposure to natural light and views . . . to provide an orientation to time of day and season."

Program spaces, such as larger activity rooms, should be user friendly with safe materials available for use by drop-in participants. In their study, McClannahan and Risley (1975) concluded that activity participation levels were increased when program supplies were readily available to clients. Carp (1978) also found that as more opportunities were present in an environment, residents reacted with an increase in activity levels.

Additional environmental research has been made in two areas that impact the design and implementation of your program: physical environmental design and wayfinding.

Much research has been conducted recently on the implications of environmental design in the treatment of the cognitively impaired resident.

The information is useful to all resident populations because a large number of cognitively impaired residents comprise our treatment base, and because the suggestions have practical implications for all resident levels. An important study by Brawley (1992) cites many examples of simple changes and considerations that can be made in environmental design to aid in resident enjoyment and participation. In discussing the benefits of good environmental design, Brawley states ". . . careful design planning can facilitate mental functioning, minimize some areas of confusion and allow individuals to function more independently to whatever capacity he or she is able— thereby improving the quality of life." She adds that a proper design reduces stress, agitation, and wandering. Areas to address in the physical environment include sight, light, color, sound, textures, temperatures, odor, air quality, space, floors, furniture, personal objects, and door handles.

Visually, Brawley suggests that familiar shapes be used for everyday objects, such as lamps, and that sharp contrasts between objects and background be made to assist with clarity. High-tech designs are not easily recognizable by many residents, and are, therefore, confusing. Light sources should remain constant between different areas to prevent shadows and glare. Colors alone are less important than contrasts between colors, according to Brawley. Some colors (i.e., blues and purples) may be indistinguishable to residents but could be pleasing to visitors. Background noise should be minimized and methods of absorbing sounds explored. Familiar textures in furniture coverings and bedcoverings can bring warm memories. Additionally, plants, mobiles, and other wall hangings provide other welcomed textures. Temperature extremes and odors should be monitored carefully. Fresh air and proper circulation in air systems assist in this process. In looking at the facility layout, Brawley recommends the use of shorter corridors with appropriate access to outdoor walking areas. All facility pathways should remain free of dangerous clutter, and when possible, have minimal contrasts in the floor coverings (borders on carpets may cause tripping hazards because of visual misperceptions). Design in rooms or corridor alcoves should invite interactions from the layout of the furniture. Lever-type door handles are easier for most residents to manage. Objects of a personal nature in common areas often bring feelings of warmth and calmness.

Including dining areas adjacent to activity areas or within activity areas is another way for the environment to assist in program implementation. Anderson (1993) mentions the use of nourishment centers that have multipurpose use in both activity and dining experiences. Community style dining in smaller resident groups is preferable to the large, and often, overwhelming dining room experience.

Other facilities have abandoned the corridor concept altogether, and have a minimum of walls or barriers, except those that contain resident bedrooms. All of the environmental suggestions should be closely considered. Design in the past was geared toward aesthetics and not to the users of the spaces.

Another part of the physical environment that should be addressed is the use of helpful identifications for residents called "**wayfinding**," guides or hints that help a person get from one place to another, or simply assist in locating a destination. Malkin (1992) calls wayfinding ". . . an act of spatial problem solving," or the use of techniques such as information gathering, decision-making, and decision implementation. Wayfinding is used by residents to locate their rooms, or most often, to find a bathroom when involved in activity programs. Malkin mentions that good wayfinding helps in general recognition, not necessarily in remembering specifics. Wayfinding incorporates three methods in your facility of which you may be a part: landmarks, cues, and signage.

Landmarks are obvious and identifiable objects used in relation to other surroundings. Brawley (1994) suggests that an effective landmark should be seen at a distance, and gives an example of a large clock.

Cues can be visual, such as color coding of walls, doorways, or entrances. Sensory cues can also direct residents (i.e., kitchen smells that guide residents to a dining room). Other cues, such as footprints on the floor or arrows leading to a toilet or exit from a particular room, can be helpful to some residents. Many facilities use pictures to illustrate a bathroom. Namazi and Johnson (1991), in two separate studies, found that both the use of floor arrows and a visibly identified bathroom area, assisted tremendously in helping residents make proper choices. A few of your residents may require a special identifier to locate their room, such as a photograph of their son or their first address after they got married, made into a street sign and hung on their door. Common items such as a mailbox, or kitchen or dining room, could have oversized pictoral representations with which residents can identify.

Signage also assists in wayfinding. Both Brawley (1994) and Malkin (1992) note that to be most effective, signage should be consistent in size throughout the facility. Signs at proper eye level, with easy to read, contrasting colors work best. Malkin mentions combining signs with visual images for greater recognition.

You may not have full control over the facility design or its equipment, but you must learn to adapt the internal spaces you have to maximize participation and enjoyment of the areas by residents. Using some of the suggestions for physical environmental adaptations and wayfinding ideas can help your residents by offering them easy choices. Simple things that are within your control, such as establishing uncluttered traffic patterns, are critical for resident safety. Comfortable and adequate seating, lighting, and climate help the resident to use the spaces. Many facilities have found that creating mini "home-like" spaces within a larger activity area brings warmth and comfort to residents. Areas can be created, such as a kitchen, bedroom, multipurpose area, and a living room. Any activity area should be cheerful and inviting, either by use of facility decorations or by the inventive activity staff. Figure 6–1 illustrates the kind of familiar, home-like environment areas that can improve the use of an activity space.

Equipment and Supply Usage

Using your program equipment and supplies effectively depends largely on the number and type of areas you have available in which to hold programs. If you use a centralized system, and run most of your programs from a large activities room, it is easy to administer your events with an in-room closet or adjacent closet for storage of equipment and supplies. If you use the decentralized system, used mainly in larger facilities, it is better to have storage closets or locked areas on each of the floors near your program areas, or a number of carts on which you can transport your program supplies to your work area from another storage spot.

Regardless of which system your facility space requires, carts and portable storage bins are important tools when organizing and using diverse work spaces. Use carts or storage bins for everything from serving refreshments and bringing art supplies to a second floor day room to transporting sensory materials for programs to your bedbound residents. By having a system for bringing supplies and equipment into one area from another, you are expanding the possibilities for programming. Try to obtain an adequate number of

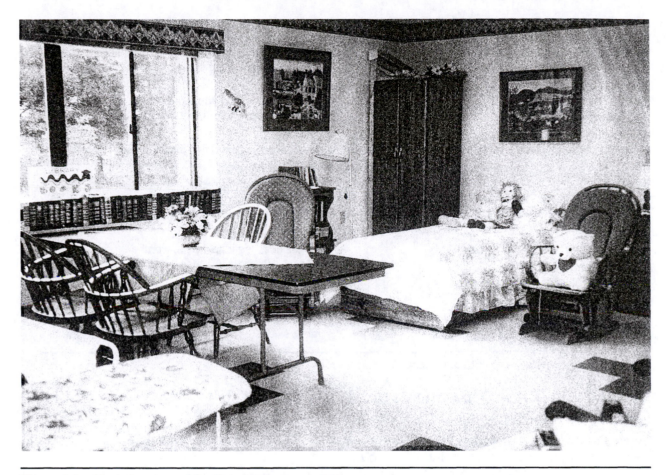

Figure 6–1 Create homey and familiar spots in your activity room.

carts or bins for your needs, and be sure to label your storage equipment with your department's name to ensure their safe return. Inexpensive plastic containers of all sizes work well to organize material on carts and in closets.

Because every facility has different resident needs and divergent activity programming, equipment and supply requirements are diverse as well. Figure 6–2 provides a basic list of some supplies you may find useful based on broad categories of resident need or use.

Remote Storage Areas

Your programming skills will increase if you have access to your supplies, and know where to find the infrequent seasonal items that are sometimes stored in a remote shed or basement area. Have all your materials as accessible as possible, but do not move seasonal items around constantly that interfere with your key program supplies. A storage system for infrequently used items works well when

the area is organized and secure, and the items in storage are rotated according to their seasonal use. Some facilities with very limited storage space use locked outdoor storage sheds or off-premises storage space to house seasonal items. Proper shelving or pallets provide your supplies with a dry and safe place. Fire codes and other regulations usually mandate that supplies be off the floor, and a minimum of clearance must exist between stored items and the ceiling. Involve other staff members, whenever possible, when setting up your storage room. Limit the access to your equipment by issuing keys (with a sign-out sheet) to any staff members in the activity department who require access. Consider the fact that this remote storage area requires at least an annual or biannual clean-up. You may opt to hold clean-up days for the entire facility to help in your efforts. Be aware that donations of equipment and supplies from community members might overwhelm you. Many "free" items may take up valuable space in your limited storage space, and you should choose wisely among donated gifts or equipment.

Large Equipment
wheelchair accessible tables and chairs, VCR, movie projector, easels, blackboard, wipe-off boards, piano, TV

Animals
feeding dish, carrier, food

Arts and Crafts
paints, markers, construction paper, brushes, glue, fabric, sewing supplies, paper bags, ribbons, woodworking items

Cooking
trays, serving utensils, baking sheets, bowls, pans, blender, toaster oven, microwave, popcorn popper

Educational
books, travel posters, resource guides

Entertainment
games, movies, videos, headphones

Horticulture
potting soil, plant containers, seeds, watering can

Life Skills
kitchen equipment, hardware and gadgets, laundry supplies, tools, grooming items, personal finance objects

Music
radio, cassette player, record player, cassette tapes and records, rhythm instruments, song books

Physical
exercise tapes, repetitive motion items, parachute, scarves, balls

Program Administration
blank calendars, carts, storage bins, microphone, decorations, signs, timer, stationery and cards, film, camera

Stimulation Items
magazines, seasonal items, weather board, bioboards, mobiles, pat mats, puzzles, games

Religious
hymn books, vestments, spiritual readings, Bibles

Sensory
fabric swatches, scented oils, rain sticks, mobiles

Figure 6–2 Activity department equipment and supply suggestions.

Working With Other Departments to Maximize Time and Space

You can enhance your programs and use your space and time more effectively by enlisting the aid of your neighboring departments. Here is a partial list of some assistance that other departments can offer:

1. *Nursing:* coordinate care schedules around special programs; assist in transporting residents to programs; lend a nursing assistant to programs; use techniques taught by activity staff to run small groups; coordinate ambulatory program; participate in information programs on health issues; encourage activity staff to participate in shift change report or attend rounds.
2. *Dietary:* plan monthly functions together that involve food; plan special food festivals; delay setting tables in the dining room to allow longer activity programs; provide informational programs on nutrition.
3. *Housekeeping:* maintain cleaning schedules of large program areas to ensure events start on time; keep hallways clear of carts to make transportation easier; lend extra staff for cleanup of large events.
4. *Social Services:* assist with resident council meetings; handle resident issues that may disrupt programs; alert activity staff to resident mood swings; train staff on handling stress and working cooperatively; cover for activity staff in case of absence.

5. *Business Office:* screen calls during activities; handle routine calls concerning programs; use paging system to notify residents of events; handle typing of newsletter and correspondence.
6. *Maintenance:* move equipment to accommodate programs; assist with trips; help with supplies in storage area.
7. *Administration:* allow opportunities to try new programs; act as a host for special functions; run an occasional activity in area of expertise.

In return for the assistance you gain from other departments, offer your help in the following areas:

1. Make announcements over the paging system to alert staff and residents of delays or changes in programs.
2. Prepare activity equipment and supplies ahead of time, and set up room and supplies on time.
3. Establish a policy for elevator use (if appropriate), and train the general staff. Transportation to activity programs will flow better when a team approach is used.
4. Use a sign-out book for facility spaces that may be used by any department (i.e., conference room or meeting rooms) to avoid conflict.
5. Notify staff of any change in routine, and if any new volunteers are assisting with programs.
6. Use a **function request form** (described in more detail in Chapter 9) to establish clearly

your time frames for assistance from other departments for each function.

7. Remove all outdated materials and information from facility bulletin boards on a regular basis.

8. Give a periodic verbal activity report to the nursing staff of the status and participation level of your residents. This enables the staff to help by encouraging or transporting appropriate clients. Provide a list to the nursing staff of possible program participants for any larger programs that you are having.

9. Use signs such as "Program in Progress" on the outside of a door to notify staff of on-going events.

SUMMARY

With proper thought and planning, environmental areas such as office, meeting and program rooms, and storage spaces can have a tremendous impact on the success of your entire program. Your relationship with peers and general staff will be determined by how well your programs succeed in the facility.

R E V I E W   Q U E S T I O N S

1. What type of materials should you keep in an accessible spot in your office?
2. Which program materials would be suitable for binder storage?
3. What is a decentralized program?
4. What is wayfinding, and why is it important in space planning?
5. Name five ways that the nursing department supports the activity department in using time and space.

O N   Y O U R   O W N

1. As the new activity director, you have discovered that the three-story facility has no closet space allotted to the activity department on any of the three floors. The only storage space exists in the activity room. Other than using carts, how will you set up an organized portable system for your programs on the three different floors?

2. What are five additional things you can think of that an activity department can do to increase cooperation from other departments and make the program spaces they have more useful?
3. Your office space is small and you share it with others. Name three ways to reorganize your space to make it more productive.

R E F E R E N C E S

Anderson, J. (1993). Nursing facility design offers residential look, feel-inside and out. *Health Facilities Management.* Nov., 62–66.

Brawley, E. (1992). Alzheimer's disease: Designing the physical environment. *The American Journal of Alzheimer's Care and Related Disorders & Research,* Jan./Feb., 3–8.

Carp, F. (1978). Effects of the living environment on activity and use of time. *International Journal of Aging and Human Development,* Vol. 9(1), 75–91.

Cohen, U., & Day, K. (1994). Emerging trends in environments for people with dementia. *The American Journal of Alzheimer's Care and Related Disorders & Research,* Jan./Feb., 3–11.

Malkin, J. (1992). Wayfinding: Are your staff and visitors lost in space? *Health Facilities Management,* Aug., 36–41.

McClannahan, L., & Risley, T. (1975). Design of living environment for nursing-home residents: Increased participation in recreational activities. *Journal of Applied Behavior Analysis,* 8(3), 261–268.

McClannahan, L. E. (1973) Therapeutic and prosthetic living environments for nursing home residents. *The Gerontologist,* 13, 424–429.

Namazi, K., & Johnson, B. (1991). Physical environmental cues to reduce the problems of incontinence in Alzheimer's disease units. *The American Journal of Alzheimer's Care and Related Disorders & Research,* Nov./Dec., 22–28.

Namazi, K., & Johnson, B. (1991). Environmental effects on incontinence problems in Alzheimer's disease patients. *The American Journal of Alzheimer's Care and Related Disorders & Research,* Nov./Dec., 16–21.

Olson, L. K. (1994). *The graying of the world.* Binghamton, NY: The Haworth Press.

Skaggs, R. L., & Hawkins, H. R. (1994). Architecture for long-term care facilities. In S. B. Goldsmith (Ed.),

F U R T H E R   R E A D I N G

Essentials of long-term care administration (p. 272). Gaithersburg, MD: Aspen Publishers, Inc.

Bailey, C., & Haight, B. (1994). The use of visual cues in mid-stage Alzheimer's disease. *The American Journal of Alzheimer's Care and Related Disorders & Research*, July/Aug., 23–29.

Carpman, J., & Grant, M. (1993). *Design that cares: Planning health facilities for patients and visitors, 2nd edition.* Chicago, IL: American Hospital Publishing.

Martin, B. (1993). Signage: Key (but not only) wayfinding element. *Health Facilities Management*, Nov., 62–66.

McClannahan, L. (1993). Recreation programs for nursing home residents: The importance of patient characteristics and environmental arrangements. *Therapeutic Recreation Journal*, 2nd Quarter, 26–31.

McClannahan, L., & Risley, T. (1974). Design of living environments for nursing home residents: Recruiting attendance at activities. *The Gerontologist*, Vol. 14, 236–240.

McClannahan, L., & Risley, T. (1974). Activities and materials for severely disabled geriatric patients. *Nursing Homes*, Vol. 24, 10–13.

Namazi, K., Rosner, T., & Rechlin, L. (1991). Long-term memory cuing to reduce visual-spatial disorientation in Alzheimer's disease patients in a special care unit. *The American Journal of Alzheimer's Care and Related Disorders & Research*, Nov./Dec., 10–15.

Namazi, K., Whitehouse, P., Rechlin, L., Calkins, M., Johnson, B., Brabender, B., & Heventer, S. (1991). Environmental modifications in a specially designed unit for the care of patients with Alzheimer's disease: An overview and introduction. *The American Journal of Alzheimer's Care and Related Disorders & Research*, Nov./Dec., 3–9.

Thomas, J., & Bobrow, M. (1984). Targeting the elderly in facility design. *Hospitals*, Feb. 16th, 83–88.

Zeisel, J., Hyde, J., & Levkoff, S. (1994). Best practices: An environment-behavior model for Alzheimer special care units. *The American Journal of Alzheimer's Care and Related Disorders & Research*, Mar./Apr., 4–21.

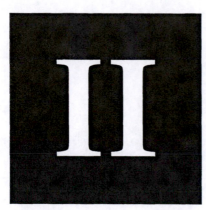

II

Activity Programming and Implementation

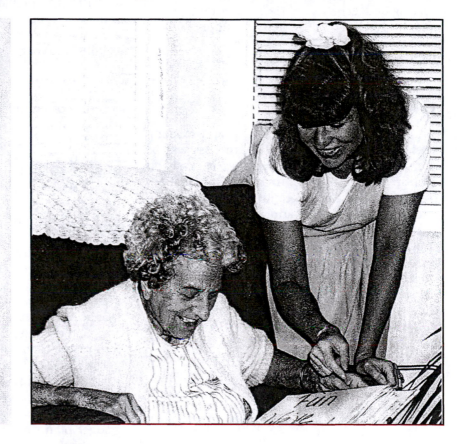

C H A P T E R 7
Budgeting

KEY TERMS..

budget	depreciate
fiscal year	payroll expenses
provider agreement	activity supply
proprietary facility	expenses
operating budget	staffing patterns
capital budget	activity supply budget
revenue	petty cash
expenses	check request

OBJECTIVES...

After completing this chapter, you should:

- ■ know how a budget is prepared in a long-term care facility
- ■ master the preparations and monitoring of an activity supply budget
- ■ establish a petty cash account
- ■ know the methods of controlling costs

INTRODUCTION

A simplified method for setting up and tracking necessary activity departmental expenses will be explained in this chapter. Guidance is given on the entire budget process, including preparation, monitoring, and recordkeeping. Suggestions on stretching your budget, and understanding the value of an activity program are also covered.

Budget preparation and supervision is an often overlooked management skill that an activity professional needs to know. Just thinking about budgets or financial planning sometimes evokes feelings of panic or dread, but learning as much as you can about budgeting is necessary to obtain the proper funding for your programs. You will not be able to fill your residents' activity needs if you do not have the appropriate money and approval. You will have the tools to succeed, however, if you have a basic understanding of how your programs are funded, and what your role is in the process.

What is a Budget? ....

A **budget** is defined as a plan that projects how you and your department allocate and spend money over a period of time to maintain its operation. A budget can be as simple as a predetermined spending limit per month, or as complicated as a detailed list of projected purchases that requires sign-offs by your administrator and board of directors each month.

Key Players in the Budget Process

In planning activity expenditures, you are the primary player, but not necessarily an expert. What you do not know already about budgets you will gain on the job, by reading the information in this chapter, and working closely with the other key players. In addition to your contribution, there are other individuals who join in the budget development process. On the management side, your administrator works with the owners of the facility to prepare a budget that reflects the needs of the residents. The owners, whether individuals or a large corporation, have a plan for spending that they then review with the administrator. The administrator, in turn, contributes ideas to the owners about facility spending. The management team, consisting of the administrator, department heads, and a bookkeeper (in larger situations, a comptroller), meet during budget planning, implementation, and monitoring. Rounding out the key players are the activity professionals employed in your department under your supervision. They should be involved in any budget planning process at some level for their input and as a learning experience for them.

Initial Budget Discussions

During your initial visit with the administrator, discuss the budget process for your department in your facility. Each facility and corporation establishes different methods of managing departmental expenses, and the procedure you were familiar with at your last facility may be quite different from the one used at this facility. If you are new to your position and facility, establish the budget guidelines with your administrator at the time you accept the position, or shortly thereafter. A smart job applicant for an activity position wants to know the budget he or she will have to work with in advance. If you know your budget already, update your administrator periodically on your department's performance, and become involved in the budgetary planning process at the designated time. A key guideline is for you, as an activity professional, to become involved in determining your budget and expenses, even if your participation is minimal!

As you prepare to meet with your administrator to discuss your budget, keep a few things in mind. First, try to limit the time you have with your administrator to a discussion of budget items only. Your conversation will have more impact if you discuss one topic, instead of interspersing your budget talk with questions about the last sensory group you held. To increase your chances of a positive encounter on this critical topic, come prepared to this (and any other) meeting. Depending on the budget you will be discussing at your meeting, arm yourself with information on the past performance of your department from the bookkeeping or financial services area of your organization. Be aware and understanding of the time constraints of your administrator, who may be interrupted by numerous phone calls, and so forth, during your conference. In order to appear professional and in control of your information, and to avoid a possible abrupt end to your meeting, document your budget request in a neat and concise memo that you can leave behind for your administrator to review at a later time. If you make a specific request for equipment or supplies, gather all the supporting documentation necessary. To accomplish this, you may need to conduct cost studies, get competitive bids, or send for catalogs to attach to your request. Do the legwork *before* you come to the meeting. Be sure to ask for a follow-up date to resolve the status of your budget request in the event that the conference is cut short.

The Budget Process ....

Some facilities have an elaborate budget planning process that goes on for months prior to the beginning of the next financial period of time, or the **fiscal year**. Other establishments keep the activity professional out of the information loop when it comes to budgetary planning. In your first meeting with your administrator, determine the involvement that is expected of you. Even in companies that prefer to provide less control to the activity department head, you should be fully aware of your financial allotments and reporting responsibilities.

A budget for the entire facility (including activities expenses) is normally prepared once a year, to coincide with the beginning of the fiscal year. A fiscal year is the annual twelve-month time frame in which expenses are planned and measured. The fiscal year budget can be based on a calendar year that runs from January 1 to December 31, or on any consecutive twelve-month time frame, often coinciding with the same time period that a facility **provider agreement** with Medicaid covers. If a fiscal year is based on the terms of a provider agreement or contract, it may run from October 1 of one year to September 30 of the next year, or any twelve-month combination. If you work in a **proprietary** facility (for profit) that participates in federal or state programs such as Medicare or Medicaid, you may experience a different planning process than if you worked in a private, nonprofit facility. Having worked in both types, I experienced greater involvement in the private, nonprofit facility because facility funds were more readily available. Proprietary facilities often work with very structured budgets that change little from year to year, and the involvement of the activity department head can be less significant.

The budget process follows four basic steps:

- Planning and estimating of expenses for the specified time period and category
- Reviewing your budget with your administrator or assistant administrator, and receiving approval for your budget
- Implementing your approved budget at the specified date
- Documenting expenditures according to facility reporting methods and monitoring your budget to ensure that limits are not exceeded

Each of the four categories will be explored in order to provide you with the knowledge you need to manage your departmental expenses.

Budget Planning

Before you can plan your budget you have to understand the whole budget framework in your facility. For each fiscal year, your administrator prepares an **operating budget** and a **capital budget** for the entire facility. The operating budget is a financial plan that guides the functioning of the facility for a specified twelve month period. It includes the projected money that comes into the facility (**revenue**) for room and board and other resident charges, and the money that is spent to operate each department or service in the facility (**expenses**). The capital budget is a special list of proposed expenditures, normally for larger facility equipment that can **depreciate**, or lose a portion of their value over time. For each service area in the facility, such as nursing or activities, a budget figure represents the projected operating expenses for the year, and in some cases, each department will be permitted to recommend or request capital expense items.

Budget Categories for an Activity Department

The two budget requirements for a typical activity department and the type of specific budget categories you may be asked to participate in are the operating budget and the capital budget.

The entire operating budget mentioned earlier consists of both revenue and expenses. Your administrator is concerned with the activity expenses that are part of the operating budget. The activity expenses in the operating budget include **payroll expenses** and actual **activity supply expenses**. A diagram, illustrating the elements of the activity department budget, is shown in Figure 7–1. Payroll expenses are simply the amount of money allocated by the facility to pay for your department staff on an annual basis. The payroll figures include salaries, and sometimes fringe benefits. From a planning perspective, you must know what your **staffing patterns** are for your department that meet your payroll budget amount. Simply put, you need to know how many staff members and departmental hours are required by regulation and approved by administration to meet your residents' activity needs on a weekly or biweekly basis.

The number of staff members, full and part time, make up your staffing pattern which is normally predetermined in a discussion with your administrator. Your payroll budget amount is derived by multiplying the hourly rate of each member of your approved staffing pattern by forty hours per week (or whatever number of hours per week your activity staff work) by fifty-two weeks per year (see Figure 7–2) This annual salary amount and staffing pattern are important to maintain. More detailed information will be given when we discuss tracking and monitoring of expenses.

The other key area of activity expenses in the operating budget is the activity departmental budget or **activity supply budget**. This budget covers the actual projection of supplies to be used, entertainers, program materials, food, decorations, and so forth, that you will require to use over the next fiscal year to effectively run your programs. Planning and developing your activities supply budget should follow these key steps:

1. If information is available from your bookkeeper or from old activity files, look at the previous activity budgets to gain a historical perspective. Old budgets may give you an idea of what was accepted in the past, but do not be limited by the information if you feel a different format or more funding is required.
2. Use a piece of scratch paper and refer to your monthly program calendars, and make headings for each month of the next fiscal year. For example, if your fiscal year is from June of one year through May of the next year, list "June," then "July," and so on. This is the first rough draft of your budget.

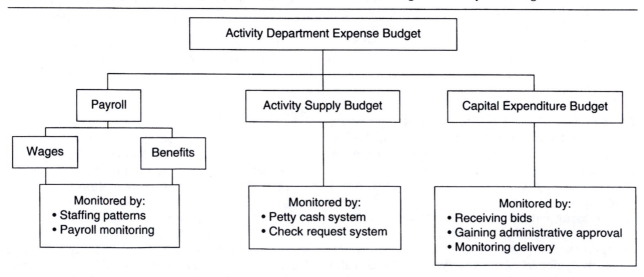

Figure 7–1   The elements of an activity department budget.

ANNUAL PAYROLL BUDGET (FISCAL YEAR 20XX-20YY) FOR THE ACTIVITY DEPARTMENT

1 full-time Activity Director @ $35.00/hour x 40 hours per week x 52 weeks per year =	$72,800.00
1 full-time Assistant Director @ $25.00/hour x 40 hours per week x 52 weeks per year =	$52,000.00
1 part-time Assistant @ $17.00/hour x 20 hours per week x 52 weeks per year =	$17,680.00
Total Annual Budget for Payroll—Activity Department =	$142,480.00

STAFFING PATTERN (IN HOURS) FOR BIWEEKLY PAYROLL FOR THE ACTIVITY DEPARTMENT

1 full-time Director @ 40 hours per week x 2 weeks =	80 hours
1 full-time Assistant Director @ 40 hours per week x 2 weeks =	80 hours
1 part-time Assistant @ 20 hours per week x 2 weeks =	40 hours
	200 hours*

*Approved amount of biweekly staff hours for the Activity Department for Chauncey Care Center. In reviewing time worked, hours should not exceed 200 for each two-week pay period.

Figure 7–2 Chauncey Care Center Activity Department—Payroll Budget.

3. Begin listing any planned programs in a particular month that require funding. You may already know that your cooking group, which meets weekly, needs to replenish supplies every other month. You are aware already that some of your other "standard" programs, such as the men's group which meets biweekly, or your monthly art therapy classes, require necessary supplies. Look at some of your popular or often repeated programs to analyze where some of your expenses might fall. List under each monthly heading the programs that you are currently projecting for the year that will most likely require some spending.

4. Next, think about all the special events that are enjoyed by your facility annually or programs that you have planned based on significant days or months throughout the year. List all of the family nights, entertainment required for holiday parties, volunteer recognition dinner, theme barbecues, National Nursing Home Week celebrations, festivals, bazaars, guest speakers, fund raisers, and the like. Refer to Chapters 8, 9, and 10 for ideas on programming.

5. Include decoration and other supply replacement as part of your budget planning for each month of the fiscal year. Take an inventory of your supplies in all of your storage areas. Do you need new holiday lights? Consider putting them on your January budget when you can get the best prices. Plan to replace some of the paper decorations and other holiday or seasonal reminders that have a limited shelf life. Try to spread out your replacement purchases throughout the year to avoid impacting your budget too severely in one or two months.

6. Keep in mind that in many facilities, expenses are often highest in October, Novem-

ber, and December because of heavier holiday programming. Another traditionally busy month for an activity department is May because of Mother's Day and National Nursing Home Week. If you do not have all your programs solidified for those months, be sure to

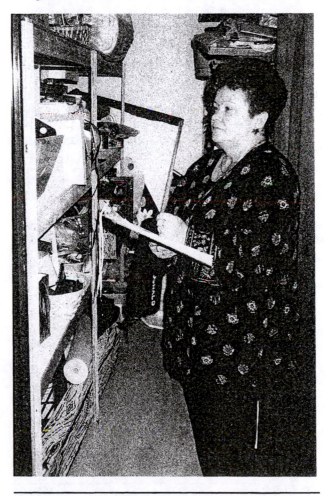

Figure 7–3 Keeping inventory will help in budget preparation.

allocate some *extra* funds for unexpected things such as refreshments for performers, flowers, and last minute gifts. These "hidden" expenses can be frustrating if you have not planned for them.

7. Translate your program needs into estimated dollar figures by using your catalogs, and contacting your supply vendors to get rough pricing on potential purchases for supplies and entertainment performances. Some items require you to approximate the expense. Remember that although your budget is an educated assumption of your upcoming spending, focus on educating yourself as much as you can. The assumption part is easy! Look into discounts on any quantity purchases. For example, some of your musical entertainers may give you a break on individual performance prices if you elect to pre-book four events a year. The same principle applies to quantity purchasing of many of your supply needs.

8. Check with your administrator on the status of any budget item that may involve more than one department. For instance, if you plan a cooking class for your residents, will the food costs be charged to the dietary budget or the activity budget? Ask about any special program where another department participates. Also, discuss your role in planning and administrating any staff activities. If you are involved with this function, find out how to budget for these programs. Should you prepare a separate budget? Are staff programs self-funded? If so, there is no formal funding from administration, but instead exist solely through fund raising. Each facility is different and your administrator will clarify this so you can complete your budget.

9. Review the rough cost projections you have made, and run a subtotal for each month and totals for the year. Is your overall annual budget figure in line with past budgets and your administrator's expectations? Are expenditures for the months uneven or is there some logic from month to month? This your opportunity to juggle items among months or to make cuts, if needed. If you decide that your budget is too high, look for areas to eliminate that will not directly impact your program. For example, ask your volunteer team to assist you in making decorations, thereby saving some costs. Be sure to let your administrator know where you were able to cut costs when you submit your final budget.

10. Review your rough budget draft with your staff and another department head for input. You are now ready to put your ideas into final proposal. Be sure that your final version is neat and easy to read. Figure 7–4 illustrates a typical annual supply budget.

In a separate budget planning phase, you may be asked to contribute ideas for capital purchases for the facility. A capital budget amount, if available, is set in advance by the administrator after

I. Supply Budget

January		March	
Special events:		Special events:	
Snowflake Ball	$125.00	St. Pats. Party	$150.00
Bell Ringers	$135.00	Family Council	$45.00
Supplies		Spring Bakeoff	$75.00
New Year's Eve Decor.	$17.00	Supplies	
Crafts (gifts for bell ringers)	$32.00	Seedlings, Soil	$29.00
Sensory Cart Restock	$83.00	Cognitive Equip.	$93.00
Flower Bulbs	$69.00	Calendars	$49.00
Misc.	$75.00	Misc.	$50.00
Total January:	**$536.00**	**Total March:**	**$491.00**
February		April	
Special events:		Special events:	
Val. Day Dance	$135.00	Passover Guests	$50.00
Health Fair	$85.00	Volunteer Lunch	$125.00
Supplies		Pets/Kids Easter Parade	$75.00
Doorway Decor.	$35.00	Supplies	
Candy Raffle	$20.00	Bed-bound Stock	$95.00
Exercise Tape	$225.00	Decorations	$45.00
Misc.	$125.00	Misc.	$100.00
Total February:	**$425.00**	**Total April:**	**$490.00**

Figure 7–4 Activity Department Expense Budget—Fiscal Year 20XX–20YY (*continued on next page*).

May

Special events:	
Mother's Day	$130.00
Nursing Hm. Wk.	$300.00
Supplies	
Invitations	$35.00
Printing	$80.00
Helium Rental	$65.00
Film	$30.00
Misc.	$50.00
Total May:	**$690.00**

June

Special events:	
Theme BBQ	$75.00
Father's Day	$100.00
50s Dance	$90.00
Supplies	
Program Books	$60.00
Sun Hats	$45.00
Misc.	$110.00
Total June:	**$480.00**

July

Special events:	
Family BBQ	$75.00
PJ Party	$115.00
Supplies	
Storage Bins	$27.00
Flags	$42.00
Patriotic Tapes	$20.00
Decorations	$69.00
Calendars	$48.00
Misc.	$80.00
Total July:	**$476.00**

August

Special events:	
Blueberry Fest.	$150.00
Swim Meet	$65.00
Twilight Party	$50.00
Supplies	
Park Fees	$50.00
10 Songbooks	$100.00
Film Develop.	$64.00
Misc.	$65.00
Total August:	**$544.00**

September

Special events:	
Theater Night	$95.00
School Program Kick-off	$65.00
Painting Party	$50.00
Supplies	
Paint (re-do reality wall)	$110.00
VCR tapes	$20.00
Misc.	$165.00
Total September:	**$505.00**

October

Special events:	
Fall Carnival	$150.00
Employee Recognition	$75.00
Halloween Party	$50.00
Supplies	
Mums	$100.00
Planters	$30.00
Prizes	$40.00
Misc.	$100.00
Total October:	**$545.00**

November

Special events:	
Wing Dedication	$200.00
Food Bank Donation Party	$75.00
Supplies	
Holiday Cards	$65.00
Woodworking	$50.00
Decorations	$35.00
Misc.	$75.00
Total November:	**$500.00**

December

Special events:	
Gift Wrap Party	$35.00
Holiday Parties	$250.00
Gifts	$100.00
Supplies	
Paper Goods	$135.00
Bakeware	$25.00
Misc.	$150.00
Total December:	**$695.00**
Total Annual Activity Supply Budget:	**$6,377.00**

II. Capital Budget

(2) 60" round tables w/pedestal base @ $300.00 ea. =	$600.00
(1) Umbrella for patio area (replacement) =	$300.00
Total Capital Budget:	**$900.00**

Figure 7–4 Activity Department Expense Budget—Fiscal Year 20XX–20YY (*continued*).

consulting with the owners of the facility. The capital budget is used for larger items, such as equipment, that depreciates over time. Depending on your administrator's directive, you may be requested to submit a capital budget request for items in this category for your department or for use in the general facility. For example, a capital expenditure specific to the activity department could be new tables and chairs for your activity room, or a new barbeque grill for your outdoor parties. If the administrator has a limited capital expense budget, he or she may ask you and fellow department heads to recommend one key item needed in the facility. One year in a particular facility where I worked as administrator, the department heads agreed that we most needed improved parking lot lights. That joint request was approved. Refer to Figure 7–4 for an example of a capital budget request. Even if the capital expenditures are limited, you should still prepare your activity requests and submit them. Be reasonable if you are told of the limitations of your "wish list," and cooperate with other team members to address and recommend items to meet the needs of the whole facility. You will get another chance next year for your activity recommendations.

Budget Preparation, Submission, and Review

After researching and thinking about your departmental needs in the three categories of payroll, activity supply, and capital budgets, you are now ready to put your ideas on paper and submit them for review. Before you do, ask your staff to look at your final proposal and make suggestions. Take the time to present your request to your administrator in a neatly printed or typed format with a memo attached to the request explaining your submission. Your chances of having your prepared budget looked at seriously increases with a neat and professional presentation. Be sure to submit your proposal within the time period your administrator gave you, and remember to retain a copy of your budget proposal for future reference.

Budget Implementation

After you receive an approval for your budget, you can begin using the money for your programs. If you have not received full approval, speak to your administrator and determine the areas that need retooling. Review the approved budget with your departmental staff, and let them know their involvement and your expectations of them in using the departmental budget. If you are the activity department head, you will most likely be handling the management of the payroll budget as well as your capital budget requests. Department staff members should be involved in understanding proper recordkeeping for the activity supply budget because they will be managing this budget with you.

What method will you use to manage your activity supply budget? The system utilized is often predetermined by your administrator, but you may be able to make a recommendation if you prefer one system over another. The most common ways to manage the activity supply budget are:

- Petty cash system
- Check request system
- Combination of both the petty cash system and the check request system

Petty cash is defined as a separate expense fund primarily used for minor expenditures. In his work, Kravitz (1990) indicates that a petty cash account ". . . requires strict control . . . " as a protection against misappropriated cash, and should be kept apart from other accounts. It is also preferable that, for safeguarding and accountability, only a limited number of staff members use the account. A petty cash system allows your department to receive an allotment of money per month (your budget) to be managed and used for all necessary expenses. A monthly budgeted amount of $200.00, for example, will demonstrate how you can manage your activity supply budget using a petty cash system. The petty cash arrangement can be set up in one of two ways. The first petty cash system provides you with a budgeted amount of $200.00 per month in a check which you receive at the beginning of the month, in cash, and then place in a strong box in a locked area in your office. You or your staff then use the cash to make the preapproved departmental purchases. Every purchase must have a receipt, and the information about the purchase written on each receipt and initialed by the purchaser. At the end of each month, the receipts are logged on a petty cash sheet (see Figure 7–5), totalled, and submitted to the administrator for approval. Once your petty cash log sheet, with receipts, is submitted to the bookkeeping department, a replenishment check for the used portion of the $200.00 is issued to you and the process begins again for the next month. A second petty cash system involves a written list of projected expenditures, prepared monthly, that meet your $200.00 monthly budget allotment. This detailed list of projected expenditures is submitted to your administrator. Once approved, you receive a check, use the money, and submit receipts. Of the two petty cash systems, the former one is preferred because it allows the activity department more control and accountability for money management.

A **check request** system involves making use of your bookkeeping department to request checks for vendor services in advance, or according to pre-established payment terms (i.e., thirty or sixty days). In many facilities, the method of choice for payment for all services is by check, almost eliminating the need to have cash on hand. A check for a specific purchase is requested using a check request form (see Figure 7–6), submitted to the administrator for approval, and then forwarded to the bookkeeper for processing. The bookkeeping department prefers this method because it provides a "paper trail," and there are no piles of receipts to sort

Month:_____

Beginning Balance: $ _____

Date	Item	Amount Used	New Balance
		$	$

Total Cash Remaining on Hand: $ _____

Total Petty Cash Reimbursed: $ _____

Submitted by: Activity Director Signature _____Date _____

Approved by: Administrator Signature   _____ Date _____

Figure 7-5   Activity Department—Monthly Petty Cash Form.

through. The downside to this system is the delay factor. The approvals needed and the wait for the bookkeeping department to actually write the checks can hold up your program. The procedure can also be difficult for activity professionals because of the need for some available cash for unexpected purchases or prompt handling of residents' personal needs. Facilities that offer small personal touches (i.e., a tradition of bringing residents a cupcake or other baked goods on their birthday or special day) would definitely want to use petty cash for these purchases. The baked items each cost sixty-five cents or less, and the event days occur randomly throughout the year. Using a check for this purchase would prove to be very impractical and would drive the bookkeeping staff crazy!

The best method of managing your activity supply budget is to combine both a petty cash system with the check request system. The ideal is to have a set amount allowable each month for petty cash, but use the check request system for items such as entertainers or craft supplies ordered from catalog. It is your responsibility to ensure that between the petty cash system and the check request system, you have not exceeded your monthly budgeted amount.

A check in the amount of $ _____ is requested for the following reason: _____

An order form or other information is attached.

The check should be made out to: _____

The check should be:

_____ mailed out no later than _____

(date)

to: _____

_____

_____

or _____ forwarded to the Activity Department by _____

(date)

Thank You! _____   _____

Activity Director Signature   *Date*   *Administrator Signature*   *Date*

Figure 7–6   Activity Department—Check Request Form.

Tracking and Monitoring Expenses

Good management of your departmental expenses for activity payroll, activity supplies, or capital expenditures related to your department requires constant tracking and monitoring of expenses by all members of your department. Establishing procedures that alert you to possible situations that may cause you to exceed your budget or other issues of budget mismanagement are critical to solving problem areas before they escalate. There are a number of methods of tracking your expenses that can help you stay within your approved budget limits; find a system that works for you and stick with it. The consequences of not maintaining your budget can be disastrous.

To track your weekly, biweekly, or monthly payroll (depending on how often you are paid in your facility), start by checking your employees' time cards or worksheets against the approved number of hours that each staff member should be working in that time period. Any discrepancies should be explained to the administrator in writing. Most facilities have policies requiring that all overtime or time exceeding normal work time, be approved by either the departmental supervisor, administrator, or other designated person before the extra time can be worked. Check with your administrator to ensure you are following the procedures for your facility. In working as an administrator, I found a good method of monitoring the expenses of all departments was the use of a payroll monitoring form that lists each department, the total approved hours for the department for each pay period, and the actual hours worked by each department per pay period. Any discrepancies required an explanation by the individual department head. This practice of closely watching payroll is very important to monitoring the staffing patterns that you have committed to maintain.

Managing your activity supply budget will likely be your biggest budget challenge. You may opt, depending on the size of your department, to delegate the job of overseeing the activity supply budget to one of your staff. You are responsible for the proper management of all departmental funds, however, and should check the status of spending on a frequent basis. You also have the responsibility of reviewing all petty cash expenditures, ensuring that receipts are properly documented, attached to all expenses, and signed-off for a finalized petty cash reconciliation that is forwarded to your administrator and to bookkeeping. Any check requests for catalog supplies, entertainers, and so forth, should be thoroughly reviewed

by you, and signed off before sending them in for payment or reimbursement. When receiving shipments of supplies, all packed items should be checked against the packing slip for accuracy of the order, and the presence of damaged materials noted. Packing slips should be dated, signed, and marked "received" before forwarding them to bookkeeping for processing. Depending on your relationship with the bookkeeping department in your facility, you may also be able to access copies of a monthly accounts payable report that can tell you if your check requests have been processed.

Controlling your capital budget expense is usually the easiest area to monitor. First, you will most likely be limited in the capital areas for which you have received approval. Additionally, you will probably be required to obtain three written bids from approved outside vendors for each capital item that is slated for purchase. You will work from some detailed specifications, and should share the same specifications with each vendor to be sure your bids are comparable. Once the bids are obtained, submit them to your administrator, along with your recommendation. Remember that the low bidder may not be the best recommendation. Your role in monitoring the capital purchases occurs when the final bidder is selected, and you check the final delivery of the product to ensure that it meets both the bidding specifications as well as normal quality standards.

Reporting Requirements

Each administrator is different in his or her approach when reporting your budget status. Some administrators want to dig into detail and discuss every purchase; others are content to know that you have not exceeded your budget, and they do not have to hear the details. One thing they all agree on, however, is that no one likes to be surprised by seeing an expense report that shows a particular department exceeding their allotted budget. Your administrator may ask you to submit a monthly or quarterly report on your spending, including projections for the upcoming months. He or she may want to see you personally to discuss progress. In any case, if you are practicing good tracking and monitoring techniques, you will be prepared for either scenario.

Stretching Your Budget

This is an area that should top your list because no matter what your budget allotment is, you certainly can use more funds. Over the years, activity professionals have done more to stretch a dollar than most groups. Many professionals share their ideas on finding new sources for "free-bies." Here are some ideas that may work for you:

1. Become an expert on all the free services from local, state, and federal organizations. There are a number of good books in the marketplace that can guide you to free items of which you may not have thought.
2. Use your people resources (staff, volunteers, and so on) to help think of creative ways to get things done and to save money. You will be surprised at the good ideas that arise from a "think session!"
3. Fund raise when you can (and are permitted). Fund raising is often a part of the nonprofit environment and is increasing in importance as funding sources decline. In larger facilities, fund-raising efforts may be chaired by someone in administration, but the activity department will be involved at some level. Warner (1975) lists numerous fund-raising ideas, ranging from auctions and book sales to concerts and luncheons. Set your own fund-raising goals with administration and make an appropriate plan for accomplishing them.
4. Ask for free help, services, and so forth, from anyone you think may be able to sponsor a program or donate time.
5. "Beef up" your volunteer program. Invite local civic groups to hold their meetings in the facility in return for a "free" program. Review Chapter 16 on volunteers for more good ideas.
6. Barter for services and supplies.
7. Attend garage sales for inexpensive supplies, game prizes, or raffle items.
8. Ask staff members to head groups based on their particular hobby or interest.
9. Check with your local or county library for free ideas on programming.
10. Get to know your resident's family; they often have many hidden talents or can suggest good ideas.
11. Think before you buy. Ask yourself if you can make the item or substitute something else in its place.
12. Develop a relationship with a local college or other school that may have a recreation or activity curriculum. Often, these schools look for field placement for their students who can complete internships while assisting with your programs.
13. Work with local vendors to take advantage of special situations. For example, an arrangement might be made with a local bakery to pick up surplus baked goods when they have a slow day. These fresh-baked items might normally be discarded but would be welcome in your program.
14. Join your local activity professional group and exchange services with the membership.
15. Ask video stores, travel agencies, and cinemas to give you their posters and banners after events are over.
16. Hold decorating contests with your staff and residents, if they are able. You will save staff time and some decorating expenses, and gain staff involvement.
17. Do programs without a lot of extras. Some of the best programs involve very few supplies!
18. Seek quantity discounts whenever possible.

Budgets and the Value of Activities

A budget represents the funding that your department has been granted to execute programs, but how does this figure relate to your value as an activity professional and the worth of your program?

The benefits of participation in activity programs are numerous in terms of meeting resident needs, decreasing anxieties, and improving resident satisfaction, to name a few. Some additional benefits of activity programming can be attributed to the area of budgeting and cost containment. Jackson and Lilly (1990) suggest that as a result of activity participation, it may be expected that fewer resident medications are necessary, staff interventions in resident care are decreased because of improved resident satisfaction and independence, and resident focus on health conditions and problems may also be decreased. All of these projected benefits can equal cost savings for residents as well as administrative staff.

Translating your value as an activity professional into financial terms may be more difficult to imagine. In her article on perceived value, Palmer (1992) describes the visible merit of an activity program by stating "Unfortunately, too often it is seen as something that is diversional, recreational, . . . but NOT essential." Palmer goes on to say that program planning should be based on ". . . real value . . ." in meeting higher level psychosocial needs, and that this value must be shared with the rest of the health care team. In another similar study, Parker (1991) uses Maslow's theory to conclude that lower level needs, such as physiological and safety needs, are met by other staff professionals, but only the activity professional ". . . has the ultimate responsibility of providing the environment whereby each individual can potentially fulfill all his/her higher needs to the point of becoming self-actualized." Parker also calls for higher educational requirements for activity professionals that should cause an increase in salaries and benefits to match other health care professionals.

Salaries and budget discussions are often uncomfortable for any manager, but the activity professional faces additional hardship because of a program perception of being less than vital, with limited educational requirements, regulations, and reimbursement from federal and state programs. To counter this, activity professionals should become familiar with salaries for similar positions in their area. Additionally, submit any supportive documentation you can to your administrator on measurable quality of life improvements that your programs have made to your residents. These efforts, along with the lobbying by activity organizations, may eventually make a difference in increasing salaries and budgets. Until that time comes, it is in your best interest to continue to improve your programs.

SUMMARY

Budget planning is a requirement for the management of activity supplies, capital expenses, and petty cash allocation for effective funding of programs. The budget planning process includes projection, preparation, meetings with administration, submission, execution, monitoring, and reporting. Mastery of the budget process techniques, as well as cost containment tips, will prove to be invaluable for the activity professional.

R E V I E W   Q U E S T I O N S

1. What is a fiscal year?
2. In which three budget areas will you be most involved with planning?
3. How are staffing patterns determined?
4. What is petty cash used for, and how is it maintained?
5. What are the advantages of the check request form?
6. What financial benefits can be derived from activities?

O N   Y O U R   O W N

1. Based on the regulations in your state, determine an adequate weekly staffing pattern for a 143-bed facility including full- and part-time staff.
2. Using the fictitious ABC nursing home (120 beds, thirty of which are in an Alzheimer's unit), plan an annual activity budget for this new facility.
3. Brainstorm to come up with ten additional ways you can stretch your budget.

R E F E R E N C E S

Jackson, T., & Lilly, J. (1990). The value of activities: Establishing a foundation for cost-effectiveness. *Activities, Adaptation and Aging,* 14 (4), 5–20.

Kravitz, W. W. (1990). *Bookkeeping: The easy way.* Hauppauge, NY: Barron's Educational Series Inc.

Palmer, M. D. (1992). Perceived value: What is an activity program worth? *Activities, Adaptation and Aging,* 16 (3), 19–25.

Parker, S. D. (1991). A new perspective on the value of activity directors. *Activities, Adaptation and Aging,* 16 (2), 81–85.

Warner, I. (1975). *The art of fundraising.* New York, NY: Harper & Row Publishers.

F U R T H E R   R E A D I N G

Annand, V. (1977). A review of evaluation in therapeutic recreation. *Therapeutic Recreation Journal*, 11(2), 42–47.

The Bowman Gray School of Medicine of Wake Forest University. (1994). *Board must participate in fund raising.* (Respite Report, Summer, 6.) Winston-Salem, NC: author.

Edginton, C., & Hayes, G. (1976). Using performance objectives in the delivery of therapeutic recreation services. *Leisurability*, Vol. 3(4), 20–26.

Olsson, R. (1986). The prospective payment system: Implications for therapeutic recreation. *Therapeutic Recreation Journal*, 1st Quarter, 7–17.

Powell, L. (1984). Fiscal management in therapeutic recreation: A perspective on educational preparation. *Therapeutic Recreation Journal*, 4th Quarter, 37–41.

Reitter, M. (1984). Third party reimbursement: Is therapeutic recreation too late? *Therapeutic Recreation Journal*, 4th Quarter, 13–19.

Touchstone, W. (1984). Fiscal accountability through effective risk management. *Therapeutic Recreation Journal*, 4th Quarter, 20–25.

West, R. (1984). Productivity analysis as a method of fiscal accountability for therapeutic recreation. *Therapeutic Recreation Journal*, 4th Quarter, 27–36.

CHAPTER 8

Program Development

KEY TERMS

need
motivation
therapeutic recreation process
service delivery
medical-clinical model
wellness model
long-term care model
therapeutic milieu model
therapeutic recreation service model
treatment
leisure education
recreation participation
leisure awareness
social interaction skills
leisure skills development
leisure resources
program
activity assessment
interest checklist
risk awareness profile

OBJECTIVES

After completing this chapter, you should:

- understand the important benefits and goals of activity programming
- differentiate the service delivery options available to activity professionals today
- comprehend the components of the activity programming process

INTRODUCTION

The reflection of your training and knowledge comes through to your residents and staff by the programs that you plan and present. Your activity program, a complex and individualized design, is the backbone of your department, and should effectively illustrate your strategy in meeting your residents' needs and interests. There is an abundance of information on programming ideas, but first we will present the foundation for programming needs.

The Basis for Activity Programming

To understand the importance of activity programming, a rationale for this service must first be discussed. Activity programming exists as a major service in a long-term care facility, but why is this service important to the overall treatment goals for an individual resident? When we first discussed the aging process in Chapter 3, time was spent in understanding the physical, psychological, and psychosocial aspects of aging. Two of the key psychosocial components that have great impact on activity program planning are **need** and **motivation**. Psychosocial needs, defined by Maslow (1968) in his "hierarchy of needs," range from the most basic physiological needs for food, shelter, and clothing to the highest level of need, self-actualization (see Figure 8–1). The basic physiological needs on the lowest level must be met in order for safety needs, on the next level, to be addressed. Once the need for protection from harm and danger is met, an individual is free to satisfy higher needs of being loved and accepted by others. When these needs are met, higher needs still, such as esteem (respect from self and others) and actualization (the experience of developing full creativity and self-expression) can be met.

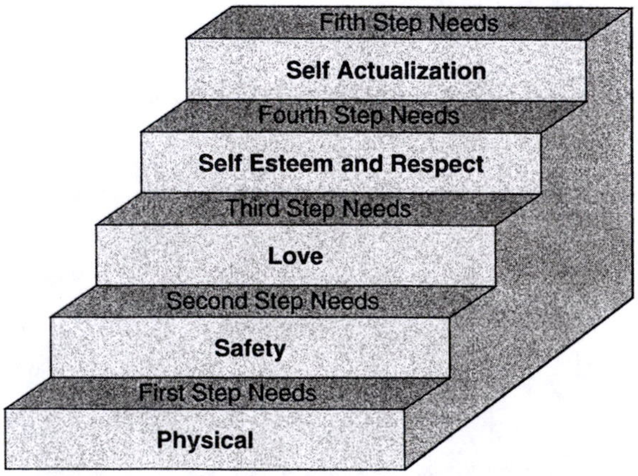

Figure 8–1 Maslow's hierarchy of needs.

Motivation, defined as the reason for an action or choice, has strong links to human needs, and is a factor to take into account when planning programs. Farrell and Lundegren (1991) discuss motivation in terms of the gain from participation in a program. Examples of external rewards are a medal or trophy, and internal rewards, joining in a group activity. Human needs act as motivators for some actions as long as needs are unsatisfied. For example, a new resident who is experiencing pain and may have come from a dysfunctional environment will probably not show interest in being part of a group (love/belonging needs), or express himself or herself creatively (self-actualization needs) until the basic needs for food, relief from pain, and shelter are fully met. Once the lower level needs are met, this resident will be motivated by other factors.

Understanding the motivation behind resident behavior, and responding to the needs of individuals, must be taken into account during the entire program planning process.

Why are Activities Needed? Benefits and Objectives of Programming

With a projected increase in the elderly population expected in the next century, more people will be living longer and could be experiencing larger amounts of leisure time. Godbey and Parker (1976) point out that the enjoyment of any leisure time by the general elderly population is governed by their health status and mobility factors. The elderly in poor or declining health, such as those in institutional long-term care, have large quantities of diversional time, but are often prevented from taking full advantage of this leisure time because of physical and mental limitations. This problem leads to challenges for the activity or recreation professional in dealing with delivery of activity services in this setting.

A few decades ago, activity planning in institutional settings was provided to give a resident ". . . diversion from an otherwise dreary existence. . ." according to Stein and Sessoms (1977). In recent years, a more positive and evolving view of activity programming has gained momentum; the notion that activity and recreation programming is part of the entire rehabilitation process. A discussion of the advantages of activity programming follows.

The numerous benefits of activity and recreation programming have been researched and analyzed over the last few decades. Lucas (1962) stated that recreation may suggest companionship to one person whereas another individual may derive the "built-in" recreation benefit of socialization. In a study on the effect of activity programs, Reichenfeld, Csapo, Carriere, and Gardner (1973) noticed that patients actively participated in formally led programs that included ". . . encouragement and repetition. . . ." Verhoven (1977) suggests that participation in recreation in an institutional setting keeps a person engaged with the community and often improves his or her ". . . physical, emotional and mental health. . . ." He cites additional examples of benefits such as enjoyment, release of tensions, assistance in the development of social relationships, increasing awareness, and establishing a feeling of purpose. Peckham and Peckham (1982) offer these additional benefits of activity programming: increasing alertness, making social opportunities available, providing choices and areas for contributions, and increasing physical health.

The therapeutic recreation research studies of Kelly, McNally, and Chambliss (1983) mention that maintaining established levels of activity participation can have increased benefits in the areas of physical and psychological health. Their work also shows that participation in certain activity programs may increase positive behaviors. Psychological needs were a focal point in the work of Incani, Seward, and Sigler (1975) when they postulated that certain of these needs can be met at least partially through programs that include "life activities." Singleton, Makrides, and Kennedy (1986) reviewed and commented on the past literature that includes reports that activity participation may increase life satisfaction and act as a resistor to stress factors in the environment. In discussing the value of taking part in recreation programs, Shiver and Fait (1985) comment that those individuals who may be ill have greater needs and, therefore, may benefit more from participation. These benefits of participation include positive changes in physical fitness, social interactions, and mental health.

Using obvious benefits to formulate program goals and objectives was another issue covered in the literature. Incani, Seward, and Sigler discuss that general program objectives might include providing cognitive stimulation, satisfying health and wellness goals, and assisting in the formation of "wholesome life attitudes." Hisek (1978), in his piece on recreation planning, offers "re-awakening of creative impulses" as a recreation or activity goal. To illustrate goals from the orientation of therapeutic recreation service, MacNeil and Teague (1983) proffer guidelines for program planning, such as the prevention of further decline in mental or physical skills, assistance in restoring resident function to optimum levels, and support in adjustment to the new institutional environment. Goodman (1983) elaborates on a review of the literature that lists the relief of loneliness or boredom, and the provision of a "happy, home-like environment" as some of the designated objectives for an activity program. Other researchers, such as Mobily (1985), have weighed in on this issue of recreation or activity programming goals, and cite objectives such as "improve functional behaviors" or "provide opportunities for acquisition of skills."

Who are We Serving?

Learning about the aging process, the body systems, and the changes that can be anticipated during acute or chronic illnesses provide a framework for understanding the needs of the residents with whom we will deal. But what do we know about the general characteristics of these residents?

Projections for population growth of older members of the demographic pool will continue to increase over the next thirty years, according to the United States Senate Special Committee On Aging (1984). Their research shows that by the year 2050, over ten percent of the total population will be over seventy-five years of age, and over five percent of the total population will be in the "old old" category of eighty-five years of age or older. In terms of gender, a shorter life expectancy for men accounts for three women for every two men in the age group of sixty-five and over, with expectations for this trend to continue into the next century.

In the area of ethnic diversity, the nonwhite elderly population continues to be the largest growing segment, with a projection of eighteen percent of the total population in 2050. In 1982, the sixty-five and over population was represented by eight percent blacks, six percent Asians and/or Pacific Islanders, five percent American Indian and/or Hispanic, and twelve percent whites.

The top four chronic illnesses of the population group sixty-five years or older were reported as arthritis, hypertensive disease, hearing impairments, and heart conditions. In discussing limitations to activity participation due to chronic conditions, close to fifty percent of the over sixty-five population experiences some limitations. The projections for the future suggest that limitations in activity because of chronic conditions will significantly increase over the next few decades, especially in the seventy-five-year-old and over category.

In this study, approximately twenty-five percent of the elderly population is reported to have mental health problems. The most significant finding is that the primary mental health problem of the older population is cognitive impairment, with mild impairment rates being slightly higher than severe impairment rates. Related to this finding, approximately twenty-three percent of all nursing home residents have a primary diagnosis that involves a "mental disorder" or "senility." One of the leading reasons for admission to a long-term care facility is because of problems in cognitive functioning.

Participation in religious activities was also studied, with the elderly population demonstrating the highest spiritual commitment of all age groups. More than eighty percent of the over sixty-five age group feel that religion is an important influence in their lives, and provides them with personal comfort.

These findings, as well as other research in the field, should assist you in planning for the general type of clients you can expect. Your residents' characteristics may not fit the statistics above, but you should look at the general statistics in your facility to help improve your programs.

What are the Program Processes Used to Meet Needs?

Armed with the information of who we are serving and the reasons for it, we must next look at an organized methodology to address resident needs. Completing a sequence of steps to meet resident needs is identified as a **therapeutic recreation process** by O'Morrow and Reynolds (1989). The goal of this process is to move an individual from a role of nonparticipant in the environment to one of participant at the highest possible level. O'Morrow and Reynolds describe four theoretical models by researchers, Berryman, Ball, Frye and Peters, and Gunn and Peterson that illustrate the application of a therapeutic recreation process. In Frye and Peters' (1972) work, Doris Berryman proposes a theoretical model for recreation processing, and suggests that "experiential bonds" develop between activities and the environment through repetitive exposures to experiences. After numerous bonds are formed, the resident can begin to establish activity experiences of his or her own. In another theory, Ball (1970) proposes a continuum model that describes recreation experiences in four different ways: activity for the sake of activity, recreation education, therapeutic recreation, and recreation. According to Ball, an individual can undergo many stages simultaneously, with time and motivation as the factors that change one experience to another. A five-stage clinical model for handling the recreation process was proposed by Frye and Peters (1972). Their model mentions developing an organized program that conforms to physician orders, marketing the program to interest the resident, building a unique program between resident and professional, notifying resident and staff of program choices, and allowing the resident to make his or her own choices in participation. Peterson and Gunn (1984) tailored a systems approach to the recreation process that involves setting purposes and goals of programming, fashioning a program based solely on defined goals, planning a delivery method, implementing the program, and evaluating or revising the program, if required.

The processes listed above are suggested methods, but you must find your own approach. Austin (1982) mentioned the "eclectic" approach that often characterizes therapeutic recreation as ". . . the utilization of approaches and techniques drawn from several sources". O'Morrow and Reynolds (1989) support that statement by noting that the therapeutic recreation process is open to interpretation and individualization by activity and recreation professionals.

How are We Delivering Services?

Service delivery, or the way in which activity or recreation services are brought to long-term care residents, does not have one accepted and standardized procedure, but rather comprises a few models for delivery. According to O'Morrow and Reynolds (1989), there are two significant reasons why a standardized service delivery method should be accepted within the recreation field: professional accountability and "right-to-treatment" litigation. Accountability issues concern justifying, through documentation, the individual plans for specific residents. The "right-to-treatment" idea deals with the rights of those confined to hospitals or institutions who are entitled by law to receive all necessary treatment that improves their condition, including interventions to humanize the psychological and physical environment. The service delivery methods that will be described are the medical-clinical model, the wellness model, the long-term care model, the therapeutic milieu model, and the therapeutic recreation service model.

Medical-Clinical Model. A traditional, illness-centered approach to treatment is the **Medical-Clinical Model**, described by O'Morrow and Reynolds (1989). Considering the treatment of a disease as the focus, rather than the person, specific departmental disciplines follow the physician's guidelines to resolve the medical issues. The thrust of medicine as the dominant force over the other professional disciplines to drive treatment is still an accepted method in hospitals, rehabilitation centers with short-term clients, and other clinical settings. It may, however, be limiting to activity or recreation professionals. A conflict between defining acute medicine and rehabilitative medicine can also effect treatment. Acute medicine has a cure as the objective, and may wait for an acute phase to pass before rehabilitative measures are taken, whereas the rehabilitative field works on restoring function through integration with all phases of care. West (1979) provides these goals for recreation personnel who work within this medical model: offer diversional programs, counsel residents on using activities following discharge, use recreation programs to provide psychological outlets for negative emotions, promote independence, and relieve loneliness or boredom through programs. The therapeutic recreation process traditionally begins with a referral or physician's order for activity or recreation treatment.

Wellness Model. An approach that focuses on humanistic concepts is described by Austin (1982) as a **wellness model**. In this view, residents are seen as whole persons composed of ". . . a unique biological, psychological and social background from which to react to the environment as a total person. . . ." A step up in this theory, described by Austin, is "high level wellness" that views a person as propelled toward ". . . maximizing the potential which the individual is capable". Holistic medicine, which views the entire person in treatment plans, has a similar basis to the wellness model. In the illness and/or wellness continuum illustrated by Austin, where illness is at one end of the spectrum and wellness is at the other, activity and recreation professionals should be concerned with clients along the entire spectrum. McDowell (1986) states that a wellness approach requires these three assumptions of an individual: body, mind, and spirit are "integrated" and "interdependent," potential exists for responsibility with care, and the highest level of wellness is sought, based on capability.

Goals for activity professionals who work within the wellness model might include increasing functional ability, understanding and applying leisure concepts to assist in coping with illness or disability, and developing new skills or techniques.

Long-Term Care Model.   Although we have already covered many of the aspects of long term care in Chapter 1, this model is based on the unique features of institutional long-term care. O'Morrow and Reynolds (1989) recall that few facilities today are reflective of the custodial model of care of the 1960s in which most components of life, such as sleeping and eating, were handled in a "controlled manner." The rigidity of the facility routines and loss of touch with the community outside the facility led to "institutional neurosis," that included apathy with the surroundings, withdrawal, and personality changes.

The **long-term care model** of today involves quality of life issues as part of the planning process. Although individuals who are candidates for long-term care have medical needs that require nursing care, they usually do not experience acute episodes of illness that could be handled by hospital care. Subacute care is the exception, where higher levels of care may be anticipated. Their conditions are primarily chronic, and may involve physical disabilities, mental disorders, or both. Studies cited by O'Morrow and Reynolds (1989) show that over seventy-five percent of nursing home residents have levels of impairment that are considered "extreme," and, of course, impact the planning and participation strategies devised by the activity professional. The objectives and goals of the long-term care model are summarized in their work as: providing ongoing care for recovery from medical conditions, guiding the resident in meeting goals of optimal mental and physical health through all key disciplines, assisting the residents where needed to achieve care in grooming and the like, and meeting the overall needs of residents in such areas as "physical, emotional, social and spiritual." The classification levels of nursing care and supervision, such as skilled nursing care, intermediate care, and residential care impact the type of activity program that is provided.

Because of the wide variety of settings in which long-term care residents receive care, and the special characteristics of long-term care life, activity or recreation professionals should be aware of the unique features of their individual treatment setting, and plan for meeting the needs of their residents accordingly. The goals of the activity professionals working in the long-term care model involve identifying and making treatment plans with the rest of the interdisciplinary care plan team to meet individual needs, scheduling and implementing diversional programs to aide in adjustment to the facility, and addressing physical, emotional, intellectual, spiritual, and other needs. Referrals are sometimes made by the attending physician to the activity or recreation professional that begins the assessment process, but often a simple physician order such as "may participate fully in activity programs" is the only reference an activity professional sees that requests his or her services. In contrast to the other delivery models, federal and state guidelines dictate that every resident must be provided with appropriate activity programming so the physician's order may be either a referral or a medical clearance for active participation. If there are questions as to the amount or type of participation that a resident can endure, a request for clarification should be made to the attending physician.

Along with the therapeutic recreation service model discussed later in this chapter, the long-term care model is the primary focus of this text, and incorporates all the elements of planning, implementing, and evaluating that comprise the therapeutic recreation process.

Therapeutic Milieu Model.   A model that has origins in the provision of service to primarily mentally ill clients is called the **therapeutic milieu model** of delivering services. A number of negative factors, such as improper staff training, overcrowded facilities, and use of a purely medical orientation in treating the mentally ill led in the past to a condition, documented by O'Morrow and Reynolds (1989), as "social breakdown syndrome." Symptoms of clients with this syndrome include lack of interest in activities and appearance, extreme withdrawal, and aggressive behavior. Along with other approaches, such as innovative drug therapies, a therapeutic milieu approach to treatment developed, and looked at all components of the recovery process: rehabilitation, recreation, client opinions, staff-client relations, and medical input. The therapeutic milieu service concept provides for clients to participate, as well as assume personal control for participating in diversional or other activities. For many activity professionals, this approach has validity because setting situations exist where long-term units are designated for psychiatric geriatric residents.

The goals for the activity professional in the therapeutic milieu model are to assist clients in re-establishing their emotional health through increasing functioning and skill development, arranging and encouraging participation in diversional programs, and allowing for client participation in the entire planning and treatment process. Because discharge is part of the expected process, activity planning includes opportunities to participate in appropriate life skills and exposure to community life.

Therapeutic Recreation Service Model. A popular approach to service delivery that incorporates many aspects of service is the **therapeutic recreation service model**, developed by Peterson and Gunn (1984). The model is a client-centered technique related to his or her amount of leisure involvement, and outlines three areas of service that address specific needs: **treatment, leisure education**, and **recreation participation**. The service classifications applicable to a particular situation relate to factors such as the need of the client (described as the purpose of the intervention), the role of the "specialist" or professional (defined as the nature of the intervention), and the amount of control that the participant has in making a choice. The authors note that for programs developed by activity or recreation professionals, each program should focus on only one service category.

The treatment category of service, described by Peterson and Gunn, is defined as "some specifically planned process to bring about desired positive change in behavior or pathology." They mention that terms such as rehabilitation or therapy, used in other clinical settings, usually have the same meaning. Assuming the role of a therapist and using proper techniques, the recreation professional uses the treatment service category to address the behavioral areas of ". . . physical, mental, emotional and social functioning" through the use of the therapeutic recreation process. In the three-stage therapeutic recreation service delivery model, Peterson and Gunn view this treatment phase as providing an opportunity to increase functional skills in a highly controlled setting, usually within the traditional medical model. In this treatment category, the client has minimal freedom in this part of the delivery system. An example of an application of the treatment component of service may occur in settings such as work with the severely developmentally disabled.

The second area of the therapeutic recreation service delivery model concerns leisure education, defined as a general category that assists clients with information and the formation of new skills and feelings toward leisure. The basis of leisure education concerns the concept of play, which is considered a core behavior. Peterson and Gunn make the argument that disabilities and chronic ailments often put individuals at a disadvantage from routine opportunities to experience play and other social outlets. Using an educational model (rather than the medical model used in treatment), the recreation professional, referred to as the "instructor" or "counselor," attempts to alter and enhance behavior by assisting the client in gaining new skills and abilities. The leisure education process can be achieved through one of four areas: **leisure awareness, social interaction skills, leisure skills development**, and **leisure resources**. Leisure awareness, the element that Peterson and Gunn feel has been absent in many past recreation programming efforts, concerns the development of an understanding of the benefits of leisure and the choice to begin involvement. The most common type of participation in leisure is through social interaction skills. Lack of skills, such as conversational abilities or cooperation and competition in all size group settings, can lead to unsatisfactory experiences. The third part of the leisure education process, leisure skills development, attempts to help a client to choose and enhance skills in specific areas that will increase enjoyment and satisfaction. Leisure resources, the last category in leisure education, relies on the client's awareness and ability to utilize all available information to maximize leisure potential. In all aspects of the leisure education model, it is important to note that the recreation professional and the client share the planning and control of the experience, as opposed to the earlier treatment model that offered little control by the client.

The last area, recreation participation, represents an arranged program that ". . . provides opportunities for fun, enjoyment, and self-expression within an organized delivery system." This program assumes that certain skills and "participatory ability" exist for the experience to be enjoyable. In this area, the client has the most control over participation, but the "leader" or group "facilitator" provides the recreation opportunity. Use of the recreation participation area can be found in both community-based settings and in clinical settings, such as a rehabilitation center or long-term care facility. Peterson and

Gunn comment that the differences in handling recreation participation in a long-term care setting are because of the increased length of treatment. They suggest that using the concept of "leisure lifestyle," activity or recreation professionals ". . . must carefully plan a full range of program and service offerings that adequately address the specific interests, preferences and skills of the clients." Programming should also include more variety to divert from "stereotype" programs such as bingo and bowling.

What is Therapeutic?

Although training and experiential expectations vary by state and country, two questions arise about the activity services we deliver: are they considered therapy? and should we consider ourselves therapists? There probably will not be clear answers to these questions until a solution is found among the primary groups that currently credential individuals in the activity and recreation field for work in long-term care settings.

Because the activity professional works almost exclusively with physically or mentally disabled persons, the activity goals of providing relaxation and diversion are replaced with a more therapeutic intent of using ". . . recreation as a treatment vehicle . . . " that Halberg (1985) and Howe-Murphy (1979) suggest follows the "therapy orientation" perspective mentioned by Meyer in the early 1980s. Mobily (1985) also identifies one of the therapeutic aspects of recreation to be ". . . identify recreational activities with the client that will divert attention, relax the clients and act in a cathartic way so that the client will avoid unnecessary stress and anxiety." Mobily adds that by viewing recreation as therapy, it suggests that

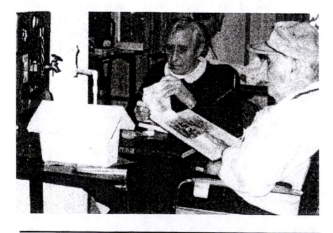

Figure 8–2 Programs offered should address resident interests, life skills, and physical/mental abilities.

". . . recreation is a means rather than an end. . . ." In their work, Mobily, Wissinger, and Hunnicutt (1987) ask the questions: "If recreation is therapy, is it any longer recreation? And if therapy is recreational, can it possibly be therapy?" They suggest that to view recreation as a way to experience change and as a goal in itself may be the most logical way to explain the therapeutic impacts of activity and recreation programming.

The Program Planning Process ......

With a theoretical structure in place to understand how activity services can be delivered, a look at the program planning process is the next step.

What is a Program?

As defined by Edginton, Compton, and Hanson (1980), an activity **program** is a ". . . vehicle for service delivery" and ". . . a purposeful plan of intervention. . . ." A program is a structured method for providing an experience to a resident or for producing specific outcomes. When beginning the process of program planning, the authors suggest that the professional consider the kind of service that is to be presented, the manner in which the program is established, and what expected impact the program has on the resident.

Program Design

Planning an entire program that takes into account the specific needs and requirements of all your residents, as well as the unique features of your facility, takes patience. The method you use to integrate all the elements is your own, but should be based on a variety of factors.

Kraus, Carpenter, and Bates (1981) mention that any selection of activities should include consideration of the potential participant's age, physical and mental state, time and space available for participation, and any previous activity experiences that the participant may have had. These factors become even more critical when you choose appropriate programs for groups. Another view on program planning is offered by Farrell and Lundgren (1991) who suggest that program planning involves "classifying" activities by the following criteria: the facilities that are needed, the staff or others who are needed to assist, age-based, interests and desires of the participants, amount of time allotted, and the predicted results. The reasons for using a classification system to program plan include ensuring that variety and balance are provided, and allowing an easy way to evaluate the program. Reviewing some of the program design factors these researchers present may help you in considering your overall program.

Role of Assessment and Interest Inventories. As you followed the guidelines in Chapter 4 about how to get to know your residents, you began your knowledge base of the assessment process. The **activity assessment** process is the act of collecting vital pieces of information about your resident, through individual interviews, observations, and family discussions, to plan for activity programming needs. The needs and desires of your residents should dictate the general direction of your program. The activity assessment is one segment of the total assessment process made up by all members of the interdisciplinary care planning team. Gathering your assessment information is done on an individual basis because activity needs are met on a personal level for each resident. But faced with the task of program planning for a large population of residents, the use of an **interest checklist** (see Figure 8–3) is necessary to look for obvious overlaps in resident backgrounds, hobbies, and so forth. The checklist is compiled by listing each resident's name in the left-hand column, and noting any past, current, or potential interests in general categories in the right-hand column. The information is totalled for each category, thereby giving the activity professional a broad idea of some repetitive desires of the resident population. For example, if your checklist shows that eighty-five percent of your clientele previously enjoyed gardening, that would be valuable information for your planning. The interest checklist should be completed by you as a new employee, to familiarize yourself with your residents and their interests on a frequent basis, as required by the changes in your resident population. You should review the interest inventory each month, and make changes to include new admissions, prior to beginning your upcoming monthly program.

Another helpful tool that can be completed after you have conducted your activity assessments is the **risk awareness profile**. A thorough activity assessment provides you with much data including resident limitations and other cautionary risk information that you should be aware of to properly plan a program. Using the format shown in Figure 8–4, prepare a risk awareness profile for the facility to alert you, your staff, and volunteers to the challenges and potential limitations of your resident population. Knowing medical information about residents, such as restrictive diets, those in geri-chairs, and behavior issues, will not only help you plan programs, but also will assist in monitoring potential problems.

An activity assessment holds information about interests and potential needs. Using your

PAST/CURRENT INTERESTS

NAME OF RESIDENT	ART	CARDS/BRIDGE	COOKING	DANCING	DECORATING	DRAMA	FISHING	FOOTBALL	GAMES	GARDENING	GOLF	HISTORY	HOMEMAKING	HOME REPAIRS	LANGUAGES	MUSIC	PAINTING	PARTIES	PETS	PHOTOGRAPHY	POLITICS	RADIO	READING	SEWING	CRAFTS	SOCIAL CLUBS	SPORTS	SWIMMING	TELEVISION	TRAVEL	WRITING				OCCUPATION	CULTURAL

Figure 8–3 An activity interest checklist will help you plan appropriate programs.

RISK CHECKLIST

NAME OF RESIDENT	ALCOHOL/ DRUG USE	ALLERGIES—FOOD	ALLERGIES—OTHER	COMBATIVE	DIABETIC DIET	FREQUENT FALLS	PSYCHOTROPIC DRUG USE	RESTRAINT USE	TRANSFER PROBLEMS	UNSTEADY GAIT	WANDERING/ ELOPING	WEIGHT GAIN/LOSS	OTHER

Figure 8–4 Knowing the risk factors and precautions for residents will aid in planning safe programs.

information carefully helps you work with your residents to satisfy their needs and assist in progress toward goals.

Age of Participants. Your setting usually dictates the age range of your residents, but many facilities have multiple units with different client needs. Additionally, facilities may have wider age variations because of admission policies, and these differences have to be addressed as you plan your program.

Physical and Mental Abilities. Participation levels vary according to the physical and mental status of your resident group. Some programs work well with many ability ranges combined, whereas other group settings are not appropriate for all residents. A balanced program considers the fluctuating ability levels and will be the most successful.

Facility Space. The physical environment of your facility is another factor to consider when planning your overall program. As we discussed in Chapter 6, the layout of your facility is crucial to the way you organize and administrate your program. A plan that calls for three programs to go on simultaneously will not be possible if your facility scheduling allows only two open areas at a time. Work creatively with the space you have, and be on the hunt for new, untapped program spots.

Equipment. Your supplies and equipment are often dictated by your budget and the "age" of

your program. For example, if your facility has been in existence for ten years and your predecessors shopped wisely, you may have inherited substantial equipment. Regardless of what you have available, find a method of obtaining the basics to hold your programs. Plans for elaborate, expensive programs are often unnecessary to meet individual needs.

Staff. The resourcefulness and creativeness of your staff is actually a more fundamental requirement than supplies, equipment, or space. An energetic and well-trained staff person can work wonders with limitations in other areas. Proper program planning requires you consider the staff and volunteers you have available before you can solidly plan your full program.

SUMMARY

Developing a comprehensive activity program begins with an understanding of the needs of residents and how activities can benefit them. Various service delivery methods are available as a resource to activity professionals who are program planning. The process for designing a full activity program involves many factors including resident assessment, tabulating interest inventories, and considering variables such as participant ages, health status, space, equipment, and staffing.

R E V I E W   Q U E S T I O N S

1. Why is Maslow's hierarchy of needs important in program planning?
2. What are three of the benefits of activity programming?
3. Describe the steps in the therapeutic recreation process, proposed by O'Morrow and Reynolds.
4. What are the three components of the service model for therapeutic recreation designed by Peterson and Gunn?
5. What is an interest checklist, and why is it important in program planning?

O N   Y O U R   O W N

1. Compare and contrast the medical service delivery model and the wellness service delivery model in your setting, and give specific reasons for supporting one model over the other.
2. What five creative methods can you use to keep your staff and volunteers informed about changes in risk awareness?
3. If your setting includes multiple age groups (such as pediatric and geriatric), different levels, and varied staffing patterns, how would you begin an overall activity program plan for your facility?

R E F E R E N C E S

Austin, D.R. (1982). *Therapeutic recreation processes and techniques.* New York, NY: John Wiley & Sons.

Ball, E. (1970). The meaning of therapeutic recreation. *Therapeutic Recreation Journal,* 14(1), 17–18.

Edginton, C. R., Compton, D. M., & Hanson, C. J. (1980). *Recreation and leisure programming: A guide for the professional.* Philadelphia, PA: Saunders College Publishing.

Farrell, P., & Lundegren, H. (1991). *The process of recreation programming: Theory and technique,* 3rd edition. State College, PA: Venture Publishing.

Frye, V., & Peters, M. (1972). *Therapeutic recreation: Its theory, philosophy and practice.* Harrisburg, PA: Stackpole Books.

Godbey, G., & Parker, S. (1976). *Leisure studies and services: An overview.* Philadelphia, PA: W.B. Saunders Co.

Goodman, M. (1983). "I came here to die:" A look at the function of therapeutic recreation in nursing homes. *Therapeutic Recreation Journal,* Third Quarter, 14–19.

Halberg, K. J. (1985). The leisure service professional. In G. G. Maguire (Ed.) *Care of the elderly: A health-team approach.* (p.185–193) Boston, MA: Little, Brown & Co.

Hisek, D. D. (1978). Recreation planning for a nursing home. *Therapeutic Recreation Journal,* Second Quarter, 26–29.

Howe-Murphy, R. (1979). A conceptual basis for mainstreaming recreation and leisure service: Focus on humanism. *Therapeutic Recreation Journal,* Fourth Quarter, 11–18.

Incani, A. G., Seward, B. L., & Sigler, J. E. (1975). *Coordinated activity programs for the aged: A how-to-do-it manual.* Chicago, IL: American Hospital Publishing Inc.

Kelly, G. R., McNally, E., & Chambliss, L. (1983). Therapeutic recreation for long-term care patients, *Therapeutic Recreation Journal,* First Quarter, 33–41.

Kraus, R. G., Carpenter, G., & Bates, B. J. (1981). *Recreation leadership and supervision: Guidelines for professional development.* Philadelphia, PA: Saunders College Publishing.

Lucas, C. (1962). *Recreational activity development for the aging in homes, hospitals and nursing homes.* Springfield, IL: Charles C. Thomas, Publisher.

MacNeil, R., & Teague, M. (1982). *Perspectives on leisure and aging in a changing society.* Columbia, MO: University of Missouri.

MacNeil, R. D., & Teague, M.L. (1983). Bingo and beyond: A rationale for recreation services within nursing homes. *Activities, Adaptation and Aging,* Vol. 3 (3), 39–45.

Maslow, A. H. (1968). *Toward a psychology of being.* 2nd edition. New York, NY: Van Nostrand Reinhold.

McDowell, C. F. (1986). Wellness and therapeutic recreation: Challenges for service. *Therapeutic Recreation Journal,* Second Quarter, 27–38.

Mobily, K. E. (1985). A philosophical analysis of therapeutic recreation: What does it mean to say "we can be therapeutic"? Part I. *Therapeutic Recreation Journal,* First Quarter, 14–26.

Mobily, K. E. (1985). A philosophical analysis of therapeutic recreation: What does it mean to say "we can be therapeutic"? Part II. *Therapeutic Recreation Journal,* Second Quarter, 7–14.

Mobily, K. E., Weissinger, E., & Hunnicutt, B. K. (1987). The means/ends controversy: A framework for understanding the value of potential of TR. *Therapeutic Recreation Journal,* Third Quarter, 7–13.

O'Morrow, G. S., & Reynolds, D. R .P. (1989). *Therapeutic recreation: A helping profession,* Third edition. Englewood Cliffs, NJ: Prentice-Hall.

Peckham, C. W., & Peckham, A. B. (1982). *Activities keep me going.* Lebanon, OH: Otterbein Home.

Peterson, C. A., & Gunn, S. L. (1984). *Therapeutic recreation program design.* Englewood Cliffs, NJ: Prentice-Hall Inc.

Reichenfeld, H. F., Csapo, K. G., Carriere, L., & Gardner, R. C. (1973). Evaluating the effect of activity programs on a geriatric ward. *The Gerontologist,* 305–310.

Shivers, J. S., & Fait, H. F. (1985). *Special recreational services: Therapeutic and adapted.* Philadelphia, PA: Lea & Febiger.

Singleton, J. F., Makrides, L., & Kennedy, M. (1986). Role of three professions in long-term care facilities. *Activities, Adaptation and Aging,* Vol. 9 (1), 57–69.

Stein, T. A., & Sessoms, H. D. (1977). *Recreation and special populations,* 2nd edition, Boston, MA: Holbrook Press Inc.

U.S. Senate Special Committee on Aging (1984). *Aging America: Trends and projections* (In conjunction with the American Association of Retired Persons, 2nd printing) Washington, DC: Author.

Verhoven, P. J. (1977). Recreation and the aging. In T. A. Stein & H. D. Sessoms (Eds). *Recreation and special populations,* 2nd edition (387–422), Boston, MA: Holbrook Press Inc.

West, R. E. (1979). Therapeutic recreation services as a component of optimal health care in a general hospital setting. *Therapeutic Recreation Journal,* 13, No. 3, 3–5.

F U R T H E R R E A D I N G

Bachner, J. P., & Cornelius, E. (1978). *Activities coordinator's guide: A handbook for activities coordinator in long-term care facilities.* (HCFA-HSQB, 78–004) Washington, DC: US Government & Printing Office.

Blair, C. E. (1994). Residents who make decisions reveal healthier, happier attitudes. *The Journal of Long-Term Care Administration,* Winter 1994–95, 37–39.

Burrows, B. A., Jason, L. A., Quattrochi-Tubin, S., & Lavelli, M. (1981). Increasing activity of nursing home residents in their lounges using a physical design intervention and a prompting intervention. *Activities, Adaptation & Aging,* Vol. 1(4), 25–33.

Caplow-Linder, E., Harpaz, L., & Samberg, S. (1979). *Therapeutic dance movement.* New York, NY: Human Service.

Crepeau, E. (1986). *Activity programming for the elderly.* New York, NY: Little Medical Division/Little Brown & Co.

Cunninghis, R. N. (1986). *The activity programming handbook.* Holmes Beach, FL: Geriatric Educational Consultants.

Curley, J. S. (1983). Letting the inmates run the asylum: Another point of view. *Activities, Adaptation & Aging,* Vol. 3(3), 13–15.

DeCarlo, T. J. (1974). Recreation participation patterns and successful aging. *Journal of Gerontology,* Vol. 29, No.4, 416–422.

Deichmann, E. S., & O'Kane, C. (1985). The activity program: Its purpose and relationship to daily life. In E. S. Deichman & M. V. Kirchhofer (Eds.) *Working with the elderly* (p. 1–4), Buffalo, NY: Potentials Development.

Dixon, J. (1978). Expanding individual control in leisure participation while enlarging the concept of normalcy. *Therapeutic Recreation Journal,* Third Quarter, 20–24.

Foster, P. M. (1980). A multi-dimensional activities program. Activities, adaptation & aging, Vol. 1(2), 35–39.

Gillespie, K., McLellan, R. W., & McGuire, F. M. (1984). The effect of refreshments on attendance at recreation activities for nursing home residents. *Therapeutic Recreation Journal,* Third Quarter, 25–29.

Greenblatt, F. S. (1985). *Drama with the elderly.* Springfield, IL: Charles C. Thomas Publishing.

Gould, E., & Gould, L. (1978). *Arts and crafts for physically and mentally disabled.* Springfield, IL: Charles C. Thomas.

Gubrium, J. F. (1975). *Living and dying at murray manor,* New York, NY: St. Martin's Press.

Halberg, K. J., & Howe-Murphy, R. (1985). The dilemma of an unresolved philosophy in therapeutic recreation. *Therapeutic Recreation Journal,* Third Quarter, 7–16.

Harrington, C. (1992). Quality of nursing home care. In M. Johnson (Ed.) *Series on nursing administration,* (Vol. 3. p. 132–149), St. Louis, MI: Mosby Yearbook.

Hastings, L. (1981). *Complete handbook of activities and recreational programs for nursing homes.* Englewood Cliffs, NJ: Prentice Hall Inc.

Hemingway, J. L. (1986). The therapeutic in recreation. An alternative perspective. *Therapeutic Recreation Journal,* Third Quarter, 59–67.

Hoppa, M. E., & Roberts, G. D. (1974). Implications of the activity factor. *The Gerontologist,* Vol. 14(4), 331–335.

Iso-Ahola, S. E. (1980). Percieved control and responsibility as mediators of the effects of therapeutic recreation on the institutionalized aged. *Therapeutic Recreation Journal,* Third Quarter, 36–43.

Keller, M. J. (1983). Selecting activities for older adults. *Activities, Adaptation and Aging,* Vol. 4(1), 11–18.

Kennedy, D., Smith, R., & Austin, P. (1991). *Special recreation: Opportunities for persons with disabilities,* 2nd edition. Dubuque, IA: William C. Brown Publishers.

Langer, E. J., & Rodin, J. (1976). The effects of choice and enhanced personal responsibility for the aged. A field experiment in an institutional setting. *Journal of Personality and Social Psychology,* Vol. 34., No. 2, 191–198.

Leary, S. (1994). *Activities for personal growth.* Sydney, Australia: MacLennan & Petty Pty Limited.

Lemmon, D. K., & Pieper, H. G. (1980). Leisure pursuits and their meaning for the institutionalized elderly population. *Journal of Gerontological Nursing,* Vol. 6(2), 74–77.

Lewthwaite, N. (1992). *Mental aerobics.* Cornish, NH: J & J Enterprises.

McCormack, D. & Whitehead, A. (1981). The effect of providing recreational activities on the engagement level of long-stay geriatric patient. *Age and Ageing*, 10, 287–291.

McGuire, F. A. (1985). Recreation leader and co-participant preferences of the institutionalized aged. *Therapeutic Recreation Journal*, Second Quarter, 47–54.

Miller, D. B. (1979). Case studies to challenge the nursing home activity coordinator. *Therapeutic Recreation Journal*, Third Quarter, 22–32.

National Association of Activity Professionals (1990). *Program standards and the role of the activity professional*. [Brochure]. Washington, DC.

Parker, R. A. (1981). Recreational therapy, A model for consideration. *Therapeutic Recreation Journal*, Third Quarter, 22–29.

Parker, S. D., Will, C., & Burke, C. L. (1989). *Activities for the elderly: A guide to quality programming*. Owing Mills, MD: National Health Publishing.

Perschbacher, R. (1989). *Stepping forward with activities*. Asheville, NC: Bristlecone Consulting Co.

Quilitch, H. R. (1974). Purposeful activity increased on a geriatric ward through programmed recreation. *Journal of the American Geriatrics Society*, Vol. 12, No. 5, 226–229.

Rabinovich, B. A., & Cohen-Mansfield, J. (1992). The impact of participation in structured recreational activities on the agitated behavior of nursing home residents: An observational study. *Activities, Adaptation and Aging*, Vol. 16 (4), 89–98.

Robertson, R. D. (1988). Recreation and the institutionalized elderly: Conceptualization of the free choice and intervention continuums. *Activities, Adaptation and Aging*, Vol. 11(1), 61–73.

Rodin, J., & Langer, E.J . (1977). Long-term effects of a control-relevant intervention with the institutionalized aged. *Journal of Personality and Social Psychology*, Vol. 35, No. 12, 897–902.

Sessoms, D. H., Meyer, H. D., & Brightbill, C. K. (1975). *Leisure services: The organized recreation and park system*. Englewood Cliffs, NJ: Prentice Hall Inc.

Shivers, J. (1993). *Introduction to recreational services*. Springfield, IL: Charles C. Thomas Publishing.

Spector, W. D., & Takada, H. A. (1991). Characteristics of nursing homes that affect resident outcome. *Journal of Aging and Health*, 3(4), 427–454.

Szymanski, D. J. (1980). An index for determining trends in selected leisure journals and publications. *Therapeutic Recreation Journal*, Third Quarter, 42–49.

Sullivan, J. V. (1984). *Fitness for the handicapped*. Springfield, IL: Charles C. Thomas.

Teaff, J. D. (1985). *Leisure services with the elderly*. St. Louis, MI: Times Mirror/Mosby College Publishing.

Voelk, J. E., Fried, B. E., & Galecki, A. T. (1995). Predictors of nursing home residents' participation in activity programs. *The Gerontologist*, Vol 35(1), 44–51.

Wallach, F. (1993). Trends that affect quality of life: Recreation as a tool for enhancement. In M. Lahey, R. Kunstler, A. Grossman, F. Daly, S. Waldman, and F. Schwartz (Eds.) *Recreation, leisure and chronic illness: Therapeutic rehabilitation as intervention in health care*. (p. 1–5). Binghamton, NY: Haworth Press.

Wechsler-Linden, D. (1994). Here, they don't have to compete. *Forbes*, January 102–103.

Weiss, J. C. (1984). *Expressive therapy with elders and the disabled: Touching the heart of life*. Binghamton, NY: Haworth Press.

Williams, J., & Downs, J. C. (1984). *Educational activity programs for older adults*. Binghamton, NY: Haworth Press.

Witt, P., & Groom, R. (1979). Dangers and problems associated with current approaches to developing leisure interest finders. *Therapeutic Recreation Journal*, 1st Quarter, 19–31

CHAPTER 9
Program Implementation

OBJECTIVES..

After completing this chapter, you should:

- establish an understanding of the activity classifications accepted in the federal regulations, as well as other organizations
- develop activity planning by looking at the methods of scheduling programs
- view the medical aspects of programming

INTRODUCTION

Continuing the building blocks of program design occurs in this chapter on program implementation. During the development phase of programming in the last chapter, the foundational reasons for programming were discussed. With that information in mind, the process of reviewing, categorizing, and selecting appropriate activity programs for your residents becomes the focus. Activities based on program type, resident interests, and seasonal ideas are many of the areas to pursue before a final program design can be determined.

Activity Classifications by Needs ....

There are a few ways to classify activities that simplify the major task of reducing multiple resident interests and needs into one comprehensive program. The first method of classifying activity programs by need comes from federal guidelines, followed by the Medicaid or Medicare programs. The only exception to this are states that have regulations more stringent than federal guidelines. A third method of categorizing activities based on need comes from a national organization.

Federal Regulations

The specified requirements for activity programming are mentioned in the Federal Register (1991) as part of the Quality of Life requirement,

#483.15, under the heading (f) Activities, that states: "(1) The facility must provide for an ongoing program of activities designed to meet, in accordance with the comprehensive assessment, the interests and the physical, mental, and psychosocial well-being of each resident." Under the "guidance to surveyors for long-term care facilities," developed by the Health Care Financing Administration (HCFA) and published by American Health Care Association (1995), the surveyors are told that, in order to interpret requirement 483.15, they should see a program that is "multifaceted and reflect each individual resident's needs." Additionally, surveyors are asked to ensure that the program ". . . provide stimulation or solace; promote physical, cognitive and/or emotional health; enhance to the extent practicable each resident's physical and mental status; and promote each resident's self-respect by providing, for example, activities that allow for self-expression, personal responsibility and choice."

From this regulation and interpretative surveyor guideline, many activity professionals derive breakdowns of activity classifications to ensure that their program is "multi-faceted," and echoes the resident's needs. Some of the category names that represent resident need include physical, cognitive or educational, social, spiritual, affective and integration, and awareness. You may have created other names for these basic classifications, but these are some that are most usually associated with planning.

Physical needs are desires for exercise, movement, and general stimulation of the body parts. Examples of activity programming that meet physical needs include dance therapy, exercise programs, fitness trails, and swimming.

Cognitive and educational needs are requirements for stimulation of the mind and mental growth through learning. These needs are met through activity programming, such as word games, formal classroom learning, trivia, and current events.

Social needs are defined as the longing to be part of a group or have companionship with others. Activity programming that addresses social needs includes parties, room visits, and any group programs such as cooking, crafts, and so forth.

Affective needs involve the yearning for emotional outlets or expressions of feelings. Activity programming to meet affective needs involve art therapy, sensory stimulation, reminiscence, and entertainment.

Integration needs or **awareness needs** are concerned with observing or learning something that results in your resident's increased self-esteem or self-acceptance. Programming to meet integration needs includes life review, phototherapy, poetry therapy, and resident's council.

Spiritual needs are described as the desire for fulfillment in religious or other values that affect a person's disposition or outlook. Spiritual needs can be met through activity programming similar to reading, formal attendance at religious gatherings or services, and quiet contemplation of nature.

Although many of the other needs were discussed in the chapter on aging, religion as a part of understanding spirituality needs must be covered here in more detail. Religion, which McGuire (1985) defines as ". . . the central value or philosophy of life that guides the behavior of an individual. . ." is viewed broadly as in the definition, or narrowly as the activity of worship or other church/synagogue activities.

In his review of religion in old age, Moberg (1965) found that many studies indicated that the elderly were more likely to be members of a religious body than any other voluntary or community association. He also discovered that participants with conservative religious beliefs had an increased feeling of serenity, and were less fearful of death. Religious attendance may decline because of physical problems, but religious beliefs and feelings increase with age. Lemmon and Pieper (1980) report that religion was ranked as the most important activity to the institutionalized members of their study. In research concerning the perceptions of religion and its relationship to health, Bearon and Koenig (1990) reported that religious beliefs among older adults are related to their feelings about health and medical symptoms. Many of the study participants felt that their medical status could be related to the deity they worshiped. Koenig, Kvale, and Ferrel (1988) discovered that life satisfaction was impacted positively by active religious participation of individuals over age seventy-five.

The benefits of religious participation and practice are well documented. Steinitz (1981) suggests that participation in religious activity positions a church or house of worship as a "surrogate family." Maintaining that family relationship in later years remains important. General benefits of spirituality and religious practice include good personal adjustments to life, according to Moberg (1965). Sullivan (1993) suggests that for the mentally challenged, religion can act as a "buffer" from negative events, such as loss. It is also purported to function as a means of social support, and to give meaning and guidance to life. Use of religion as a coping mechanism for stressful situations is also a noted trend in almost half of a resident sample, reported by Koenig, George, and Siegler (1988).

In viewing religion and the potential value in programming, consider that religion and leisure have some similar characteristics, as proposed by Godbey and Parker (1976). First, both religion and leisure have goals of "personal well-being and self-realization." They are situations that afford chances to use choice and decision-making, and can add a sense of control to one's life.

National Association of Activity Professionals (NAAP) Categories

The NAAP (1990) refined the idea of activity classifications by providing the following three categories in their organizational standards of practice: supportive activities, maintenance activities, and empowerment activities.

Supportive activities are defined as those which ". . . promote a comfortable environment while providing stimulation or solace to clients/residents who cannot benefit from maintenance or empowerment activities." These programs are geared to residents with mentally and physically limiting conditions who have a low tolerance for formal group situations. Programming examples in this category include sensory stimulation, use of mobiles, or exposure to the sounds of nature.

Maintenance activities are designed to ". . . provide a resident with a schedule of events that promotes the maintenance of physical, cognitive, social, spiritual and emotional health." Multiple ability levels are reached in this category by activities such as dance and movement programs, group discussion, social gatherings, religious services, and pet therapy.

The last category, **empowerment activities**, advocates ". . . self-respect by providing opportunities for self-expression, choice, and social and personal responsibility." Residents in this classification find purposeful gains through programs such as the arts, horticultural therapy, life skills, and resident advocacy.

Activities Based on Resident Interests

Having activity classifications as parameters adds balance to the task of program planning. The focus is the selection of specific programs governed by the past and current interests of the resident. Using the activity assessment to produce an inventory checklist and risk awareness profile for your entire resident population guides your directions for programming. With your work completed on the inventory checklist, the risk awareness profile, and totals done, look at this information for programming guidance. You should be asking yourself the following questions: 1. Where do my residents' interests lie? 2. What generalities can I draw from this information? 3. What precautionary measures do I have to take in planning programs to address potential risks?

Medical Aspects of Programming..

Although your resident population varies in their reasons for needing the skilled care of a long-term care facility, some of the common medical conditions you encounter will be important to understand because of their impact on program planning. Miller (1979) offered that some of the greatest challenges an activity professional faces in programming is to be cognizant of the changes that occur with age, especially those of sensory or perceptual functions. As discussed earlier in Chapter 3, one of the most frequently seen medical conditions, according to the 1985 National Nursing Home Survey, is disorders of the nervous system, such as Alzheimer's disease, which we will review from a program planning viewpoint.

Dementia Related Disorders

Dementia is one of the commonly seen medical conditions in a long-term care facility, and because of its prevalence, it requires special programming adaptations. The definition of dementia, given by the National Institutes of Health Consensus Department (1987), is ". . . a clinical state with many different causes, characterized by a decline from a previously attained intellectual level."

The cause of dementia is a type of brain dysfunction with thought, perception, or other processes disrupted. Although the onset of dementia is a slow process, it usually begins with small problems in normal living, such as forgetfulness, restlessness, or repeated actions. As the disease progresses, an individual may not recognize family, can get lost in familiar areas, and exhibits other disruptive or unsocial behaviors. Impairments also occur in sensory, motor, and perception skills to a varying degree. At the time of death, which may be many years after onset of the disease, the only way to confirm many of the key dementing diseases is by means of an autopsy.

There are two main types of dementia: reversible and irreversible. **Reversible dementias** may be improved over time, because they are a result of a condition or disease. Some examples of causes of reversible dementia include infections, intoxication, disorders of the metabolism, depression, reactions to medications, nutritional disorders, and heart or lung problems that deprive the brain of oxygen. **Irreversible dementias** are characterized by a progressive pathological disease in which no secondary cause is identified. The best known of the irreversible dementias are **Alzheimer's disease** and **multi-infarct dementia**.

Alzheimer's disease, identified in 1906 by Dr. Alois Alzheimer, is reported by Alzheimer's Disease Education & Referral Center (1994) to be the most common form of dementia. Thought, language, and memory are effected in the specific parts of the brain by abnormal deposits and bundles of twisted plaque material. Other nerve cells and chemicals required for complex message transmission appear to be damaged during the disease process. The disease is thought to begin after age sixty-five. Increased age appears to have a direct bearing on the chances of developing Alzheimer's. By age eighty-five, over half of all persons have the potential to develop the disease. Treatment options are limited because the disease has no cure, but treatment interventions include making individuals comfortable, containing symptoms, and modifying behaviors.

Multi-infarct dementia, the second most common form of irreversible dementia, is found by the Alzheimer's Disease Education & Referral Center (1994), to afflict individuals between the ages of sixty and seventy-five. Men develop the disease more than women. The dementia is thought to be caused by a group of strokes that cause brain tissue to be destroyed. Some of the initial causes of the strokes that may, in turn, cause the multi-infarct dementia, are diabetes, heart disease, and high blood pressure. The symptoms of the disease are similar to those of Alzheimer's disease, but also include a rapid, shuffling walk, incontinence, and inappropriate laughing or crying. No cure is available as yet but the ADEAR center suggests that caregivers, ". . . encourage patients to keep up their daily routines and regular social and physical activities."

Understanding how a diagnosis is made and how the different stages in each disease progress is important in program planning. The diagnosis of a dementia disease is an involved process that requires participation by both patients and caregivers. An example of the type of diagnostic process involved is demonstrated by the research of Coyne, Meade, Petrone, Meinert, and Joslin (1990). In order to make an accurate diagnosis among the many types of dementing diseases, they look at the following components:

- patient medical history and lifestyle factors
- full physical examination
- blood profile
- urinalysis
- EEG (electroencephalogram)
- EKG (electrocardiogram)
- an assessment of social issues
- participation in activities of daily living
- an MRI (magnetic resonance imaging) test
- cognitive test results.

Testing to determine the level of cognitive functioning is part of the diagnostic process conducted by the medical team. Ramsdell, Rothrock, Ward, and Volk (1990) list the steps involved in determining a diagnosis, and a management plan:

- recognition of the cognitive impairment
- selecting a diagnostic category for the patient's impairment
- determining a management approach
- setting up a follow-up

One of the most commonly used tests to determine mental status quickly during a complete physical is the **Mini-Mental State Examination**, devised by Folstein, Folstein, and McHugh (1975). This test is administered by a clinician, and eleven questions concerning the year, season, day, month, date, state, country, and town are asked. Other cognitive skills are tested, such as backwards counting by sevens, recall of information, language abilities, following instructions, and sentence construction. Points are awarded

and scores are tallied. The total available points are 30; a score of 20–24 indicates mild impairment, a score of 16–19 shows moderate impairment. Those with scores of 15 or less show a severe cognitive impairment. The test has the advantage of being easy and quick to administer, and can be used in subsequent visits for notes on progress of dementia. The drawback is the variation in experience and education levels of participants that can impact the results.

Another method of ranking cognitive impairments is through the use of the **Global Deterioration Scale**, developed by Reisberg, Ferris, DeLeon, and Crook (1982). Using "clinical characteristics," such as the amount of memory loss or confusion detected, and some test scores, patients are ranked into seven stages. The stages with corresponding descriptions are:

- *Stage 1 (no cognitive decline):* no memory complaints and no evidence of problems during the examination.
- *Stage 2 (very mild cognitive decline):* forgetfulness of names and familiar objects.
- *Stage 3 (mild cognitive decline):* performance declines, concentration problems, some denial, loss of items, or loss of direction.
- *Stage 4 (moderate cognitive decline):* memory deficits in task completion and events. Time and person orientation may still be present, but the ability to travel or function alone may be difficult. Denial of condition is strong.
- *Stage 5 (moderately severe cognitive decline):* early dementia when patients need assistance to manage. Disorientation to time, place, and person is present, but information about personal facts may be intact. Clothing choices may be a problem, but toileting and eating are usually done independently.
- *Stage 6 (severe cognitive decline):* the middle stage of dementia evidenced by a lack of ability to remember key people or recent events. Dependence on caregivers is acute and most activities of daily living require assistance. Emotional upheavals and personality changes are noted in this category.
- *Stage 7 (very severe cognitive decline):* loss of verbal and speech abilities. Incontinence is present, and there is a need for feeding. Brain connections needed for skills such as walking may no longer be present.

The advantages of the Global Deterioration Scale is that cultural and educational differences are taken into account during the test. The disadvantage are that the testing takes longer, and requires much more information than the Mini-Mental State Examination.

Other cognitive scales exist for categorizing the impairment levels of individuals, such as the **Rancho Los Amigos Scale of Cognitive Functioning** described by Hagen, Malkmus, and Durham (1985). This scale lists rankings from level 1, labeled as "no response" and characterized by an unresponsive state given to stimuli, to level 8, in which the individual is thought to be "purposeful and appropriate," and is independent in skills. Hartmaier, Sloane, Guess, and Koch (1994) suggest using the cognition data collected on the Minimum Data Set as a simple way to rank residents appropriately according to cognitive function. One of the negative factors associated with use of the MDS data is the fact that in order to be useful, the cognitive data has to be collected uniformly and according to accepted practices.

The reason these tests are important in activity programming is because of the framework they provide for properly staging residents into programs. Before the existence of testing and ranking, determining adequate programming for the many categories of dementia among residents was a difficult task. The tests and rating scales are only tools to use in planning; they do not substitute for activity assessments and observations. A physician may have ranked a person in one category, but through your experience and observation with the resident, you may have seen some different behavior. When faced with a large number of residents with varying degrees of cognitive impairment, having a means of beginning to manage the program offerings is important.

What kind of activity programming is appropriate for this large portion of the resident population? For those residents with reversible dementia, traditional programs based on individual interests, coupled with reality orientation may be appropriate. For residents with irreversible dementia, other programming options are necessary. In research on environmental modifications for the cognitively impaired, Namazi, Whitehouse, Rechlin, Calkins, Johnson, Brabender, and Hevener (1991) commented that individuals develop "patterns of activity" during their lives that may have no outlet in the institutional environment. They propose that boredom would be decreased and behaviors such as wandering reduced if activity development centered on the reinstatement of familiar tasks. Sabat (1994) adds "it is clear that aspects of social and personal life can still flourish to some degree despite losses in a variety of individual cognitive functions." Life-long activities and interests should be integrated into programming for maximum benefits to this population.

Beginning activity research on programming for the cognitively impaired has been documented independently by Zgola, Sheridan, Lucero, Jones, Hommel, and Bowlby. Zgola (1987) suggests that a functional evaluation be conducted on each resident with questions such as: What can the client do? How does he do it? Which parts of the task is he unable to do? and When or where does he perform the best? Once that information has been determined, Zgola proposes "programming to the client's strengths" in the areas of habitual skills, primary motor function, primary sensory function, emotions, remote memory, and preservation. Habitual skills are defined as those abilities that have been done so frequently that given cues, a response is almost automatic. An example is seeing a dust pan and broom, and knowing that sweeping the floor is required. Primary motor and sensory function relate to skills in organization, dexterity, and use of senses. Expression of feelings and tapping into long-term memories are also important. Turning repetitive activities into a comfortable and familiar situation can also be a positive in programming.

Lucero (1994) suggests that during the assessment phase of program planning for your residents, tallies should be completed for all residents in each of the Global Deterioration Scale categories. Armed with that information, programs can be designed with the specific needs of each group in mind. Lucero talks about capitalizing on "universal strengths" and adds the sense of rhythm and sense of humor to Zgola's list of skills. In planning for individual and group programs, Lucero suggested developing kits or items to use for interactions. Some of the categories she suggests for kits include familiar female tasks, specific occupations, familiar male tasks, specific life periods, specific hobbies, and specific geographic locations. An example of a kit item for a familiar female task might be sewing supplies, whereas an example of a specific life period object might be a wedding album. For reaching the needs of residents in the higher ranges (i.e., Stage 7) of the Global Deterioration Scale, Lucero discusses interventions of providing materials that residents can explore, trace, or fiddle with, and other examples of manipulative but safe tasks.

In her work, Bowlby (1993) advocates the theory that ". . . the most meaningful and successful activities are those that enable the continuation of lifelong roles." She feels that the activities most beneficial are those that are adult in nature, contain overlearned tasks, emphasize gross motor skills, and present a chance for active participation and immediate feedback. Bowlby postulates that because the institutional environment is often lacking familiar cues that trigger behaviors, individual involvement in activities of daily living should be the primary focus of activities. She suggests using a daily routine and familiar tasks that conform to the personal habits and past memory of the participants. Activity programs set up with this purpose in mind have the benefits of using familiar tasks that have a high probability of success, increase self-esteem, and give the opportunity for individual routines and interactions. Another advantage is the team approach required to plan and deliver activity programs. In this model, all departments are involved in planning the daily routine and schedule to maximize resident goals and ultimate success. Some of the many tips that Bowlby gives for setting up activities of daily living for the cognitively impaired residents include reducing tasks to smaller steps, starting programs at a point where a resident can achieve a successful experience, using familiar cues, decreasing distractions, and integrating personal routines whenever possible. Almost all programs are adaptable, but Bowlby mentions the use of handicrafts, horticultural therapy, food programs, intergenerational events, movement, music, pets, spiritual, and the creative arts as possible sources for programming.

Jones (1996) proposes the concept of Gentlecare®, ". . . based on the premise of accurately defining the deficit the person is experiencing, and organizing the macro-environment (people, programs, and physical space) into a prosthesis to compensate for the deficits in functioning, to support existing or residual function and to maximize the quality of life." Developed as a twenty-four hour model of dementia care, Gentlecare suggests that programs be driven by "client initiatives and rhythms" and be set up to avoid "null behavior," which Jones defines as the absence of stimulation or activity. Instead, Jones suggests preparing an individualized program schedule that has a mix of "core" activities (i.e., eating and toileting), "necessary" activities (i.e., sleep and privacy), "essential" activities (i.e., touch and movement), and "meaningful" activities (i.e., work, play, and recreation). She suggests avoiding practices that she terms "parachuting in," where activity professionals or others come onto a specialized unit for a brief program or try to integrate dementia residents into ongoing, large activities. Her effective program guidelines include making activities physical, simple, repetitive, one-step, and related to past experience or roles. Jones also mentions positive programming tips such as being

prepared, reducing glare and noise, monitoring fatigue, and communicating clearly as vital to success in working with this population.

Hommel (1995) has developed a successful intervention program called "diversional activity zones" for working with cognitively impaired residents. Using a program model based on learning center concepts normally used in educational settings, Hommel field-tested a system for presenting a variety of activities and tasks to residents with cognitive deficits in a group setting. The diversional activity zones, categories of tasks or activities grouped by theme at small tables, are designed to meet the individual interest and functional levels of residents. After staff members identify life interests and functional abilities of the cognitively impaired residents in their population, materials or props are selected, and an area is established for the diversional zones. Residents are placed at appropriate tables with activity staff members acting as facilitators to motivate and respond to a resident's changing needs or interests. The learning center concepts such as independence, smaller groups within a larger group, and pacing of individual abilities are applied easily. Some examples of appropriate zones mentioned by Hommel include life skill tasks such as laundry, gardening, gift wrapping, business, or baby care, and sensory and/or manipulative tasks such as puzzles, tactile pillows, and pat mats. Examples of active stimulation zones are areas for pacing, velcro dart games or punching bags. Passive stimulation through the zone concept is exemplified by the use of bird feeders, visually stimulating books, and environmental areas. Hommel suggests documenting the tasks that the resident enjoys in the care plan, but also noting any unusual responses in the interdisciplinary episodic notes.

The primary benefit of the use of diversional activity zones is the increase in attention span and engagement in diversional tasks, according to Hommel. Traditional group programs, although still useful for certain events, had not previously allowed residents the chance to use their remaining skills in programs with successful results. Additional benefits of the zones include the reduction of negative behaviors and the increase in self-esteem.

Sheridan (1987) concurs with the other researchers by offering a breakdown of specific suitable programs for the cognitively impaired in the categories of music, exercise, food preparation, crafts, gardening, solo activities, family games, and reminiscence. Dowling (1995) offers programming ideas in similar categories with the addition of humor, art, television, and videotapes.

Presenting an environment that allows freedom and uninterrupted movement may help reduce some behaviors such as restlessness or pacing. Creating activity spaces like rummaging areas or homey, familiar spaces may make residents comfortable, and decrease the anxiety that leads to difficult behaviors. Other activity projects that work well with this population for both residents and staff are memory boxes and biography boards. Memory boxes, which many facilities are using with success, are containers that hold special items of significance for a particular resident. Used with an activity professional, going through the memory box acts as a reminiscence and memory-triggering activity, and has positive effects. The biography boards are a collage of information about a particular resident that is available in an album, a box, or a picture hung in or near the resident's room. The purpose is to give the staff and other visitors clues and cues for conversations with, and understanding of, the resident.

Other tips that may be helpful in working with this resident base include using simple phrases and specific questions, giving individual instructions, using touch and eye contact in a slow, deliberate way, monitoring body language and emotions for cues, using validation techniques, removing distractions, and remaining focused on the needs of the residents with whom you are working.

Timing with the cognitively impaired resident may be altered due to confusion, but all efforts should be made to conform to personal schedules. As discussed in earlier chapters, an appropriate time for an activity intervention may be at an odd hour of the day or night. Schedules must be tailored to specific residents' needs.

Should residents with dementia be housed in their own unit, when possible? Professionals and researchers are not in full agreement on this issue. Ohta and Ohta (1988) feel that not enough research supports the idea of segregated units for the cognitively impaired. They do mention that some of the factors that should be present in a special unit for the cognitively impaired include unique environmental design, wandering space, training for staff members, and special therapeutic features. Ohta and Ohta suggest that activities ". . . should be designed to exercise each patient's physical, cognitive and social skills." Other researchers, such as Zeisel, Hyde, and Levkoff (1994) offer that a unit designed for cognitively impaired residents should take into account the environmental influences on behavior (discussed in Chapter 6) and make adjustments. They suggest consideration of environmental factors such as exit control, wandering options, privacy, personalization, freedom in outdoor space, safety, and sensory features, such as noise control.

There are many other medical conditions that have impact on programming, but the high frequency of cognitively impaired residents in the long-term care setting makes it necessary to be aware of the special considerations and planning requirements. Figure 9–1 illustrates some examples of programs that can be selected based on group size, type of stimulation, and cognitive level.

SAMPLE ACTIVITIES BY GROUP TYPE AND COGNITIVE ABILITIES

Group Type	Minimal Cognitive Impairment	Minimal to Moderate Cognitive Impairment	Severe Cognitive Impairment
Individual-Mobile	Life Interests/Independent programs	Crafts, Manual Arts	Walking Path, Rummaging Areas
Individual-Bedbound	Reading, Games, Visiting	Pet Therapy	Sensory Stimulation
Small Group—Passive Stimulation	Religious Services	Life Skills Programs	Music Therapy
Small Group—Active Stimulation	Horticultural Therapy	Exercise	Tactile Stimulation
Large Group—Passive Stimulation	Lecture/Presentation	Movies/Videos	Musical Entertainment Program
Large Group—Active Stimulation	Dance/Movement Programs	Social Clubs	Sing-along

Figure 9–1 An example of activity choices based on group type, stimulation level, and cognitive abilities.

Activities Based on Seasonal and/or Community Ideas

Resident needs and interests are the driving force behind your programs, but another aspect of programming orientation has to do with seasonal adaptations and developing a sense of community.

In everyday life, you function with a twenty-four-hour day and a twelve-month calendar that reflects the seasonal changes through the year, variable depending on the area of the world you live in. Adding the dimensions of the changing seasons over the months expands the overall program significantly. Bringing the seasonal adaptations to programming in a mature way should be viewed as a positive step, because it adds an extra layer of reality to an already busy schedule.

In a larger sense, the long-term care facility is its own community and within that community, are special events and programs unique to that facility. Perhaps there is a health fair every year, or maybe twice a year there is a particular contest to which the whole facility looks forward. These are examples of differentiating factors that make your long-term care community unique. These elements should be incorporated into your programming plan to maintain and foster the sense of community that has already developed. Residents of all cognitive and ability levels can anticipate and participate in the community-based programming particular to your facility.

Therapeutic Rituals

There are many memories tied up in the ways that celebrations were handled in the past by all residents that it becomes important to maintain those ties to the past through the incorporation of various therapeutic rituals.

Gubrium (1975) uses the term "ceremonials" to describe the events that are considered planned and special around the facility; typically that which would be included on an activity calendar. Similarly, Johnson (1987) mentions therapeutic rituals to include special acknowledgement of significant events such as achievements or even death. All rituals, like important holidays, serve many purposes according to Johnson. Rituals are a method for expressing and coping with certain life experiences. Through rituals, group members bond, and maintain a relationship with one another as they see each other at repeated intervals. The rituals found in the nursing home environment brings a decrease in anxiety for residents by presenting familiar events in a new setting. Cultural variations within rituals are important to note so all residents are comforted in the manner in which they have been accustomed. Consider the proper placement of rituals in your program schedule as you plan.

Activities by Program Type

With many factors to ponder as you begin to formulate your activity schedule, the number of participants who will attend your program and in what format you will present your program become as important as what you offer. There are a few program types that you should be familiar with:

- group programs
- individual activities
- bedside programs
- special events
- trips

Hastings (1981) actually suggests that too much emphasis has been placed on programs at both extremes (large groups or individual programs) in terms of number of participants, whereas the socialization benefits of small group programs has been overlooked.

In each program category, **active stimulation** or **passive stimulation** can exist. Active stimulation refers to an activity established to promote a reaction or some participation from the resident. An example of an activity with active stimulation goals is a music therapy program that uses rhythm band instruments. Passive stimulation makes reference to activity programs that require little in the way of participation from attendees. Listening to an entertainer is an example of a passive stimulation activity. In each program type, the active and passive stimulation examples are given to demonstrate how many different factors should be considered as you plan programs.

Groups

Groups are a common setting for many of your programs. In addition to the benefits of group dynamics (discussed in Chapter 11), socialization and the ability to reach many residents at the same time are some of the key benefits. Bachner & Cornelius (1978) list three categories of group activities: independent group activities, interdependent group activities, and independent/interdependent group programs. Independent programs are those in which each member works as a group, but on individual projects. Interdependent groups require each member to carry out a specific part of the whole task. In independent/ interdependent groups, members work independently for a common goal.

Size is a factor in group planning and structuring. A group can be as small as two participants or as large as your entire resident population. You have the advantage of more control with smaller groups, but participation may be less because the situation is not stimulating enough. In a large group, too many people can become a problem if some group members are impaired or the noise level or group purpose is actually a hindrance. Small groups may be appropriate for programs such as reminiscence or discussion, whereas larger groups are useful for special events, entertainment, or parties.

The similar needs and goals of group participants is important to think about when planning. Mismatching group members for certain programs or within programs can spell disaster. For example, a life skills program can be stimulating and enjoyable to members when seating at tables is based on interests, compatibility, and cognitive functioning. However, group programs that require a situation where one large table and members partaking in a shared project around it, should probably be restricted to a compatible group of residents with similar skills and needs. Hosting more than one version of horticulture therapy for different ability levels at different times, or planning two different groups to meet simultaneously but in opposite ends of the same room, is your job to determine as the group leader. Some people will say "everyone should be welcome at all activity programs." That may be true, but consideration for the experience of all members of a group should be the driving force as you plan your program.

Your ability as a leader to prepare and manage a group properly is another function of the process of using groups as an activity setting. Prepare for your group by bringing the necessary materials and supplies to avoid abrupt departures to find equipment or locate items. Transportation of residents to group programs should be within a window of time so that the program begins on time, group members are not straggling in, and you do not have to leave to gather missing residents.

Group programs fall into either the active or passive stimulation category. Active stimulation group programs include a cooking class, a sing-along, drama therapy, or bowling. Passive stimulation group programs include videos, poetry reading, and religious services.

Individual Programs

Individual programs should be encouraged, and account for a large part of your responsibility.

There are two types of individual programs: self-directed resident programs and individual activity sessions that you have arranged for the resident. In self-directed programs, a resident makes decisions to participate in a diversional or hobby activity. For programs that you have suggested, or helped plan for a resident, you take supplies or materials to a resident's room. Or the resident may come to you for guidance. In either case, your role is one of facilitator to ensure the resident has what he or she needs, is moving forward with the activity, and is satisfied.

An example of an individual activity is reading, making reassurance phone calls to other elderly residents, or doing crossword puzzles. Passive stimulation programs include watching the weather change from the front porch, listening to the radio, or sitting in the sensory garden.

The demand of offering one-to-one programming is very challenging. DeBolt and Kastner (1989) describe it by saying "the one-to-one activity is the most intense, time-consuming, energy-consuming and free-wheeling type of activity we can devise." Respecting the wishes of residents who do not wish to participate in formal group activity situations is something you must do regularly. DeBolt and Kastner offer these tips in working on a one-to-one relationship: avoid rushing, do not act superior, share and use humor, be confidential and respectful, listen, and assist the resident in "remembering who he is." Your responsibility is to assess and document needs and provide residents with the materials they require to have a positive activity experience in whatever setting they choose.

Bedside Programs

One of the special categories in individual programming is the provision of adequate programs for residents at bedside. Bed-bound residents are those who are unable (and in some cases unwilling) to participate in most programs offered in the facility.

Bedside programs are especially appropriate for severely cognitively impaired residents or those with limiting medical conditions. Stimulation, via sensory techniques, is often an option. In describing some of the residents you may encounter, DeBolt and Kastner mention that "so many people seem trapped inside their bodies and minds. It is the task of the activity director to help them get out." They suggest stimulating the residents through senses, emotions, and memories with *one-to-one* programs instead of *one-on-one* programs because of the relationship factor. DeBolt and Kastner offer that relationships are built on equal standards and one-to-one phrasing is more appropriate.

How should individual bedside programming be accomplished? After an assessment of needs and interests, the activity professional must determine an effective method for service delivery to the resident. Four factors must be assessed:

- room or area environment
- personal resident comfort
- program supplies
- timing

Can the environment in which you will be presenting a program to a resident be modified to accommodate your needs?

- Is there enough light, or too much light?
- Is the temperature acceptable?
- Are there any background noises that may interfere?

When considering the personal comfort of the resident, ask these questions:

- Is the resident positioned properly in the bed or chair?
- Are tubes, restraints, and pillows in place?
- Can the resident see, hear, and manipulate adequately from his or her position?

In terms of program supplies and equipment:

- Are the supplies easy to pack and unpack?
- Are they prepared so the program can begin promptly?
- Are there any hazardous items to be concerned about?
- Can the supplies be put away quickly if the program ends abruptly?

Concerning timing:

- Has the time for the session been selected around the schedule of the resident?
- Are there other conflicts?

Depending on resident needs, most programs can be adapted to the bedside. Forsythe (1988) suggests appropriate bedside programs as music, grooming, games, reading, pet therapy, seasonal activities, crafts, exercise, and social programs. All the above are examples of active stimulation in bedside programs except reading. Passive stimulation at the bedside includes entertainment or sensory stimulation programs. The sensory programs mentioned in detail by DeBolt and Kastner (1989) will assist you greatly as you plan your bedside programs.

Special Events

Special events are just that—special occasions marked by a significant program. These events can be tied into rituals or ceremonials, such as holidays, or they can be thought up by you and your staff to spark interest and participation. What you do for a special event depends on the facility and the interest level. Some facilities have special events for every possible major and minor holiday, whereas other homes have entertainment as their special event once in a while.

In trying to achieve a balance in programming, special events work well because they offer an opportunity for any and all residents who are physically able to attend to gain some benefit from the function. During a special event, you may have active stimulation occurring for some residents and passive stimulation happening for others. For a big band entertainment night, some residents may sit in chairs in the front row and sing along or clap in active stimulation. Other residents who may attend the function might be passively stimulated, content to sit quietly and enjoy the music.

There are many books on the market to give you ideas on special events planning. Strive for the balance that allows you at least a few special events programs each month.

Trips and Outdoor Programs

Using the outdoor areas around your facility and in the neighboring community is a resource tool that many activity professionals overlook. Your calendar should include trips for different groups to outside destinations as frequently as possible. Participating in trips gives residents a sense of anticipation, a change of scene, and a bond to the community. Transportation can be arranged by use of a facility van (if you are lucky enough), a community supplied van, or personal cars. Be sure

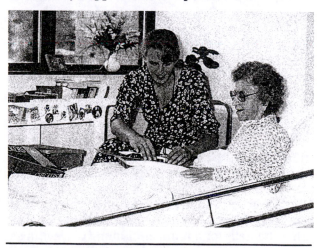

Figure 9–2 Residents who may be roombound or bed-bound by choice or condition should have specialized programs brought into them.

to check your facility's insurance policy with your administrator to ensure that all staff members and volunteers are adequately covered in case of an accident. Simple trips can be planned to the local mall, lunch, to see the changing seasons, a local spot of interest, or a particular event such as a play. Allow plenty of time for loading and unloading everyone at each end of the trip. Comfort stops for resting and toileting should be preplanned, and know where bathrooms are located all along the route in case of emergency. Medications must be handled by the nursing staff prior to the departure and any restrictions or contraindications, such as special diets, must be known ahead of time. Rotate the individuals that you take on trips to give everyone possible a chance to get out.

Using your own outdoor areas frequently should be another option of your programming. When talking with other administrators, some have expressed a desire to see more use of outdoor space in regular daily programming. Being outside in the fresh air is uplifting to almost everyone. Walking, for those who can ambulate, is a wonderful motivator when done outdoors. Gueldner and Spradley (1988) found that nursing home residents walk infrequently, and thirty-six percent of nursing home residents report that they never go outside. A surprising eighty-one percent of nursing home residents reported that they never walked outside. Their study also indicates that regular outdoor walking actually lowers fatigue and should be recommended for health as well as emotional benefits. When traffic or other safety reasons make setting up an outdoor walking program impractical, Gueldner and Spradley suggest using "borrowed space" such as skylights, plants, and greenhouse areas to substitute indoor walking for outdoor.

Many of your normal programs can be adapted to the outdoors with some advanced planning. Issues with exposure, wind, and sun should be considered as you tailor your programs. Other outdoor programs, such as fitness trails and sensory gardens, can also add much to your program. Fitness trails provide improvements in mobility, flexibility, increased cardiovascular abilities, and muscle strength. A fitness trail is an organized walkway with stops for exercise or other activities. A study by Gissal, Ray, and Smith (1980) showed that fitness trails improved health, provided more energy, and generally improved residents' activities overall after using the trails for a number of months. Devising a fitness trail can be accomplished with the collaboration of your nurses, physical therapists, occupational therapists, and other team members.

Horticultural techniques can be used to create a sensory garden that has horticultural benefits as well as sensory stimulation applications. Taking a space and turning it into a spot for visually viewing of the beauty of plants, enjoying the scents of flowers, and for spiritual reflection can be very uplifting. Even a small space can make a difference in programming options.

Putting Your Program into Action..

Gathering the base of knowledge about programming can be overwhelming, but your focus should remain on two very important points: *1. Program planning must be based on interests and needs*, and *2. The residents always come first*. With that said, we need to look at other ways to ensure that your programs are successful.

Master Calendar

The first order of business for you, now that your monthly, quarterly, and yes, even some of your annual events have been roughed out, is to make up a master calendar. Before we talk about how to use a master calendar, we must know how to put one together. A master calendar is your guide to the activities that you plan to offer for a particular time period, usually a month at a time.

To begin the process, take a blank calendar book, such as a blotter or desk calendar, or make your own, as shown in Figure 9–3. Armed with the list of programs you have decided to offer in response to your resident needs, you are ready to begin making your master calendar.

Types of Programs.   Although your residents are individuals, your program planning on the master calendar often reflects group activities. After carefully weighing the needs of your residents individually, you may have drawn some conclusions about groups that can be formed. For example, your interest inventories and other work sheets have told you that you need a daily workshop for the high number of cognitively impaired residents. You may also realize that a small component of more alert residents has requested an area for a morning discussion group. You need time allotted for room visits, entertainment, and other programs that have universal appeal. You also need to tie in key cultural, ethnic, and seasonal events. Some programs will be offered once a month, others once a day, or once a week. Consider all the kinds of activities by reviewing those discussed in the last three chapters. This should greatly assist you.

ACTIVITY DEPARTMENT MONTHLY CALENDAR					Month: _____ Year: _____	
Sunday	Monday	Tuesday	Wednesday	Thursday	Friday	Saturday

Figure 9–3   A blank calendar is one of the starting points for program planning.

Now you have a list of programs that will be included on your calendar, along with the names you will use to refer to them. A few words of caution about naming programs: use dignified names that have meaning to both residents and staff. Also, use of certain therapy terms to describe a program (i.e., "music therapy" for a sing-along program) is not acceptable unless it is hosted by a professional therapist.

Your experiences during the month may cause you to change many of the programs that you offer. Your calendar is deliberately a "work in progress," with each month having variations based on what has worked and what has not, new residents admitted with new needs, and so on.

Timing of Programs.   Before you put pencil to paper, make your master calendar planning easier by eliminating any time periods unsuitable for programs. For example, you should not schedule a make-your-own-sundae party at twelve noon when lunch is in session. Most facility meal times can be blocked out as unusable because most activity programs would be in conflict with the goals of good nutrition. The time it takes to transport residents to and from dining areas must also be considered. There are, however, many new concepts of using life skill adaptation at meal time that involve forming joint efforts among the nursing, activity, and dietary departments to offer a dining experience to some residents who can participate in the preparation, serving, and clean-up of meals (similar to life in their own homes). Your facility may have the capabilities that warrant a look into this type of programming.

Other time constraints that are a reality to your program calendar involve things such as scheduled physician rounds (often a good time for room visits because many residents are waiting there!), staff availability, and facility visits from the hairdresser or other professional services. Like it or not, you have to make programming allowances for them.

Traditional activity time scheduling of the past tells us that we should plan one or two morning activities starting between 9:30 and 10:00 a.m., then one or two (or more, depending on your facility's size and needs) afternoon programs starting at 2:00 or 2:30–3:30 p.m. and then an evening program, most days of the week, beginning at 6:30–7:00 p.m. This traditional time scheduling was the way we built our calendar in the past, but it is not necessarily the best format for today's residents when you consider that quality of life is not bound by a time schedule! You may find the best success if you abandon the traditional format and look to your residents and their needs to dictate the best schedule for your program.

It is important to remember that facilities are open "24/7" (twenty-four hours a day, seven days a week). When we think of taking advantage of leisure time activities, we sometimes think of specific times for some programs. For example, theaters usually do not schedule movies for 3:00 a.m. because it is a nontraditional time for viewing. But many facilities, especially those with special needs groups such as an Alzheimer's unit, may be looking at a whole new concept in traditional time scheduling. Residents are not always able to conform to clear time delineations because of medical reasons, and have needs at all hours. Some facilities are addressing this by stretching their calendars to accommodate them. Your residents may need a breakfast program at 7:30 a.m. or they may be in need of some form of intervention at 10:30 p.m. How do you respond to the increasing demands and changing needs of the residents you serve? Focus on what your residents tell you, your assessment and observations, and listen to what other staff members have observed and say. A change in program schedule, of course, requires a change in staff schedule. An activity professional who works 9:00 a.m. to 5:00 p.m. may serve your particular residents better by working 7:30 a.m. to 3:30 p.m., with another staff member filling in the evening hours. Some facilities with higher need clients are realizing that the traditional time scheduling must be abandoned, and programs do need to be held in different time periods, such as during the 11:00 p.m. to 7:00 a.m. shift.

Calendar Presentation.   Using the blank calendar you have made or purchased (many of the vendors sell calendars of all sizes), you are ready to finalize your calendar for the upcoming month. Be sure to designate locations for all of your programs, such as "upper living room" or "second floor dayroom." Make an office copy; this is your master to which you can refer and make adjustments. This master copy can also be filed after the month is completed so you have a reference for the future. Once it is completed (and this should be done a week or two in advance of the start of the next month), review it with your administrator if you are new, or if this is part of the requirements for your position at the facility.

Once your calendar is approved, if an approval process exists, you are now ready to market your program. The way in which you present your calendar to residents, families, staff, and the community is the first step, and a decision that you need to make based on the people involved.

Most facilities have a large print or oversized calendar made from their master calendar, and post it in a few strategic locations throughout the building, such as the nursing stations, resident dining areas, and the lobby or entrance area. This is useful for reaching some residents, most of the staff, and family members who come in at odd hours and want to know what new programs there are. Having the large calendars in many places in the facility also helps the infrequent visitor locate a possible program of interest around which to plan their next visit. By using the big calendar, you are demonstrating to your staff and residents that your program is important, and that you took the time and care to plan and "announce" it. No one can say that he or she "did not know about it" when the calendar on the wall is larger than life!

Key staff members and other department heads will appreciate receiving a photocopy of your master calendar in their mailboxes with key events highlighted or even a note attached that brings attention to something in particular. Some facilities like to distribute photocopies of the calendars to each resident or hang them in some of the other activity areas. Placing take-home copies of your calendar in the entrance area is also a good idea.

In addition to the standard large print calendar, innovative facilities have tried other approaches to notify and sell programs to their residents. Some facilities publish a weekly or daily activity sheet that may be color coded. This is done to draw emphasis to the specific upcoming programs, and to make things easier by limiting the amount of information presented to residents at one time. Other facilities publish a small weekly magazine (similar to the TV Guide) of their upcoming activities to which residents can refer on a daily basis.

In addition to posted or distributed copies of calendars, draw attention to your programs by highlighting the day's events on your big hallway calendars. Use wipe-off boards to further emphasize special programs. You might make an arrangement with the dietary department to post an abbreviated version of their daily resident menu. This information could also be included in your daily or weekly "magazine." Announcements via an intercom system, if you have one, can also be a good reminder to residents and staff. Or, involve one of your more active residents in a volunteer capacity to make the announcements for you.

Do not forget the best marketing tools of all: you and your staff. If you are enthusiastic and confident about your program, you will win over many people. Allow extra time in your morning routine to visit residents, and sell your program to them through encouragement and support.

Emergency Program Ideas

An easy thing for activity professionals to forget is that the day will come when illness or emergency keeps them and/or their staff home. Left without direction, how will the other departments cope with residents in need of activity programming for the day? Establishing a policy and procedure for an emergency program (the specifics of policy writing will be covered in Chapter 13) and reviewing it in advance with other department heads and key staff will provide the assistance that other departments will need. Your policy and procedure plan should include detailed directions to staff for at least two or three group programs each day that can be run in your absence. A day of emergency programs is not the same as a day with your staff, but at least you will not be leaving programming options to chance.

Working With Other Departments

If you were to question the most successful activity professionals, they would tell you that having a thriving and integrated facility program is dependent on a supportive and educational relationship with the other departments. Being supportive of other departments simply means a realization that your department often requires the services of another department to meet its full potential. For example, starting a large afternoon program in your activity space without the cleaning services of the housekeeping department following lunch, would make for a difficult start. In Chapter 6, we discussed how to work with other departments to make the best use of time and space. To meet your programming requirements, the services of many departments are often needed to bring the whole program together. In addition to the cleaning situation, other examples of interdepartmental assistance include:

- a nursing staff member may be required to accompany residents on a trip
- a special cart of cooking supplies is prepared by the dietary staff
- your administrator is the keynote speaker at a special program
- a maintenance department staff member may be required to help install new decorations for a party
- a business office worker may help by taking reservations for a large function.

All of these requests for help from other areas can be made easier through the interdepartmental use of a **function request form** (see Figure 9–4). When used properly, this form improves relationships and streamlines the request process. The initiator of the form (an activity professional, nursing director, dietary manager, and the like) completes the top section with the particulars of the event, and makes specific requests of individual departments. The form is then dated and signed by the initiator with copies to each department involved, and the administrator. Depending on the scope of the event, some function request forms should be completed in advance, and with the prior approval of the administrator if the requests are unusual or break any normal facility routines. Always keep a copy for your records. It goes without saying that even if items or services are requested in advance, it would benefit you to

FUNCTION REQUEST FORM

To: All Departments
From: The Activity Department
Date of Request: _____

A function has been planned for:
Date:_____ at _____a.m./p.m.
in the _____.   Expected guests:_____
　　　room/area/location　　　　　　　　　　　　　　number
Name of function or description _____

We are requesting your assistance with the following:
Dietary
—— Please prepare the following food items: _____
_____
___ Please deliver by cart no later than _____ a.m./p.m.
—— Someone will pick up the cart by _____ a.m./p.m.

Housekeeping
__ Please have the room/area cleaned and ready no later
　　than _____ a.m./p.m.
___ Special Instructions: _____
_____

Nursing
—— Please provide assistance in ambulating/transporting
___ Special Instructions: _____
_____
Miscellaneous
__ _____
_____
_____
_____

cc: Administrator　　　　　　　　　　　　　　　　　*Thank You!*

Figure 9–4　The Function Request Form.

check a few days ahead of time with the other departments to ensure that your request did not get lost at the bottom of a mailbox, and a spot check should be made before an event begins to ensure that key items are not missing. The easiest way to submit function request forms to departments for the activity programs for the upcoming month is to attach copies of the function request forms to a copy of your monthly calendar, and submit these to the various departments prior to the beginning of a calendar month so your colleagues can properly schedule their time and staff. Following a program that relied on interdepartmental help, give verbal and written thanks for all the assistance you received. By so doing, you are setting the stage for a successful encounter the next time.

From an educational standpoint, there is much you can offer other departments that will have a positive spin on your programs. Your in-service programs, discussed in Chapter 18, are very important when addressing formal educational needs, but you also need to keep the other departments informed on a more casual basis. When you make major programming changes, or when you see a problem that requires handling, request a meeting with the departments involved. You cannot expect other departments to know what is required of them if you have not had the courtesy to tell them! Review of new policies, changes in existing programs, trip schedules, and other changes in routines all sound trivial, but are crucial issues in which face-to-face dialogue is important in order to avoid future problems.

SUMMARY

Basing programs on resident interests and needs is the basis of solid programming. Considering medical aspects and the role of seasonal and ritual events is also part of individual scheduling. Identifying programs by the number of participants, and planning programs accordingly is of paramount importance.

R E V I E W   Q U E S T I O N S

1. What are some of the techniques for running individual programs?
2. What is the difference between active and passive stimulation?
3. Define an affective need, and suggest an activity that may meet that need.
4. What are the activity classifications proposed by NAAP?
5. What special program adaptations must be made for residents with Alzheimer's disease or related disorders?

O N   Y O U R   O W N

1. Write a list of ten program interventions you can think of, based on the medical needs of your residents.
2. Think of five ritual events that are not typical holidays; plan a program for a day-long celebration for each, and include programs for all levels.
3. If you observed that fewer residents were benefiting from large group programs because of divergent needs, how would you tailor your individual visit and bedside program to meet the demands?

R E F E R E N C E S

Alzheimer's Disease Education & Referral Center and National Institutes of Health (1994). *Alzheimer's disease: A guide to federal programs.* (NIH publication No. 93–3635), Silver Spring, MD.

American Health Care Association (1995). *The long term care survey.* Washington, DC: American Health Care Association.

Bachner, J. P., & Cornelius, E. (1978). *Activities coordinator's guide: A handbook for activities coordinator in long-term care facilities,* (HCFA-HSQB, 78–004). Washington, DC: US Government Printing Office.

Bearon, L., & Koenig, H. (1990). Religious cognitions and use of prayer in health and illness. *The Gerontologist,* Vol. 30, No. 2, 249–253.

Bowlby, C. (1993). *Therapeutic activities with persons disabled by Alzheimer's disease and related disorders.* Gaithersburg, MD: Aspen Publishers Inc.

Coyne, A., Meade, H., Petrone, M., Meinert, L., & Joslin, B. L. (1990). The diagnosis of dementia: Demographic characteristics. *The Gerontologist,* Vol. 30, No. 3, 339–334.

DeBolt, N., & Kastner, M. E. (1989). *"I'm in here": Strategies for one-to-one activities.* Torrington, WY: Lutheran Health Systems.

Dowling, J. R. (1995). *Keeping busy: A handbook of activities for persons with dementia*. Baltimore, MD: The Johns Hopkins University Press.

Federal Register (1991). Vol. 56, No. 187., *Part 483–Requirements for long term care facilities*.

Folstein, M. F., Folstein, S. E., & McHugh, P. R. (1975). Mini-mental state: A practical method for grading the cognitive state of patients for the clinician. *Journal of Psychiatric Research*, 12, 189–198.

Forsythe, E. (1988). One–to-one therapeutic recreation activities for the bed and/or room bound. *Activities, Adaptation & Aging*, Vol. 13 (1/2), 63–76.

Godbey, G., & Parker, S. (1976). *Leisure studies and services: An overview*. Philadelphia, PA: W.B. Saunders Co.

Gruetzner, H. (1992). *Alzheimer's: A caregiver's guide and sourcebook*. New York, NY: John Wiley & Sons Inc.

Gubrium, J. F. (1975). *Living and dying at Murray Manor*, New York, NY: St. Martin's Press.

Gueldner, S. H., & Spradley, J. (1988). Outdoor walking lowers fatigue. *Journal of Gerontological Nursing*, Vol. 14, No. 10, 6–12.

Hagen, C., Malkmus, D., and Durham, P. (1985). *Levels of cognitive functioning*. Rancho Los Amigos Hospital, Clinical Management, Vol. 5 (5).

Hastings, L. (1981). *Complete handbook of activities and recreational programs for nursing homes*. Englewood Cliffs, NJ: Prentice Hall Inc.

Hartmaier, S., Sloane, P., Guess, H., & Koch, G. (1994). The MDS cognition scale: A valid instrument for identifying and staging nursing home residents with dementia using the minimum data set. *Journal of the American Geriatric Society*, 42, 1173–1272.

Hommel, D. (1995). *Diversional activity zones*. Unpublished manuscript. Brookville, NJ: DH Special Services.

Johnson, D. R. (1987) . Therapeutic rituals in the nursing home. *Activities, Adaptation and Aging*, Vol. 9, No. 3, 151–169.

Jones, M. (1996). *Gentlecare: Changing the experience of Alzheimer's disease in a positive way*. Burnaby, British Columbia: Moyra Jones Resources.

Koenig, H., George, L., & Siegler, I. (1988) . The use of religion and other emotion-regulating coping strategies among older adults. *The Gerontologist*, Vol. 28, No. 3, 303–310.

Koenig, H., Kvale, J., & Ferrel, C. (1988) . Religion and well-being in later life. *The Gerontologist*, Vol. 28, No. 1, 18–28.

Lemmon, D. K., & Pieper, H. G. (1980). Leisure pursuits and their meaning for the institutionalized elderly population. *Journal of Gerontological Nursing*, Vol. 6(2), 74–77.

Lucero, M. (1994). *"Comfort Care". A dementia capable program*. Presented at American Health Care Association Convention, Las Vegas, NV.

McGuire, F. A. (1985). Recreation leader and co-participant preferences of the institutionalized aged. *Therapeutic Recreation Journal*, 2nd Quarter, 47–54.

Miller, D. B. (1979). Case studies to challenge the nursing home activity coordinator. *Therapeutic Recreation Journal*, 3rd Quarter, 22–32.

Moberg, D. O. (1965) . Religiosity in old age. *The Gerontologist*, 5, 78–112.

Namazi, K., Whitehouse, P., Rechlin, L., Calkins, M., Johnson, B., Brabender, B., & Heventer, S. (1991). Environmental modifications in a specially designed unit for the care of patients with Alzheimer's disease: An overview and introduction. *The American Journal of Alzheimer's Care and Related Disorders & Research*, Nov/Dec, 3–9.

National Association of Activity Professionals (1990). *Program standards and the role of the activity professional*. [Brochure]. Washington, DC.

National Institutes Of Health Consensus Development Conference Statement (1987). *Differential diagnosis of dementing diseases*. Vol. 6, No. 11, July 6–8. Bethesda, MD: National Institutes Of Health.

Ohta, R., & Ohta, B. (1988). Special units for Alzheimer's disease patients: A critical look. *The Gerontologist*, Vol. 28, No. 6., 803–808.

Ramsdell, J., Rothrock, J., Ward, H., & Volk, D. (1990). Evaluation of cognitive impairment in the elderly. *Journal of General Internal Medicine*, Vol. 5., 55–64.

Reisberg, B., Ferris, S., DeLeon, M., & Crook, T. (1982). The global deterioration scale for assessment of primary degenerative dementia. *American Journal of Psychiatry*, 139(9), 1136–1139.

Sabat, S. (1994). Recognizing and working with remaining abilities: Toward improving the care of Alzheimer's disease sufferers. *The American Journal of Alzheimer's Care and Related Disorders & Research*, May/June, 8–16.

Sheridan, C. (1987). *Failure-free activities for the Alzheimer's patient: A guide for caregivers*. San Francisco, CA: Cottage Books.

Steinitz, L. (1981). The local church as support for the elderly. *Journal of Gerontological Social Work*, Vol. 4(2), 43–53.

Sullivan, W. (1993). "It helps me to be a whole person": The role of spirituality among the mentally challenged. *Psychosocial Rehabilitation Journal*, Vol. 16(3), 125–134.

Zeisel, J., Hyde, J., & Levkoff, S. (1994). Best practices: An environment-behavior model for Alzheimer special care units. *The American Journal of Alzheimer's Care and Related Disorders & Research*, Mar./Apr., 4–21.

Zgola, J. (1987). *Doing things: A guide to programming activities for persons with Alzheimer's disease and related disorders*. Baltimore, MD: The Johns Hopkins University Press.

FURTHER READING

Aver, S., Sclan, S., Yaffee, R., & Reisberg, B. (1994). The neglected half of Alzheimer's disease: Cognitive and functional concomitants of severe dementia. *Journal of the American Geriatrics Society*, 42, 1266–1272.

Arrigo, S., Lewis, A., & Mattimore, H. (1992). *Beyond bingo: Innovative programs for the new senior.* State College, PA: Venture Publishing Inc.

Basmajian, J. V. (1984). *Therapeutic exercise,* 4th edition. Baltimore, MD: Williams and Wilkins.

Cable, T., & Udd, E. (1988). Therapeutic benefits of a wildlife observation program. *Therapeutic Recreation Journal,* 4th quarter, 65–70.

Edginton, C., Compton, D., and Hanson, C. (1980) . *Recreation and leisure programming: A guide for the professional.* Philadelphia, PA: Saunders College.

Elliott, J., and Sorg-Elliott, J. (1991). *Recreation programming and activities for older adults.* State College, PA: Venture Publishing Co.

Filinson, R. (1988). A model for church-based services for frail elderly persons and their families. *The Gerontologist,* Vol. 28, No. 4, 483–486.

Foster, P. (1980) . A multi-dimensional activities program. *Activities, Adaptation and Aging,* Vol. 1 (2), 35–39.

Gissal, M., Ray, R., & Smith, E. (1980). Fitness trails: A healthful activity for older adults. *Therapeutic Recreation Journal,* 2nd quarter, 43–48.

Helgeson, E., & Willis, S. C. (1987) . *Handbook of group activities for impaired older adults.* Binghamton, NY: Haworth Press.

Hoffman, M. (1981). Recreation therapy: A prescriptive approach. *Therapeutic Recreation Journal,* 3rd quarter, 16–21.

Hoppa, M., and Roberts, G. (1974) . Implication of the activity factor. The *Gerontologist,* Vol. 14, 331–335.

Lesser, M. (1978). The effects of rhythmic exercise on the range of motion in older adults. *American Corr. Therapy Journal,* Vol. 32, No. 4, 118–122.

Lunchins, D., & Hanrahan, P. (1993). What is appropriate health care for end-stage dementia? *Journal of the American Geriatrics Society,* 41, 25–30.

McClannahan, L. (1993). Recreation programs for nursing home residents: The importance of patient characteristics and environmental arrangements. *Therapeutic Recreation Journal,* 2nd Quarter, 26–31

McClannahan, L. E. (1973). Therapeutic and prosthetic living environments for nursing home residents. *The Gerontologist,* 13, 424–429.

McClannahan, L., & Risley, T. (1974). Design of living environments for nursing home residents: Recruiting attendance at activities. *The Gerontologist,* Vol. 14, 236–240.

McClannahan, L., & Risley, T. (1974). Activities and materials for severely disabled geriatric patients. *Nursing Homes,* Vol. 24, 10–13.

McClannahan, L., & Risley, T. (1975). Design of living environment for nursing-home residents: Increased participation in recreational activities. *Journal of Applied Behavior Analysis,* 8(3), 261–268.

McGowin, D. (1993). *Living in the labyrinth: Personal journey through the maze of Alzheimer's.* San Francisco, CA: Elder Books.

Namazi, K., & Johnson, B. (1991). Physical environmental cues to reduce the problems of incontinence in Alzheimer's disease units. *The American Journal of Alzheimer's Care and Related Disorders & Research,* Nov/Dec, 22–28.

Namazi, K., & Johnson, B. (1991). Environmental effects on incontinence problems in Alzheimer's disease patients. *The American Journal of Alzheimer's Care and Related Disorders & Research,* Nov./Dec., 16–21.

Namazi, K., Rosner, T., & Rechlin, L. (1991). Long-term memory cuing to reduce visuo-spatial disorientation in Alzheimer's disease patients in a special care unit. *The American Journal of Alzheimer's Care and Related Disorders & Research,* Nov./Dec., 10–15.

Parsons, V. (1993). *A year of holidays: A planning and idea book for holiday activities in nursing homes.* LaGrange, TX: M&H Publishing Co.

Perkins, K., Rapp, S., Carlson, C., & Wallace, C. (1986) . A behavioral intervention to increase exercise among nursing home residents. *The Gerontologist,* Vol. 26, No. 5, 479–481.

Sullivan, J. (1984). *Fitness for the handicapped.* Springfield, IL: Charles C. Thomas Publisher.

Waynant, L., & Wilson, R. (1974). *Learning centers: A guide for effective use.* Minneapolis, MN: Judy/Instructo Publishers.

C H A P T E R   1 0
Program Implementation—Beyond Traditional Programming

KEY TERMS ....

developmentally
  disabled
leisure counseling
aromatherapy
art therapy
bibliotherapy
dance therapy
drama therapy
horticultural
  therapy
milieu therapy
music therapy

pet therapy
phototherapy
poetry therapy
reality orientation
remotivation
validation therapy
reminiscence
life review
sensory stimulation
humor
touch
therapeutic touch

OBJECTIVES ....

After completing this chapter, you should:

- realize the program adjustments that are necessary to work with residents in different treatment settings
- understand the variety of therapies and treatment modalities that exist to enhance programming
- recognize the methods of incorporating activity programming into other facility projects

INTRODUCTION

Awareness of the structural components of program planning will lead you to seek innovative methods of meeting resident needs in various congregate settings. Reviewing selected activities through activity analysis and making adaptations for your resident or setting is a critical step in the planning process. The use of alternative therapies and treatment modalities offer additional methods of reaching residents as your total program is finalized. Finally, integrating activity goals into other facility projects is an important step in interdepartmental relationships.

Program Variations Based on Resident Settings ....

Facility space is a factor in planning, but having multiple client settings in your facility presents you with additional scheduling challenges. The common practice for residents with different needs is to provide a semisegregated environment for cohabitation. This choice is considered a positive one, and allows the members to receive the specialized services and attention that are tailored to their respective needs. In most cases, however, the unit or area is still connected to a "main facility." The core services (nursing, activities, dietary, housekeeping, and so forth) are administrated from the main facility, but the amount and kind of services delivered to each long-term care unit

varies. You may be in a facility that is free-standing (not attached to a main facility) and provides a subspecialty within the institutional long-term care setting. In either case, you have planning considerations to make as your review your program.

AIDS Residents

Residents with AIDS, commingled with your elderly residents or in a separate unit, may be placed in long-term care for the end stage of their disease. The progression of the disease may not require intensive, skilled medical care until the late stages. With long-term care opportunities in community-based or home based facilities remaining limited, some individuals with AIDS may eventually need care in a long-term care facility

The needs of AIDS residents may be greater than your traditional elderly long-term care clients. The disease does not discriminate by age, financial background, or circumstance, whereas your elderly residents have some common experiences because of their age. The client mix of the AIDS residents may be so diverse that proper activity planning is a challenge. Characteristics vary among AIDS residents, but you may find that some feel estranged from family and friends, put their affairs in order, strive to do certain activities "one more time," or feel shame or loneliness. The commonality of experience that you draw from your elderly residents is impossible with AIDS residents. In working with AIDS residents, look to maintain interests. Set up specialized and important projects, and help the resident put his or her affairs in order, if requested. Caroleo (1988) suggests programs such as stress reduction and volunteering as important. Nutritional issues are also a large concern. Turner and Keller (1988) add that program planning should include those programs that have immediate gratification. Time frames for offering programs or interventions should not be bound by a clock, since you may have a resident who would like to hear classical music in the middle of the night. Providing spiritual resources is useful. Some holistic approaches, such as aromatherapy and massage therapy, may be helpful in pain management. Working with the hospice team is another link for the activity professional. Familiarize yourself with healthcare resource materials, such as Kubler-Ross' (1987) book, and in-services concerning the AIDS experience. Turner and Keller caution activity professionals about the possibility of burnout in working with this population.

Assisted Living, Boarding Home, and Residential Clients

Residents who have a higher level of independence and no need for skilled care services are individuals served in residential settings that are called assisted living, boarding homes, personal care homes, or many other variations. Because of their independence and nonlimiting medical needs, an activity program for this segment is diverse and very active. Individual hobbies and interests are continued with attempts to plan for new interests. A large number of diversional and entertainment programs are also encouraged. Trips, for both recreational and personal needs, are planned and implemented each week. Resident involvement as volunteers, either in the long-term care component of the facility or in the community, remains important, but the resident's physician should be consulted before he or she begins to volunteer. Residents can make their own activity schedule, and prefer to be segregated from long-term care residents in the same building. The view of the potential next step in their aging process is often not appealing to them. Activity programming and implementation with residential clients may be overseen by an activity professional, but carried out by a personal care assistant or other trained staff member.

Day Care Clients

Adult day care has been available since the late 1970s and is unique because it is not part of home-based long-term care or institutional long-term care, and is not necessarily part of a community long-term care offering. Adult day care is a program of recreation and meal activities offered to qualified individuals during the day at a center or as part of another program.

Weissert, et al. (1989) found that the average age of day care participants was almost seventy-eight years, with over fifty percent of the clients having some functional dependence. In addition, they discovered that over forty percent of day care clients had some cognitive difficulties or mental problems. The study by Weissert et al. comments that the elderly who participate in day care are most likely to be considered a subcategory of the elderly residing in a community. In contrasting day care residents with nursing home residents, their study showed that day care clients were more likely to be married and less dependent in activities of daily living. The time frame of operation in a typical center is 9:00 a.m. to 3:00 p.m., with two or four activity programs scheduled each day. In addition to diversional and skill building activities, the centers also offered assistance with nutrition, transportation, and counseling. Staffing at the centers varied from social service workers to nursing personnel and activity professionals.

Program planning by activity professionals who have an adult day care center on premises in the long-term care facility is best served by maintaining separate programs. Try different versions of the same programs with your two different groups. Document hobbies and interests of participants, and incorporate it into program planning. Thews, Reaves, and Henry (1993) suggest developing a calendar of "parallel activities" so that options exist for the participants. They also mention the importance of having numerous back-up plans for programs that may not be of interest, and of keeping the level of programs simple at first. The objective of programming in adult day care is "participant fulfillment, not project completion."

Developmentally Disabled Residents

According to Riddick and Keller (1991), the term **developmentally disabled** refers to individuals with one of the following conditions: autism, mental retardation, cerebral palsy, or neurological affliction. Their research estimates that a growing adult population with developmental disabilities has not been met with adequate research concerning their activity needs.

The developmentally disabled elderly population receives care and assistance in numerous settings, including institutional long-term care. Riddick and Keller suggest that activity services for developmentally disabled elders should be provided in the least restrictive environment with "interagency collaboration," so that residents get the benefits of all possible services. The planning model that Riddick and Keller present includes four steps: assessment, design, implementation, and evaluation. During assessment, how free time is spent, and in what setting, is important. Determining abilities is also crucial. The other steps are similar to other recreation planning models previously discussed although adaptions in equipment, supplies, and program length may be necessary.

Time frames for programming should be structured and based on previous routines and desires. Integration of the rest of the population is also important, as well as the individualization of programs.

Mental retardation, one form of developmental disability, is seen the most frequently in institutional long-term care. Planning staff in-services to address the special needs will certainly help in the delivery of services. Some states have separate regulations for the mentally retarded developmentally disabled (MRDD). Check with your state agency to see if additional guidelines apply to your facility.

Head Trauma Residents

Handling an activity program for traumatic head injuries or **head trauma** residents may be a part of your job in your facility. The effect of a profound injury to the head, usually from an accident, results in physical, behavioral, cognitive, and emotional problems. Although the physical trauma is obvious, Fazio and Fralish (1988) mention that the social aspects and cognitive impairment components actually require more attention. Luczak (1980) states that the two major consequences of head trauma are partial paralysis and lack of skills to socialize properly.

The study by Fazio and Fralish (1988) illustrates that the general age of head trauma clients falls between eighteen and thirty-five, with fifty percent of facilities having mixed disability situations instead of a facility that handles head trauma residents only. Their research also shows that the top five areas for recreation and leisure goals for head trauma residents are developing social skills, decreasing withdrawal and isolation, reintegration into the community, forming independent leisure

participation, and self-expression and verbalization. Additionally, because of the age range of clients, appropriate programs that meet personal goals and are age-specific are the most effective. The time frames for residents must conform to therapy and other medical schedules. Much of the program takes place at the bedside during the initial months of recovery. After that, a combination of group and individual programs are appropriate.

Pediatric Residents

Working with children in long-term care is a challenging situation. Some children, because of congenital problems, injury or accident, require long-term, skilled medical care, and are probably in a separate unit of your facility. The age range may vary from infants to young adults, and programming cannot be generalized to the needs of one age group. Specific and individual programs at the bedside or in age-appropriate groups may work best, with larger entertainment programs to round out the schedule. Because of the intense nature of some medical conditions, activity or recreation goals may be geared toward diversion or skill development. A pediatric wing of a long-term care facility is most likely segregated from an elderly long-term care wing because the needs of both groups are so divergent. The time frame for activity programs probably follows the therapy and medical calendar. Family and friends will be a large and important part of any activity program.

Psychiatric Residents

Residents with psychiatric needs are becoming more commonplace in long-term care facilities. A large number of institutional long-term care residents are shown to have some cognitive impairments, but often residents with true psychiatric problems may not be identified and assisted appropriately. Some facilities are forming psychogeriatric units, specifically geared for elderly long-term care residents who are facing psychiatric issues. Activity programming for this group borrows from the work with the cognitively impaired because similarities exist. Dealing with psychiatric problems of the elderly requires mental health training, as well as an understanding of the aging population. If a psychogeriatric unit is attached to your facility, it may be a locked area for the safety of both the residents contained in that unit as well as the other long-term care clients. Individual programs, geared toward the interests and goals of each resident, are important, but group work and group programs are also a focal point. Scheduling of programs will probably follow traditional time frames, although staff will need to have activity interventions to use during nonprogram hours.

Subacute Residents

Subacute care, one step down from the acute care offered in hospitals, takes place with greater frequency in long-term care facilities. Units with subacute care clients are now attached to long-term care facilities to replace the high hospital cost with high-level, skilled nursing care for such medical conditions as wound management, respirator care, ventilator care, head injuries, and other rehabilitative conditions. Typically, the resident resides in the subacute care unit for a short stay of up to ninety days. The unit may be managed by a nurse coordinator or someone with specialized training, such as a respiratory therapist working as the manager of a ventilator unit. The goals of treatment are to provide rehabilitation so that a resident is able to move down to a lower level of care as soon as possible. This means that a resident ultimately could be discharged home, to a rehabilitation facility, or to a traditional unit within the long-term care facility.

From an activity professional's standpoint, residents in subacute units have primary goals of rehabilitation. Therapy schedules have top priority. Activity programs should focus more on individual programs instead of group efforts, and evening programs may become important to plan. Consideration also must be given to the fact that residents in this unit are entering and discharging at a higher frequency than traditional long-term care residents. Assessments, goals, and implementation of plans must be made quickly. Because of the special needs of subacute patients, consideration is being given to revising the MDS to accommodate subacute care.

The view that residents have of themselves in the subacute care unit also becomes important in planning. With quick discharge as an ultimate goal, many residents do not wish to be associated with long-term care residents. It may be more sensitive to retitle the names of the activity professional's position to lifestyle coordinator, recreation services worker, or service coordinator.

Program Review and Adaptation...

Reviewing programs for their usefulness to specific residents must be an ongoing process. Activity analysis is a major process in that review

procedure. Making adaptations or tailoring programs to fit the needs of individuals is another key step.

Activity Analysis

Activity analysis, which Crepeau (1986) defines as ". . . the process by which an activity is broken down into its component parts to determine the skills required to do it," is an important part of program planning and adaptation. The analysis process begins when the activity professional makes a written draft (plan) for the activity. This involves listing all the steps to conduct the activity from beginning to end, and who is responsible for completing each step. Next, answers must be given to the physical (will standing be necessary?), social (does this activity have to be done with a group?), emotional (will this activity meet needs for belonging?), and cognitive (what is the learning environment?) aspects of the activity as they relate to a particular resident's ability to participate in the activity. Additional areas to be analyzed include cost and specific sensory areas, such as vision and hearing. Bowlby (1993) adds that the activity analysis should include information about the value of the activity to the participant (i.e., increases self-esteem).

Although activity analysis is an enlightening exercise, practicality dictates that it cannot be conducted with every program. There are certain residents or situations that make analysis of programs necessary. Bowlby (1993) wisely suggests that an activity analysis be conducted for any programs you have used that were not successful, so you can learn from the experience.

Program Adaptation

A look at programs you are planning to present to your residents may make you feel uncertain of the potential for success with your residents. At times, a program may seem too advanced or out of reach in terms of goals for some residents. Adapting programs for different levels and various residents is an ability you must acquire to help you build a solid program. For example, a cooking program means preparing, cooking, serving, and eating a special meal to one group of high functioning residents, whereas the cooking program of another group might mean mixing ingredients to make quick-set Jello™. By tailoring the level of ability required and the outcome, almost any activity you can envision can become a reality for your residents. Many activity professionals make a mistake by thinking "my residents could not do that; it would be too frustrating," instead of using activity analysis techniques to identify problem areas and scaling down the program accordingly.

Leisure Counseling

Two aspects of a recreation (or activity) professional's scope of responsibility that is often overlooked are the concepts of **leisure education** and **leisure counseling**. Due to the high level of cognitive impairments of many of our long-term care residents, leisure counseling may not be an option. Chinn and Joswiak (1981) define leisure education as ". . . a comprehensive program employed to enhance the quality of a person's life through leisure." Using leisure education, a professional may center on an individual's attitudes toward work and leisure, social skills, use of leisure resources, and ability to make choices concerning leisure; all of which ultimately bring a person closer to the goal of an independent leisure lifestyle. Leisure counseling, as discussed by Peterson and Gunn (1984), is an intervention technique of the leisure awareness component of the entire leisure education model. In assisting clients to become aware of their leisure attitudes and needs, the recreation professional acts as a counselor or instructor to help clients meet their goals. Peterson and Gunn feel that the term "leisure counseling" is too limiting because it only refers to the technique, instead of addressing the whole category of leisure education. Taking a different approach, Leitner and Leitner (1985) define leisure counseling as ". . . a helping process designed to facilitate maximal leisure well-being," and comment further that nursing home clients can benefit from leisure counseling to help structure leisure time in the facility, as well as assist in the adjustment period after discharge. With controversy surrounding the use of this term, Chinn and Joswiak (1981) suggest that practice standards be set up for the use of leisure counseling, but for now, the process should be considered, ". . . one of the tools that can be a part of the repertoire of the trained professional."

Review of the Therapies and Treatment Modalities ....

Aromatherapy

As part of an orientation to holistic healing and the wellness model of service delivery, **aromatherapy** is opening up a new dimension in programming. Rose (1992) defines aromatherapy as ". . . healing with essential oils through the sense of smell by inhalation . . .", a practice, she says, was used as far back as 400 B. C. Using essential oils, the chemical components of plants, to stimulate the sense of smell, can have a powerful effect on the mind and body. Rose postulates that inhaling certain essential oils can impact the mind psychologically, and has physiological effects, such as stimulating certain systems of the body. There are well over 100 different kinds of essential oils, all with different expected effects. Lavender, thought to reduce anxiety, and eucalyptus, proposed to aid in recovery from illness, are both examples of common essential oils and their use. To gain the benefits of aromatherapy, essential oils should be released in hot water, or misted through an atomizer or other dispenser.

The use of aromatherapy in activity programming is obvious. Residents who may be unable to communicate or actively receive stimulation in their world, can be stimulated through aromatherapy. Additionally, life review and reminiscence programs can be enhanced through the careful introduction of memory-triggering smells. Relaxing, stress releasing moods may be created to assist in relieving tensions and other problems. When combined with the skills of a professional massage therapist or other technician, the benefits of aromatherapy can be increased. The attending physician should be consulted before using any aromatherapy technique in the event of any contraindication with a resident's medical condition.

Art Therapy

Using art to express conscious and unconscious feelings was first suggested by Naumberg (1966). This technique comprises a whole field of academic study, and uses methodology that asks a resident to express, in drawings or images, what they may have trouble expressing in words. By using artwork instead of talking to communicate, residents can share their feelings. The art therapists direct and interpret the art experience.

Normally, the guidelines of **art therapy** must be conducted by a trained art therapist and often, art therapy is used in tandem with other therapies. Labarca (1979) suggests some art therapy techniques that can be scaled down for use by other professionals. She mentions that the colors and subject matter chosen by clients often reveal the feelings a person has. Another art therapy method that is useful involves the client drawing a self-portrait. The resulting portrait, what is represented, and the size of the drawing or elements, all contain interesting information for interpretation. Having experience as an art therapist, or working with one, are two ideal situations for the application of art therapy in long-term care. Activity professionals can use modified art therapy techniques to stimulate group activity or to aid in communication in individual meetings. Artistic abilities are not a prerequisite for the resident, but the ability to hold or direct a drawing instrument may limit the application to more regressive residents. Crosson (1976) mentions that a limitation of using art therapy in geriatric settings is often the problem of limited spontaneity in expression.

There is a professional association for art therapists called The American Art Therapy Association. In addition, art therapy, as a discipline, is part of the National Coalition of Arts Therapies Associations (NCATA), comprised of individual members who also belong to the following six creative arts therapy associations: The American Art Therapy Association, The American Association for Music Therapy, The American Dance Therapy Association, The American Society for Group Psychotherapy and Psychodrama, The National Association for Drama Therapy, and The National Association for Poetry Therapy. By joining in this coalition, these separate creative arts organizations can share goals and related procedures.

Sandel (1992) offers these overall benefits of any of the six creative arts therapies in assisting the elderly:

- increasing orientation and activity
- guiding reminiscence
- increasing self-awareness and acceptance
- helping form positive interpersonal relationships
- assisting in forging community spirit

Keep these benefits in mind as the discussion of the other creative arts therapies (art, music, dance/movement, drama, and poetry) continues in this section.

Bibliotherapy

A technique that is not widely used, but affords benefits to particular residents, is called bibliotherapy. The origins of this technique are unclear, but Austin (1982) mentions that the method of assisting others through examples in reading materials such as books, plays, and pamphlets can be useful in demonstrating that others may share similar problems. Austin also notes that this concept is most widely used in psychiatric environments, and may not have as many applications in other settings, such as long-term care.

Dance Therapy

The American Dance Therapy Association (1995), formed in 1966, defines dance and movement therapy as ". . . the psychotherapeutic use of movement as a process which furthers the emotional, cognitive and physical integration of the individual." Sandel (1987) mentioned the origins of dance therapy as the work of Marian Chace with psychiatric elderly in hospitals in the 1940s. Using a portable record player, she was able to reach many elderly residents through movement and music techniques. Many years later, according to Sandel, exercise and calisthenics programs for the elderly began to appear in physical education curriculums.

Through the use of basic elements, participants in dance therapy can receive many positive experiences. Leary (1994) cites the provision of healthy leisure activities and working on problems through dance as some of the primary benefits. Using expressive movement, Leary feels that self-expression is encouraged and, as a result, the physical state is improved. Additionally, self-awareness can be enhanced, emotions can be controlled through directed action, and some of the expected changes that require an adjustment period may be handled a little more easily through dance therapy methods.

The parts of movement that comprise dance include shape, space, time, and force, as reported by Fisher (1995). In terms of understanding dance therapy, shape is defined as ". . . the position of the body or any body part, such as an arm or leg." Fisher gives many examples of movement exercises that involve shape, such as "freezing" in a specific shape, using arms and legs. Space is the room or area where the movement exercises occur, and include different directional paths, various body levels (sitting, standing, or multiple positions). In movement, time is related to the speed of the movement, whether it is done quickly or slowly. Finally, force in movement relates to the type of movement: relaxed, weak, hard, or soft.

Dance therapy offers many opportunities for programming for activity professionals because, as Leary (1994) observed ". . . dance in some form is almost always possible." Sandel (1982) discusses some of the specific benefits to those elderly residents with special needs. For those with cognitive impairment, she suggests that the consistent, predictable aspects of dance therapy, even incorporating reality orientation techniques when appropriate, can offer stability to participants. Residents with physical limitations can participate in moderate dance therapy and thus prevent further deterioration of physical attributes. Depression, that effects many elderly, may be reduced by an active role in dance therapy. Sandel (1987) also mentions that programs that include singing, repetitive movements, or other "rituals," assist in communication for those residents who are limited. Linder (1982) reminds us to be reflective of the cultural backgrounds of residents in dance or movement programs, because many older adults ". . . may have a vocabulary of nonverbal gestures and a heritage of personal and ethnic movement experiences. . ." which could be the key to guiding proper participation. She also comments that reminiscence and life review programs are aided by the use of dance and movement expression that include props. Because dance and movement therapy offers a wide range of programming options, the techniques are now being used in activity programs around the country.

Drama Therapy

As one of the creative arts therapies, **drama therapy** is defined by Johnson (1982) as ". . . the intentional use of creative drama toward the psychotherapeutic goals of symptom relief . . . and personal growth. . . ." Johnson explains that the difference between drama therapy and other creative arts therapies, such as music or art therapy, is that a clear understanding exists between the client and the drama therapist of the specific goals of the drama activity. Drama therapy techniques involve role-playing and self-expression through improvisational methods or other exercises. When used by trained drama therapists, who have both creative arts and mental health education, stimulation of a person's creativity is a primary goal. Role-playing, a method used to encourage spontaneity and creativity, leads to role analysis, which Johnson explains, is the pattern of behavior that emerges during a role-playing session. Improvisation, or unscripted things that occur during role-play or other drama sessions can also be revealing. Drama therapy also encourages the formation of groups that may be threatening to some individuals. Jennings (1978)

cautions that use of drama therapy can sometimes unleash feelings that lead to conflicts among group members. Used properly, working in nonthreatening drama groups encourages comfort and assists residents to express problems during a group process.

Horticultural Therapy

The American Horticultural Therapy Association (AHTA) (1993) describes **horticultural therapy** as ". . . a process utilizing plants and horticultural activities to improve the social, educational, psychological, and physical adjustment of persons thus improving their body, mind and spirits." In discussing the background of horticultural therapy, the AHTA, formed in 1973, noted that in the early 1800s, a physician named Dr. Rush noticed the positive effects of gardening in mentally ill patients. Other practitioners used the approach in similar ways, but it was not until the 1940s that horticultural therapy became known as a significant part of the total therapy offered in veteran's hospitals. Today, in addition to many applications in all types of health settings, there are college-level training courses for degree programs in horticultural therapy.

According to Rothert and Daubert (1981), research has ranked gardening activities as one of the most popular for elderly clients. Although the benefits of horticultural therapy exist for different age levels, the elderly, especially those in institutional settings, derive many benefits from horticultural therapy because it provides a link to past life skills and gives an element of control over the environment. Other positive factors for the elderly mentioned by Rothert and Daubert include the need for caretaking of a living thing, exposure to beauty, and the observation of growth and transformation that comes from involvement in plant life. Houseman (1986) suggests that links between horticultural therapy and aging assist in promoting a sense of well-being for older adults. Some researchers have shown that life satisfaction improved through exposure to horticultural therapy, and Lewis and Mattson (1988) effectively demonstrated that gardening may actually reduce blood pressure in elderly adults. Creativity in self-expression, variety, control, independence, and opportunities for social interaction and service are also benefits of institutional horticultural therapy programs, as noted by Burgess (1990). Riordan and Williams (1988) suggest that moderate regular activity, such as gardening pursuits, may promote good health.

Planning a horticultural therapy program should be done with the needs of the residents in mind. Rothert and Daubert (1981) list general goals for institutional horticultural therapy programs, such as providing the residents with opportunities for participation in new or previously acquired hobbies, improving health, fostering social interactions, designing an environment of increased life-satisfaction, and offering programs that permit self-expression. In working with elderly clients, they suggest horticultural activities such as plant propagation, forcing bulbs, window herb gardens, indoor flowering plants, and outdoor raised-bed gardening. Program modifications include use of a magnifying glass, bright-colored tools, padded handles on tools, and large seeds or strips of seed tape. The authors provide specific cautionary notes on working with residents suffering from particular conditions. For example, in gardening programs with diabetics, Rothert and Daubert suggest avoiding exertion and exposure to sharp plants, such as roses. The American Horticultural Therapy Association (1995) offers further guidelines on adapting equipment and gardening supplies to reach a handicapped audience. Their suggestions include creating maps of garden areas by using varied pavement textures and designing sensory spaces using colorful and fragrant flowers.

For tips on beginning a horticultural experience, Burgess (1990) mentions the use of a feasibility study with residents as a way to get a program started. Other ideas include selecting an appropriate gardening spot that has adequate sun exposure and high traffic, which Burgess attributes to increase motivation and participation. Moore (1989) suggests setting goals, making a gardening schedule in advance, and researching all resources.

Cautionary guidelines, discussed by Reif (1994) during the horticultural therapy process, involves avoidance of overexposure to the sun, safety in the use of equipment, and awareness of the dangers of overexertion.

Horticultural therapy is popular with activity professionals because it is adaptable to every resident level and is universal in appeal.

Milieu Therapy

Milieu therapy is defined by Citrin and Dixon (1977) as the therapeutic interventions designed to assist in making the institutional environment healthier for residents by altering the patterns and the environment in which the residents live.

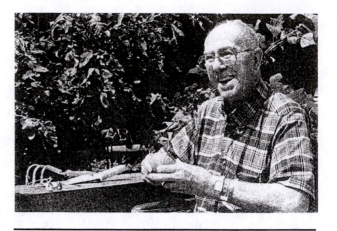

Figure 10–1 The simple benefits of horticultural therapy can be enjoyed by most residents.

The purpose of milieu therapy is to help residents avoid social withdrawal, decreased physical activity, and other negative impacts that are possible in an institution. Forsythe (1988) suggests that program approaches such as reality orientation, sensory stimulation, and remotivation are examples of milieu therapy that will be discussed in the following sections.

Music Therapy

The National Association for Music Therapy (1994) defines **music therapy** as ". . . the use of music in the accomplishment of therapeutic aims: the restoration, maintenance, and improvement of mental and physical health." The use of music in the healing process dates back to ancient cultures (Egyptian and Greek) where music was incorporated into regular medical treatment to assist in recovery. Following wartime in the late 1940s and early 1950s, the Veteran's Administration hospitals used music professionals to assist in rehabilitation. Music therapy became an academic field of study shortly thereafter, with many colleges and universities offering degrees in the discipline.

Although the benefits of music were thought to be present in modern medical practice, until recently there were no scientific studies with facts to support those claims. In her article, Avenoso (1995) postulates that music therapy has gained more recent popularity because of two factors: the greater acceptance of alternatives to traditional medicine, and the fact that more attention has been focused on the issue of music therapy through grants and research. Lynch (1987) describes the ongoing relationship of music to health by stating, "The association of music and the magic of healing begins with the fact that music is an integral part of human life through sound."

The benefits of music therapy are numerous. Clair (1994) suggests that some of the positives of music therapy for residents, and even family members, include stress relief, personal enrichment, and meaningful interactions. Other researchers, such as Lynch (1987), mention the physical benefits of music, such as "involuntary rhythmic response," release of emotional tension, increase in metabolism, changes in muscle energy, and positive circulatory and respiratory impacts. Knoll (1992) adds that music therapy assists in increasing attention span, adding motivation for increased movement, and may actually act as a deterrent to pain (by distraction). In describing the reasons why music therapy is helpful, Knoll talks about the structured nature of music that leads to predictability and familiarity, and is comforting to elderly residents.

Program applications of music therapy in activity settings can be varied, since music can reach residents in many forms. Lipe (1987) mentions that an important distinction should be made between programs that are considered diversional versus those that are therapeutic in nature. In discussing specific music therapy program applications in long-term care settings, Wade (1987) suggests one area of music/movement that could have implications in the nursing home: rhythm instruments. Using lightweight rhythm instruments such as bells, maracas, or tambourines, a layperson can integrate the instruments into an existing exercise program, or make them part of a sing-along. Wade also mentioned more advanced music therapy concepts, called orff and eurhythmics, that involve specialized training in the field of music therapy and should be presented only by a music therapist. Music programs that are easy to incorporate into any activity program are categorized by Lewallen (1987) as ". . . music listening or music appreciation groups, environmental music, musical games, including music bingo, sing-alongs, resident performance groups, and outside entertainment groups." Kartman (1980) reminds us that simple nostalgic and ethnic music reached some residents when no other treatment intervention had been successful.

Specific resident programs may benefit specific resident groups with music therapy. In working with Alzheimer's residents, Smith (1990) suggests using music to help residents establish a sense of achievement as well as keeping the brain stimulated. The relaxing benefits of music often calm agitated residents and control difficult behaviors. The phenomena of "automatic language" may work when a cognitively impaired individual is able to remember the words to a familiar song, but may not recognize his or her own name. Bumanis and Yoder's (1987) work with reality orientation groups demonstrated that the inclusion of music in groups created greater social and emotional improvement of participants. In hospice programs, Colligan (1987) found that the inclusion of musical activities can be a positive experience in managing pain, providing general comfort, and lending support to the resident and his or her family. Reminiscence programs are enhanced by memories that can be stirred through musical journeys, according to Karras (1987). Lipe (1987) suggests that music in individualized programs assists in bringing comfort, companionship, and special bedside events to those with severe mental or physical limitations. Combining music and any program certainly increases the benefits to the resident.

Pet Therapy

Another therapeutic intervention that has gained in popularity over the last decade is the application of **pet therapy**. Pet or animal therapy is defined as the use of animals to provide therapeutic effects and to illicit positive emotions. The beneficial effects of contact with animals by certain groups, such as the elderly or psychiatric residents, have been known for years despite the lack of scientific proof or research. Bustad (1980) talked about the historical uses of animals for companionship and comfort in ancient cultures. He noted that the first use of animals in therapy occurred in the 1940s in the United States. As far back as her early work on nursing, Florence Nightingale (1946) commented on the positive effects of using animals to assist in recovery from illness.

Some of the primary reasons that pet therapy is so successful has to do with the needs of the elderly population. Bustad and Hines (1983) discuss the therapeutic value that the introduction of pets in the institutional environment can provide. Residents have autonomy and dignity returned, relief from boredom. and quality stimulation offered. Studies they cite suggest that animals offer "positive, nonverbal communication signals" through love and touch. The overall presence of the pets improves morale and helps develop a community feeling.

To fulfill these needs, there are two main types of pet therapy programs: animal visiting and animal care. During animal visiting, one or more types of animals are brought into a facility for a visit of a specified length. The animals visit members of a resident group, and may go on room to room visits as well. Residents get ample time to pet and visit with animals, and the visit schedule may be repeated on a regular basis. Other facility programs, such as life review, reminiscence, and therapeutic touch can be enhanced with the use of pet therapy.

Animal care is more involved because it usually means that the facility has adopted a pet or pets, who actually live there full-time, or visit for most of each day. The positives of animal care are the opportunities that residents have to see the animals every day and establish a close bond. Negative considerations include illness and death of the pet, as well as the responsibility of the daily care of the pet that may fall on the activity department. Other factors to think about are the regulations in your state concerning the care of animals in the facility. Many states have set strict guidelines for the protection of residents, staff, and visitors. But despite this, the positives certainly outweigh the negatives. Many professional organizations, such as Therapy Dogs International and the Delta Society, can be of great assistance as you begin your pet therapy program planning. Pet therapy is an easy and rewarding addition to your program agenda because of the benefits it affords your residents.

Phototherapy

As a relative newcomer to the therapy scene, **phototherapy** uses snapshots and family photo albums as a stimulation and bridge to therapeutic communication. Weiser (1993), in her book about the technique, states that "Photographs are footprints of our minds, mirrors of our lives, reflections from our hearts, frozen memories we can hold . . . " and she refers to photographs as "therapeutic tools."

To use the techniques of phototherapy, Weiser suggests an assessment phase of learning about a client may well be aided by the use of photos to understand family relationships and dynamics. There are five techniques outlined in the phototherapy process:

- review of photos taken *of* the client
- review of photos taken *by* the client
- review of self-portraits (client taking photos of himself or herself)
- review of photos of groups of friends or family (biographical shots)
- use of the projective technique

The projective process is defined by Weiser as the act of a client placing his or her own personal values or responses to the viewing of a photograph.

When using the methods of exploring photography with the elderly, a "reproductive, communicative and creative" part of reality emerges, according to Zwick (1978). In working with the phototherapy technique, there are many elements of discovery along the way, but there are also some cautionary notes given by Weiser. Suggestions are made that, without a "therapy" piece for some interpretation, phototherapy becomes a viewing of photographs and nothing more. Weiser mentions that the process should be flexible to the situation in which the technique is being used. With a combined background in art therapy and photography, her abilities to interpret photographs with clients may be easy. For the activity professional trying to make use of some of the phototherapy concepts, a clear adaptation to the needs of residents in long-term care must be made. Although phototherapy has not been thoroughly researched with elderly residents, especially in activity programming, the strong associations and applications to life review and reminiscence help us understand its importance. Further research will be necessary to test the lasting impacts.

Poetry Therapy

Another member of the creative arts therapies, **poetry therapy**, uses a poem ". . . as a catalyst for exploring deeper thoughts and feelings," according to Reiter (1994). Reiter feels that poetry, as an art form, combines the heart, spirit, and mind in pursuit of therapeutic goals.

Often used in conjunction with life review, reminiscence, or bibliotherapy programs, poetry therapy enforces several key points that Reiter describes. First, the storytelling aspects of poetry make the resident feel validated by the fact that someone is interested in listening to their poetry. From a therapeutic standpoint, using poetry to tell his or her important story may release powerful feelings. Using images or "word pictures" to describe a story acts as a method to unlock feelings and emotions that normally would be unavailable.

The process of poetry therapy begins with a trained poetry therapist selecting an appropriate poem that meets the needs of a specific resident or residents. The reading of the poem to the resident by the therapist sets the stage for discussion afterwards. Using specific references in the poem, the poetry therapist tries to illicit a discussion that will trigger memories and release feelings. The sharing of feelings from the resident can be reworked into a poem by the therapist that may be read and discussed at length at another session.

Program challenges that exist in establishing a poetry therapy group were mentioned by Peck (1989). Some of the areas to be aware of include shy residents, fluctuating class size, and speech problems.

Many of the poetry therapy programs can be adapted by an activity professional, but the services of a certified poetry therapist is preferable. The National Association for Poetry Therapy can be of assistance in directing you or describing other program information.

Reality Orientation

Reality orientation, a term initially used to describe a program of treatment for moderate to severe cognitively impaired residents, was pioneered by Dr. Folsom in a veteran's hospital in Kansas in 1959, according to Barnes (1974). Using either a classroom approach or a twenty-four-hour method, appropriate residents, who suffered temporary memory loss or withdrawal, were presented with correct information as to time, place, and person to stimulate a recovery. The classroom method uses small groups, held two or three times a week, led by an instructor who guides participants through appropriate responses. Classroom tools, such as calendars, clocks, and other information boards are used to encourage participation. The twenty-four-hour reality orientation method has the potential for greater effect on the participants because this technique involves the staff. Each opportunity to reinforce correct time, place, and person is used in every possible interaction that staff members have with residents. Hackley (1973) offers the idea that confusion and disorientation can be combatted by ". . . continual, stimulating, repetitive orientation and by encouraging the resident . . . back into his environment."

Although research in the 1970s and early 1980s seemed to indicate that reality orientation might hold a significant answer for the large number of individuals who appeared disoriented and confused upon admission to an institutional setting, Alzheimer's disease research has shown that some cognitive impairments are not reversible, and may not respond to reality orientation techniques. Lloyd (1985) suggests that program goals, such as helping residents function at their highest level

and assisting them in obtaining a sense of self and identity, are important components of the program today. The reality orientation method is easily integrated into activity programs and is still quite useful for helping new residents, with appropriate disease process, make adjustments to their new facility and surroundings.

Remotivation

Finding new ways to ". . . provide an environment and opportunity to activate the untouched areas of a person's personality," is the way that Toepfer, Bicknell, and Shaw (1974) describe the method of **remotivation**. Developed by Dorothy Smith in the 1950s for use by nursing employees in state hospitals, this technique uses a small group format to focus residents on a particular theme, such as a season or event. The technique has five key steps:

- the climate of acceptance
- a bridge to reality
- sharing the world we live in
- an appreciation of the world
- the climate of appreciation

The group is led through this sequence by the group leader.

During the climate of acceptance phase, the leader welcomes the group, thanks them for coming, and greets each member in a friendly way. In the bridge to reality portion, a poem or article is read to the group. The leader encourages participation in group members by reading parts of the article or passing it along. This step is thought to bring an increase in response to positive stimulation from the environment. In the sharing-the-world-we-live-in stage, a theme is chosen by the leader and questions are asked that are intended to bring about a discussion. Visual aids or props, such as pictures or other objects, are used to stimulate responses. During this behavioral phase, the leader responds to answers that relate to the topic, but simply asks a new question when a nonappropriate response is given. The fourth step, appreciation of the world, is where the leader tries to relate the theme to the group's past interests. This stage is thought to center on "normal" behaviors. In the last phase, called the climate of appreciation, the leader focuses on demonstrating pleasure at the achievements of the group, thereby enforcing the positive behaviors of the session.

The techniques described are still in use in many settings: psychiatric, rehabilitation units, and long-term care facilities. Using a modified re-motivation method, Janssen and Giberson (1988) conducted a study in a community-based day care setting with clients who exhibited moderate to severe dementia. The researchers' results supported the fact that the remotivation technique still has applications and usefulness in group settings that include attempts to bridge the perceived and actual reality of residents.

Validation Therapy

Developed by Naomi Feil over a period of years and starting in 1963, the **validation therapy** technique is defined by Feil (1994) as ". . . a therapy for communicating with old-old (over 75 years of age) people who are diagnosed as having Alzheimer's disease and related dementias." Referring to Erikson's life development stages, Feil theorizes that any incomplete tasks from earlier stages of life may emerge for resolution in old age, and the old-old resident will use present day people to unleash many emotions during this resolution. By identifying behavior patterns of the old-old, Feil developed ten beliefs and values that include the concepts of understanding, the uniqueness of all people as individuals, and the value of all people, despite their level of disorientation.

In her book, Feil reports that some of the benefits of participation in validation therapy include a decrease in restraint usage, a resurgence in residents' dignity and feelings of control, and an increase in staff morale. Families of residents are also assisted by finding new ways to relate to and help their relatives.

Feil suggests that the very old who may have unresolved life tasks pass through four key stages of resolution: malorientation, time confusion, repetitive motion, and vegetation. The malorientation stage of resolution is characterized by a need to release emotions that have not been handled in earlier stages of life. Individuals in this stage have had no prior history of mental illness and have recent memories in place. They may fear a loss of control over issues in their life and may blame or accuse others of this. The time confusion stage of resolution is marked by some physical deterioration, as well as some confusion with chronological time. The individuals in this stage may have forgotten names, have little emotional control, and possess a very short attention span. The third stage, repetitive movement, involves members who may show degenerative brain damage and rely on rhythms and other movements to request their needs. Social controls are lost, and

feelings cannot be hidden: these are replaced by sounds and other repetitive movements. The vegetation stage illustrates an individual's end to the struggle within by giving up on the world and retreating inward. Characteristics such as closed eyes, lying in the fetal position, and immobility with no speech are the norms in this stage.

Each stage of resolution requires that the techniques of validation be applied. The ten techniques of validation therapy described by Feil are:

- centering
- using nonthreatening speech
- rephrasing
- use of polarity
- imagining the opposite
- reminiscing
- maintenance of eye contact
- use of ambiguity
- clear, loving tone of voice
- mirroring motions and emotions

Most of the techniques are self-explanatory and easy for professionals to be trained in the methodology. One of the distinct advantages of validation therapy is that a specific therapy background or degree is not required. A training program, however, does exist. An empathetic manner with a desire to soothe residents during these difficult transitions are the only requirements to begin training. Many activity staff and other caregivers have found great success in using this technique in both group and individual settings.

Integrating Activities into Other Facility Programs ....

Restorative

Working with the other members of the interdisciplinary team who primarily are focused on rehabilitative and restorative issues can benefit your program tremendously. Physical therapists, occupational therapists, speech therapists, and physiatrists are team members who have treatment goals for residents that involve motivating them back to a previous (or more independent) medical capacity. The therapy disciplines have different objectives and examples include learning to use an injured leg again and assisting in ADLs, such as combing the hair and improving swallowing techniques.

Their objectives may seem unrelated to your program planning, but there are benefits to be gained by teaming up with other interdisciplinary team members. First, the input from the whole rehabilitative team, in meetings and on the medical record, will be helpful to you as you conduct your activity assessment and continued reassessment of residents. Hearing and reading about the progress of each resident in areas other than yours gives you more insight into the total person and prepares you further for your interventions.

Additionally, there are a number of program opportunities that you may try with the restorative team to add to your overall schedule. Because of the physical aspects of care and the indirect emotional rewards of treatment (such as a feeling of satisfaction in progress), the therapy team may be able to work with you in formal and informal ways to increase the rehabilitative objectives for residents. Some of the joint methods of involving the therapy team with the activity staff include the formation of an ambulation program, establishing a fitness trail, setting up an enhanced dining program, and adding dimension to bed-bound exercise programs. The therapy team can also be consulted for in-service programs or to work together on the encouragement of residents in related goals.

Dining

Although not an activity, the consumption of meals is an anticipated part of the daily routine of the facility for your residents. Programs that involve dietary, nursing, and the activity department to achieve greater goals and a higher quality of life at meal time are becoming more of the norm.

When you break down the elements of the dining experience, you may see opportunities to improve the services that your residents receive as well as expanding your activity program. Remember, your activity program should not be so narrow as to occur at certain times of the day, but instead should be an integral, ongoing part of each resident's day. With that in mind, look at dining elements such as transportation to the dining area, seating arrangements, socialization, environment, assistance with feeding, and cultural considerations that may help you find ways to add to your program. The routine that your facility uses to manage transportation to the dining room may be enhanced by the activity department if you use this time to work with, or talk to, certain residents. Your ambulation or walking program may be part of this as you walk to and from the dining room. The involvement of other departments, such as activity and social services in the ongoing (and ever changing) seating arrangements in the dining room, would certainly be wise. With your knowledge of backgrounds,

hobbies, interests, cultural backgrounds, cognitive levels, and so forth, input to others would be valuable. The dining environment can be enhanced by the combined skills of many departments. Often a dining area is loud because of the commotion caused by the delivery of meals to a large number of people in a short period of time. Using barriers or dividers to create smaller areas, playing dinner music, and using soft colors and simple-to-understand table layouts can create a calming experience for diners. An activity person scheduled for dining room assignment, as a prompter for socializations and a motivator for feeding specific residents, may be a benefit.

Setting up life skill dining experiences for appropriate groups can be an offshoot of the main dining room seating, and can augment your activity program. Eating is one of the most primary activities of daily living. Some mildly cognitively impaired residents can benefit from a combined activity that incorporates the (limited) preparation, serving, and cleanup of a meal as a reinforcement of life skills within a social context. Bowlby (1993) discusses establishing meal groups for appropriate residents and assesses the benefits by saying, "The social setting of mealtime encourages social behavior, improves appetite and promotes overlearned functional responses, such as self-feeding." Setting up a meal group requires some kitchen equipment, such as a sink, at minimum, and some method of reheating foods or making toast. Bowlby suggests selecting participants who have some residual verbal and other functional abilities and identifying goals for members that can be tracked and evaluated by the activity professional over a period of time. Many facilities are experimenting with variations of this concept, and other similar ideas (multiple dining room seatings) with success.

Innovative Settings

Some researchers were unsatisfied with simply using activity programs to meet residents' needs individually, and instead, devised innovative overall facility programs to change the nursing home environment and offer the highest quality of life. Two examples of alternative settings are the Eden Alternative and the Snoezelen Environment.

The Eden Alternative, an environmental concept for nursing homes, was tested in 1991 by Thomas (1994) as an answer to the continued loneliness, helplessness, and boredom that he regularly encountered as a physician practicing in long-term care facilities. By placing ". . . too much emphasis on treatment and far too little on helping residents grow. . . ," he felt that facilities were not offering the kind of surroundings in which residents would thrive. Thomas felt that individuals need companionship, a reason to care for others, and variety in their environment. He, therefore, created the "human habitat" concept. Thinking less as managers and more as maintainers of the habitat would provide a healthier climate. Additionally, building a community of social diversity, where children and animals are involved, compliments the concept.

By "edenizing" the facility, the administrator leads other departments to revise their thinking to include ideas such as giving up the institutional framework to incorporate pets, children, and plants. Other ideas include involving the residents in daily programs and functions that help to maintain the habitat, but ". . . de-emphasizing the programmed activities approach to life. . . ."

As an experiment in progress, some of the benefits of the human habitat, as outlined by Thomas, include medication reductions, a decrease in mortalities, infection reductions, and a positive increase in employee involvement.

To bring the concepts of eden to an existing long-term care environment, Thomas suggests starting ongoing children's programs on-site, hosting regular community group meetings, having facility pets, and bringing plants and horticultural therapy programs into the facility. Perhaps elements of the Eden Alternative already are present in your activity program. The Eden Alternative is a total, facility-wide idea that requires full support of all members. States other than New York are now looking to adopt this concept, and many more are sure to follow.

The Snoezelen environment, defined as a recreational program for children and adults, offers a ". . . blend of sights, sounds, aromas, movement and sensory stimulation in a positive environment" according to Flaghouse (1994). Primarily conceived in Holland as an intervention for those with severe cognitive impairments, this technique of creating a stimulating environment may have applications with certain portions of the elderly long-term care population. For those with profound disabilities, Pinkney (1993) proposes that an environment be created that includes visual, auditory, tactile, and olfactory stimulation. In her work, a somewhat darkened room was prepared with drapes, a partially carpeted floor, rocking chairs, bean bag chairs, music, aroma diffuser, stimulation equipment such as a wall projector to display abstract images, and a bubble making machine. Residents were selected and scheduled for a block of time (thirty minutes) to use the room, making as many of their own seating and interaction choices as possible. The results of Pinkney's research indicates that residents seem to observe the stimulating environment rather than participate in it, but the setting seems to be relaxing and to decrease restlessness.

The ideas used to create the environment are sound, but there is limited available research to support the use of this system in long-term care. The high cost of the projection and other equipment also makes this a limited option for many facilities. Modified versions of a stimulating and soothing environment can be manufactured by resourceful activity professionals while research is being conducted.

Other Types of Programs

There are many other useful activity interventions which may not come under the heading of a treatment, therapy, or modality, but they are very important in the delivery of services.

Reminiscence. **Reminiscence** is defined by Butler (1936) as ". . . the act or process of recalling the past. . . ." The practice of reminiscence is considered a part of the life review process that may occur naturally as an elderly individual approaches death. Havighurst and Glasser (1972) report that two categories of reminiscence exist: oral and silent.

Some of the research concerning reminiscence shows positive results. In an exploration of reminiscence, Havighurst and Glasser (1972) noted a "syndrome" of relatedness between positive social adjustment and high frequency of reminiscence. Merriam and Cross (1981) discovered that those residents who classified reminiscence as enjoyment had higher life satisfaction scores than those residents who felt that reminiscence was used to cope. Hughston and Merriam (1982) concluded that structured reminiscence programs can improve cognitive functioning in females. They also report that reminiscence programs are an activity that most individuals enjoy while working on maintaining their cognitive skills. Lappe (1987) found that higher self-esteem was reported by participants in reminiscence groups versus those in current events groups.

This information and research can be put into application in your schedule through group or individual reminiscence programs. Burnside and Haight (1994) discuss one-on-one encounters with residents and mention that rambling, anxiety, and even catastrophic reactions can be problem areas about which to be aware in individual reminiscence sessions. Group reminiscence can be a difficult task because individual attention is required, and group dynamics need to be taken into account. Burnside and Haight remind us that a key goal of group reminiscence is to bridge new relationships that are founded on current, successful practices. As a part of life therapy, or in collaboration with other program therapy techniques, such as sensory stimulation, art therapy or aromatherapy, reminiscence is a vital program for inclusion in all activity schedules.

Life Review. Butler (1963) conducted the initial research on **life review** and concluded that the "... occurrence in older people of an inner experience or mental process of reviewing one's life" is a universal phenomena. As a potential reaction to approaching death, Butler postulates that a process takes place to deal with outstanding, unresolved

conflicts. Other researchers, such as Hausman (1980), speculate that life review is part of the last stage of development that Erikson described as ego versus despair. Burnside and Haight (1994) update the life review definition as ". . . a process of reviewing, organizing and evaluating the overall picture of one's life with the purpose of achieving integrity by seeing one's own life as a unique story."

As part of psychotherapy, Lewis and Butler (1974) feel that life review is a useful tool because it offers spontaneous and unselective information that may aid the client in an understanding of the past. Kiernat (1979) suggests using life review with cognitively impaired residents to stimulate conversations and increase attention span. In group settings, McMordie and Blom (1979) concluded life review benefits are increased when structure is imposed that includes memory enhancing methods. Some of the topics that were uncovered in life therapy projects conducted by Ellison (1981) included details about hobbies and interests, as well as discussions about loss and sadness. In looking at program enhancements for life review, Kartman (1991) discusses the ways that music therapy can augment a life review project by using songs of a particular era or year to generate certain memories.

Similar to reminiscence, Burnside and Haight (1994) mention that life therapy can be conducted individually or in a group setting, with the use of memory and reminiscence as the primary tools for exploration. They also suggest that a critical aspect of the life review process is an evaluation phase, in which an individual assesses his or her life, and then reaches acceptance.

A thought-provoking process, life review remains an important component of the program and process that an activity professional should be incorporating.

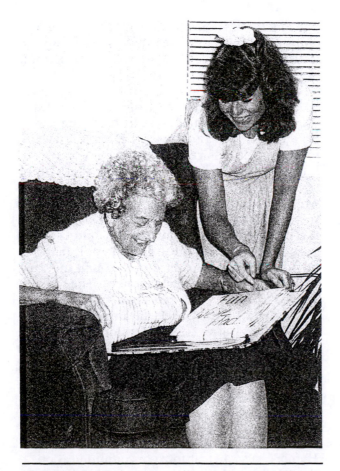

Figure 10–2 Techniques such as reminiscence, life review, or phototherapy can assist residents with their emotional needs.

Sensory. **Sensory stimulation** is a method of activating one or more of the five senses to cause a positive response. Stimulation techniques attempt to make the five senses (vision, touch, smell, taste, and hearing) react. This method uses one or a combination of stimulation ideas to work with regressed or severe cognitively impaired residents or others in which traditional programs often do not work. Oster (1976) suggests that sensory deprivation in the elderly becomes a distinct possibility in light of the increased physical and mental deterioration. Citing the purpose of sensory stimulation or training as a means of slowing the degenerative aging process, Heidell (1972) designed a program that used the stimulation of all five senses during a daily program with successful results. A discussion session resembling reminiscence concluded the program. Erickson and Leide (1992) mention the impacts that sensory stimulation has on reminiscence programs, especially with touch, smell, and taste. They suggest using props and comparisons to generate tactile activities. By showing and letting the participants feel the props (an old silk hat or quilt) memories are stirred. The use of comparisons, such as the difference between an informal housedress and a formal party outfit, can also be helpful. Bridging other program ideas can also be accomplished when starting out with a touch activity. Erickson and Leide discuss how the beginning of a touching event may lead to other programs, such as poetry, music, or art.

The use of the sense of smell is a powerful tool in programming. Earlier, we discussed aromatherapy and the application of this technique to activity programming. Programs using smell for sensory effect can be easily integrated into your calendar. In their article, Erickson and Leide cite results of a 1986 National Geographic survey that found that stronger odors help recall the most vivid memories, whereas distasteful odors are just as likely to prompt a recall as pleasant odors. They suggest such obvious smells as ". . . freshly cut grass to remember summertime or just-baked pumpkin pie for fall. . . ." for use in programs.

Integrating taste into programming can be accomplished simply. Most residents who are physically able love to eat, and will be happy to try some new things, especially if they are reminded of something they used to do. Special tasting events for groups or individuals at the bedside can be planned by using topics, themes, or specific resident interests.

Tapping into visual memories involves the use of any of the visual media: pictures, books, posters, movies, videos, filmstrips, and photographs. As we discussed in the section on phototherapy, looking at a picture often brings back powerful memories and stimulates the senses. Program materials should be large and clear enough for participants to understand their meaning. With the unending array of visual materials available, triggering of the sense of sight can be coordinated easily into an activity program.

Using the sense of hearing to stimulate emotions can be conducted by listening to music, news reports, and other taped programs. Volume, appropriateness of material, and disruptive background noises are all factors that should be considered when planning a program that uses the auditory sense.

Sensory stimulation programs are usually used specifically to meet stimulation goals of one or more of the senses. But there are numerous programs that employ sensory aspects in a diversional manner. Every program that you plan has some aspect of sensory participation of which you may or may not be aware. For example, your exercise group involves touching and listening to the group leader. A party comprises smells, tastes, and visual components. Drama groups involve auditory and visual participation. Becoming more aware of all the sensory components in programming will help you get the most from all your activities.

Humor. The application of **humor** in the treatment of illnesses, and in general, has long been understood. Humor, of course, is the universal experience of joy and laughter. Simon (1988) defines humor as ". . . a coping strategy based on an individual's cognitive appraisal of a stimulus which results in behaviors such as smiling or laughter."

Using the therapeutic aspects of humor and relating them to illness was done dramatically by Cousins (1979) when he used his own personal medical experiences and recovery to outline the positive aspects of humor. In his book, he describes how he recovered from a serious illness using a combination of good medical care, a willingness to live, and humor. He felt that surrounding himself with opportunities to see the humorous side of life would actually aid in his recovery by producing positive chemical changes within his body. Cousins documented his return to health with his well-publicized use of the nontraditional application of humor, and set off a flurry of interest. As a respected person (and former patient) he stepped forward to tout the benefits of humor, and now this knowledge can be applied in other health care areas.

Looking at some of the advantages of humor, Sullivan and Deane (1988) mention how anger or frustration can be reduced with a humorous view of events. With the elderly population facing many changes and losses at once, humor can be an antedote for increasing tensions. According to Sullivan and Deane, the use of humor has been linked to increased pain tolerance, decreases in anxiety and stress, and increases in relaxation. Humor is also a great form of communication, although the authors comment that "mental states such as confusion or depression can impair or preclude humor involvement." Despite a lack of full comprehension for the reasons for humor, the actual act of laughter has positive benefits for all participants.

Simon (1988) discusses previous research on humor that identifies four health related functions of humor: communicative, social, psychological, and physiological. The communication aspects of humor are that trust and bonding are formed in relationships. From a sociological standpoint, humor may help in handling the external pressures of health care. The psychological angle of humor can be seen in the release and reduction of negative feelings, such as anger and tension. From a physiological vantage, positive reactions are seen in heart rate and respiratory functioning when humor and laughter are present. McGuire, Boyd, and James (1992) add that through laughter, skeletal muscles become active and positive hormonal changes take place.

The results of the 1989 Clemson Humor Project, which tried to assess the impact of humor on the quality of life of long-term care residents, were discussed by McGuire, Boyd, and James (1992). Although the findings of the study were mixed, humor was identified as a tool for influencing life satisfaction and overall happiness. Pain reduction through humor intervention was not discovered, but short-term effects of feeling better about medical situations occurred when humorous movies were viewed.

How can humor be integrated into activity programming? Sullivan and Deane (1988) feel that certain circumstances have to be present in order for humor to be present. A relationship must exist between the "humor originator" and the "humor receiver" that allows for a playful atmosphere. An activity professional must account for possible visual and auditory difficulties in interpreting humor, and tailor it to individual tastes. McGuire, Boyd, and James (1992) suggest that "our primary task in setting the stage for humor programs is removal of the prohibitions against laughing." They offer that humorous touches should be added whenever possible to the physical and emotional environment to allow for uninhibited behavior. Additional suggestions, such as creating a joke board, hanging up humorous photos, and setting up a traveling comedy cart, can get the whole staff in the spirit and add much humor in the lives of the residents. New groups, devoted to laughter and humor, can supply you with more referrals and information to help you set up your program.

Touch and Therapeutic Touch. Using the sensory aspects of tactile stimulation as a starting point, **touch** and **therapeutic touch** are two related components of care that should be examined for possible use in activity programming.

Touch, a tactile method for communicating, is defined by Barnett (1972) as ". . . the reaching out to someone. . . to exchange feelings, thoughts and words. . . ." Touch is thought to be a powerful tool in communicating. Barrett explains that sense organs, such as the skin, are managed by receptors to receive signals. Touch can be used in nonverbal communication to express feelings of joy, anger, excitement, and frustration, and is the first form of language any of us knows as infants. To understand the role of touch in medical settings, Barrett proposes looking at some responses that occur during an admission to a hospital or other clinical setting. Physical responses (pain or discomfort) may give way to psychological reactions (anxiety, depersonalization, and regression). Depersonalization is defined as a feeling of removal from one's environment whereas regression is a withdrawal from responsibilities in order to concentrate on other things (in this case, getting well). Another negative, psychological reaction to illness that may occur is sensory deprivation, or the removal of a person from the normal sensory contact required to thrive. Barrett suggests that appropriate touch, used in all aspects of care, can provide a means for generating positive emotions, feelings, and comfort to clients, and prevent some of the psychological reactions listed above. Some cautions in using touch applications apply to situations where pain is present, or in cases such as schizophrenia, where touch could trigger an adverse reaction. When used properly in small doses or by a massage therapist, touch can be a very rewarding experience.

Therapeutic touch or "TT," is defined by Jaroff (1994) as ". . . a controversial form of therapy. . . which not only comforts and relaxes patients, but also relieves pain, produces chemical changes in the blood and promotes healing." Called a "pseudo science" by some, therapeutic touch involves the use of hand motions to "smooth kinks or congestion in the energy field that surrounds every human being," according to Jaroff. Already used in some nursing curriculums and in practice, therapeutic touch should undergo more research before being clinically accepted as a true form of treatment. The Touch For Health Association and other groups can provide information on touch techniques.

SUMMARY

Working with different resident settings can be challenging. Activity analysis and program adapta-tion are useful tools in program implementation. Using the available therapies and treatment modalities to integrate into program planning is vital to offer the most options possible to residents.

R E V I E W   Q U E S T I O N S

1. What program adaptations should be made for subacute residents?
2. What are some of the benefits of dance/movement therapy?
3. Why is reality orientation limited in applications?
4. What are the six areas of creative arts therapies united by NCATA?
5. Why is music therapy so popular?

O N   Y O U R   O W N

1. What are three specific programs you can think of that incorporate aspects of reminiscence, life review, and phototherapy?
2. What other improvements can you make to dining or other facility programs to incorporate activity elements?
3. Using the development of a horticultural therapy sensory garden as the proposed activity, conduct an activity analysis for one of your residents.

R E F E R E N C E S

American Dance Therapy Association (1995). [Brochure]. Columbia, MD: author.

American Horticultural Therapy Association (1993). Horticultural therapy facts. [Brochure]. Gaithers-burg, MD: author.

American Horticultural Therapy Association (1995). People & plants: Growing through horticultural therapy. [Brochure]. Gaithersburg, MD: author.

Austin, D. R. (1982). *Therapeutic recreation processes and techniques*. New York, NY: John Wiley & Sons.

Avenoso, K. (1995). Instrumental medicine: Through music therapy, patients march to the beat of a dif-ferent drummer. *The New York Daily News*, January 8th, 10–11.

Barnes, J. (1974). Effects of reality orientation class-room on memory loss, confusion, and disorienta-tion in geriatric patients. *The Gerontologist*, Vol. 12(2), 138–142.

Barrett, K. (1972). A theoretical construct of the con-cepts of touch as they relate to nursing. *Nursing Research*, Vol. 21, No. 2, 102–110.

Bowlby, C. (1993). *Therapeutic activities with persons dis-abled by Alzheimer's disease and related disorders*. Gaithersburg, MD: Aspen Publishers Inc.

Bumanis, A., & Yoder, J. (1987). Music and dance: Tools for reality orientation. *Activities, Adaptation & Aging*, Vol. 10(1/2), 23–25.

Burgess, C. W. (1990). Horticulture and its application to the institutionalized elderly. *Activities, Adaptation & Aging*, Vol. 14(3), 51–61.

Burnside, I. & Haight, B. (1994). Reminiscence and life review: Therapeutic interventions for older people. *Elsevier Science Inc.*, Vol. 19, No. 4, 55–61.

Bustad, L. K. (1980). *Animals, aging and the aged*. Minneapolis, MN: University of Minnesota Press.

Bustad, L. K., & Hines, L. M. (1983). Placement of ani-mals with the elderly: Benefits and strategies. *California Veterinarian Supplement*, 3, 32a–38a.

Butler, R. (1963). The life review: An interpretation of reminiscence in the aged. *Psychiatry*, 26, 65–76.

Clair, A. (1990). The need for supervision to manage behavior in the elderly care home resident and the implications for music therapy practice. *Music Therapy Perspectives*, Vol. 8, 72–75.

Crepeau, E. (1986). *Activity programming for the elderly*. New York, NY: Little Medical Division/ Little Brown & Co.

Caroleo, O. O. (1988). AIDS: Meeting the needs through therapeutic recreation. *Therapeutic Recreation Journal*, 4th Quarter, 71–78.

Chinn, K., and Joswiak, K. (1981). Leisure education and leisure counseling. *Therapeutic Recreation Journal*, 4th Quarter, 4–7.

Citrin, R., & Dixon, D. (1977). Reality orientation: A milieu therapy used in an institution for the aged. *The Gerontologist*, Vol. 17(1), 39–43.

Colligan, K. (1987). Music therapy and hospice care. *Activities, Adaptation & Aging*, Vol. 10(1/2), 103–122.

Cousins, N. (1983). *Anatomy of an illness as perceived by the patient*. New York, NY: Bantam Books.

Crosson, C. (1976). Art therapy with geriatric patients: Problems of spontaneity. *American Journal of Art Therapy*, Vol. 15, 51–56.

Ellison, K. (1981). Working with the elderly in a life re-view group. *Journal of Gerontological Nursing*, Vol. 7, No. 9, 537–541.

Erickson, L. M., & Leide, K. (1992). Touch, taste and smell the memories. *Activities, Adaptation & Aging*, Vol. 16 (3), 25 – 39.

Fazio, S., & Fralish, K. (1988). A survey of leisure and recreation programs offered by agencies serving traumatic head injured adults. *Therapeutic Recreation Journal*, 1st Quarter, 46–54.

Feil, N. (1994). *The validation breakthrough: Simple techniques for communicating with people with "Alzheimer's type dementia."* Baltimore, MD: Health Professions Press.

Fisher, P. P. (1995). *More than movement for fit to frail older adults: Creative activities for the body mind and spirit*. Baltimore, MD: Health Professionals Press.

Flaghouse Inc. (1994). Snoezelen: Developmentally appropriate recreation. [Brochure]. Mount Vernon, NY: author.

Hackley, J. (1973). Reality orientation brings patients back from confusion and apathy. *Modern Nursing Home*, Sept., 48–49.

Hausman, C. (1980). Life review therapy. *Journal of Gerontological Social Work*, Vol. 3(2), 31–37.

Havighurst, R., & Glasser, R. (1972). An exploratory study of reminiscence. *Journal of Gerontology*, Vol. 27, No. 2, 245–253.

Heidell, B. (1972). Sensory training puts patients "in touch." *Modern Nursing Home*, Vol. 28, 39–43.

Houseman, D. (1986). Developing links between horticultural therapy and aging. *Journal of Therapeutic Horticulture*, Vol. 1, 9–14.

Hughston, G., & Merriam, S. (1982). Reminiscence: A nonformal technique for improving cognitive functioning in the aged. *International Journal of Aging & Human Development*, Vol. 15(2), 139–149.

Janssen, J., & Giberson, D. (1988). Remotivation therapy. *Journal of Gerontological Nursing*, Vol. 14, No. 6, 31–34.

Jaroff, L. (1994). A no-touch therapy. *Time*, Nov. 21st, 88–89.

Jennings, S. (1978). *Remedial drama: A handbook for teachers and therapists*. New York, NY: Theatre Arts Books.

Johnson, D. (1982). Principles & techniques of drama therapy. *The Arts In Psychotherapy*, Vol. 9, 83–90.

Kartman, L. L. (1980). The power of music with patients in a nursing home. *Activities, Adaptation & Aging*, Vol. 1(1), 9–17.

Kartman, L. L. (1991). Life review: One aspect of making meaningful music for the elderly. *Activities, Adaptation & Aging*, Vol. 15(3), 45–57.

Karras, B. (1987). Music and reminiscence: For groups and individuals. *Activities, Adaptation & Aging*, Vol. 10(1/2), 79–91.

Kiernat, J. (1979). The use of life review activity with confused nursing home residents. *The American Journal of Occupational Therapy*, Vol. 33(5), 306–310.

Knoll, C. (1992). Music therapy: An effective tool in health care. *Focus on Geriatric Care & Rehabilitation*, Vol. 5(10), 1–2.

Kubler-Ross, E. (1987). AIDS: The ultimate challenge.

New York, NY: Macmillan.

Labarca, J. (1979). Communication through art therapy. *Perspectives in Psychiatric Care*, Vol. 17, No. 3, 118–122.

Lappe, J. M. (1987). Reminiscing: The life review therapy. *Journal of Gerontological Nursing*, Vol. 13, No. 4, 12–16.

Leary, S. (1994). *Activities for personal growth*. Sydney, Australia: MacLennan & Petty Pty Limited.

Leitner, M. J., and Leitner, S. I. (1985). *Leisure in later life: A sourcebook for the provision of recreational services for elders*. Binghamton, NY: Haworth Press.

Lewallen, M. (1987). Adding life to the place: Musical activities in the nursing home. *Activities, Adaptation & Aging*, Vol. 10(1/2), 47–62.

Lewis, M., & Butler, R. (1974). Life- review therapy: Putting memories to work in individual and group psychotherapy. *Geriatrics*, Vol. 29, 165–173.

Lewis, J. F., & Mattson, R. H. (1988). Gardening may reduce blood pressure of elderly people: Activity suggestions and models for intervention. *Journal of Therapeutic Horticulture*, Vol. 3, 25–37.

Lindner, E. (1982). Dance as a therapeutic intervention for the elderly. *Educational Gerontology*, 8, 167–174.

Lipe, A. (1987). A justification of music therapy in the nursing home setting. *Activities, Adaptation & Aging*, Vol. 10(1/2), 17–22.

Lloyd, C. (1985). Reality orientation: Its application as a ward based program for the institutionalized elderly. *Activities, Adaptation & Aging*, Vol. 7(2), 91–97.

Luczak, M. (1980). Activities appropriate for the brain-injured population. *Therapeutic Recreation Journal*, 3rd Quarter, 21–25.

Lynch, L. (1987). Music therapy: Sets historical relationship and value in programs for the long-term care setting. *Activities, Adaptation & Aging*, Vol. 10(1/2), 5–15.

McGuire, F., Boyd, R., & James, A. (1992). *Therapeutic humor with the elderly*. Binghamton, NY: The Haworth Press.

McMordie, W., & Blom, S. (1979). Life review therapy: Psychotherapy for the elderly. *Perspectives in Psychiatric Care*, Vol. 17, No. 4, 162–166.

Merriam, S. & Cross, L. (1981). Aging, reminiscence and life satisfaction. *Activities, Adaptation & Aging*, Vol. 2(1), 39–50.

Moore, B. (1989). *Growing with gardening: A twelve-month guide for therapy, recreation and education*. Chapel Hill, NC: The University of North Carolina Press.

Naumberg, M. (1966). *Dynamically oriented art therapy: Its principles and practice*. New York, NY: Grune & Stratton.

National Association For Music Therapy Inc. (1994). NAMT fact sheet. [Brochure]. Silver Spring, MD: author.

National Association For Music Therapy Inc. (1994). Music therapy and elderly persons. [Brochure]. Silver Spring, MD: author.

Nightingale, F. (1946). *Notes on nursing: What it is, and*

what it is not. Facsimile edition, New York, NY: D. Appleton–Century Co.

Oster, C. (1976). Sensory deprivation in geriatric patients. *Journal of The American Geriatrics Society,* Vol. 24, No. 10, 461–464.

Peck, C. (1989). *From deep within: Poetry workshops in nursing homes.* Binghamton, NY: The Haworth Press.

Peterson, C. A. and Gunn, S. L. (1984). *Therapeutic recreation program design: Principles and procedures.* Englewood Cliffs, NJ: Prentice Hall.

Pinkney, L. (1993). Snoezelen: An evaluation of a sensory environment used by people who are elderly and confused. Unpublished manuscript. Mount Vernon, NY: Flaghouse Inc.

Reisberg, B., Ferris, S., DeLeon, M., & Crook, T. (1982). The global deterioration scale for assessment of primary degenerative dementia. *American Journal of Psychiatry,* 139(9), 1136–1139.

Reiter, S. (1994). Enhancing the quality of life for the frail elderly: Rx, the poetic prescription. *Pride Institute Journal,* Vol. 13(2), 12–19.

Relf, P. (1994). *Gardening in raised beds and containers for older gardeners and individuals with physical disabilities.* Petersburg, VA: Virginia Tech/Virginia Cooperative Extension.

Riddick, C., & Keller, M. J. (1991) Developing recreation services to assist elders who are developmentally disabled. In J. Keller (Ed.). *Activities with developmentally disabled elderly and older adults,* (19–33). Binghamton, NY: Haworth Press

Riordan, R.. & Williams, C. (1988). Gardening therapeutics for the elderly. *Activities, Adaptation & Aging,* Vol. 11(1/2), 103–111.

Rose, J. (1992). *The aromatherapy book: Applications and inhalations.* Berkeley, CA: North Atlantic Books.

Rothert, E., & Daubert, J. (1981). *Horticultural therapy for nursing homes, senior centers & retirement living.* Glencoe, IL: Chicago Horticultural Society.

Sandel, S. (1987). Developing a movement therapy program for geriatric patients. *Activities, Adaptation & Aging,* Vol. 9(3), 41–47.

Sandel, S. (1992). Aging artfully: Health benefits of art and dance. Testimony presented at the U.S. Senate Special Committee on Aging Hearing, Washington, DC.

Simon, J. (1988). The therapeutic value of humor in aging adults. *Journal of Gerontological Nursing,* Vol. 14(8), 9–13.

Smith, S. (1990). The unique power of music therapy benefits Alzheimer's patients. *Activities, Adaptation & Aging,* Vol. 14(4), 59–63.

Sullivan, J., & Deane, D. (1988). Humor and health. *Journal of Gerontological Nursing,* Vol. 14, No. 1, 20–24.

Thews, V., Reaves, A., & Henry, R. (1993). *Now what? A handbook of activities for adult day programs.* Winston-Salem, NC: Bowman Gray School of Medicine of Wake Forest University.

Toepfer, C., Bicknell, A., & Shaw, D. (1974). Remotivation as behavior therapy. *The Gerontologist,* Vol. 12, 451–453.

Thomas, W. (1994). *The Eden Alternative: Nature, hope and nursing homes.* Shelburne, NY: Eden Alternative Foundation.

Turner, N., & Keller, M. J. (1988). Therapeutic recreation practitioners' involvement in the AIDS epidemic. *Therapeutic Recreation Journal,* 3rd Quarter, 12–22.

Wade, F. (1987). Music and movement for the geriatric resident. *Activities, Adaptation & Aging,* Vol. 10(1/2), 37–46.

Weiser, J. (1993). *Phototherapy techniques: Exploring the secrets of personal snapshots and family albums.* San Francisco, CA: Jossey- Bass Inc. Publishers.

Weissert, W., Elston, J, Bold, E., Cready, C., Zelman, W., Sloane, P., Kalsbeek, W., Mutran, E., Rice, T., & Koch, G. (1989). Models of adult day care: Findings from a national survey. *The Gerontologist,* Vol. 29, No. 5, 640–649.

Zwick, D. (1978). Photography as a tool toward increased awareness of the aging self. *Art Psychotherapy,* Vol. 5, 135–141.

F U R T H E R   R E A D I N G

Aronoson, D., & Graziano, A. (1976). Improving elderly clients' attitudes through photography. *The Gerontologist,* Vol. 16, No. 4, 363–367.

Berger, L., & Berger, M. (1973). A holistic group approach to psychogeriatric outpatients. *International Journal of Group Psychotherapy,* Vol. 23, 432–444.

Buettner, L. (1988). Utilizing developmental theory and adaptive equipment with regressed geriatric patients in therapeutic recreation. *Therapeutic Recreation Journal,* 3rd Quarter, 72–79.

Burch, M., Reiss, M., & Bailey, J. (1985). A facility-wide approach to recreation programming for adults who are severely and profoundly retarded. *Therapeutic Recreation Journal,* 3rd Quarter, 71–78.

Cable, T., & Udd, E. (1988). Therapeutic benefits of a wildlife observation program. *Therapeutic Recreation Journal,* 4th Quarter, 65–70.

Douglas, D. (1989). *Accent on rhythm-music activities for the aged,* 3rd ed. St Louis: MMB Music Inc.

Forsythe, E. (1988). One-to-one therapeutic recreation activities for the bed and/or room bound. *Activities, Adaptation & Aging,* Vol. 13(1/2), 63–76.

Gibbons, A. C. (1988). A review of literature for music development education and music therapy with the elderly. *Music Therapy Perspectives,* 5, 33–40.

Graubarth- Szyller, B., & Padgett, J. (1989). *Longevity therapy: An innovative approach to nursing home care of the elderly.* Philadelphia, PA: The Charles Press.

Gropper- Katz, E. (1987). Reality orientation research. *Journal of Gerontological Nursing,* Vol. 13, No. 8, 13–18.

Gwinnup, P. (1985). *Fragrance projects for sensory stimulation*. Buffalo, NY: Potentials Development Inc.

Hackman, R., & Wagner, E. (1988). Gardening for health. *National Gardening*, February, 56–57.

Hegland, A. (1990). Activities for low-functioning residents. *Contemporary Long-Term Care*, July.

Joswiak, K. (1980). Recreation therapy assessment with developmentally disabled persons. *Therapeutic Recreation Journal*, 4th Quarter, 29–38.

Karras, B. (1987). *"You bring out the music in me": Music in nursing homes*. Binghamton, NY: Haworth Press.

Keller, M. J., & Turner, N. (1986). Creating wellness programs with older people: A process for therapeutic recreators. *Therapeutic Recreation Journal*, 4th Quarter, 6–14.

Knoth, M. (1990). *Activity planning at your fingertips*. Lafayette, IN: Valley Press.

Koch, K. (1977). *I never told anybody: Teaching poetry writing in a nursing home*. New York, NY: Random House.

Kutlenios, R. (1987). Healing mind and body: A holistic perspective: *Journal of Gerontological Nursing*, Vol. 13, No. 12., 9–14.

Li, R. (1981). Activity therapy and leisure counseling for the schizophrenic population. *Therapeutic Recreation Journal*, 4th Quarter, 44–50.

Linden, D. (1994). Here they don't have to compete. *Forbes*, January 17th, 102–103.

Lucia, C. (1987). Toward developing a model of music therapy intervention in the rehabilitation of head trauma patients. *Music Therapy Perspectives*, 4, 34–39.

Mace, N., & Rabins, P. (1991). *The 36-hour day*. New York, NY: Warner Books.

McCandless, P., McCready, K., & Knight, L. (1985). A model animal therapy program for mental health settings. *Therapeutic Recreation Journal*, 2nd Quarter, 55–63.

Pollinque, A., & Cobb, H. (1986). Leisure education: A model facilitating community integration for moderately/severely mentally retarded adults. *Therapeutic Recreation Journal*, 3rd Quarter, 54–62.

Randall-Riley, A. (1995). Exotic animals are outstanding in pet therapy. *Animals, Exotic & Small Magazine*, Jan., 26.

Reigler, J. (1980). Comparison of a reality orientation program for geriatric patients with and without music. *Journal of Music Therapy*, Vol. 17 (1), 26–33.

Relf, D. (1981). Dynamics of horicultural therapy. *Rehabilitation Literature*, Vol. 42(5/6), 147–150.

Rosin, A., Matz, E., & Carmi, S. (1977). How painting can be used as a clinical tool. *Geriatrics*, January, 41–46.

Sandel, S., & Johnson, D. (1987). *Waiting at the gate: Creativity and hope in the nursing home*. Binghamton, NY: The Haworth Press.

Schlenger, G. (1988). *Come sit by me: Discussion programs for activity specialists*. Owings Mills, MD: National Health Publishing.

Schultz, W. (1987). Age is no barrier. *National Gardening*, March, 48–50.

Schwebel, A. (1993). Psychological principles applied in horticultural therapy. *Journal of Therapeutic Horticulture*, Vol. 7, 3–12.

Steward, J., & Croft, M. (1988). *The leisure pen: A book for elderwriters*. Plover, WI: Keepsake Publishers.

Tabourne, C. (1991). The effects of a life review recreation therapy program on confused nursing home residents. *Topics In Geriatric Rehabilitation*, Vol. 7, No. 2, 13–21.

Toughill, E. (1990). Creativity can make a difference. *Geriatric Nursing*, Nov./Dec., 276–277.

Ulrich, R. 1984). View through a window may influence recovery from surgery. *Science*, Vol. 224, 420–421.

Vanderark, S., Newman, K., & Bell, S. (1983). The effects of music participation on quality of life of the elderly. *Music Therapy Perspectives*, 3, 71–81.

Voelkl, L., & Wverch, B. (1981). A comprehensive approach to leisure education and leisure counseling for the severely handicapped person. *Therapeutic Recreation Journal*, 4th Quarter, 24–35.

Warren, A. C. H. (1994). *Into the lives of others: Moments of connection—four years with nursing home residents*. New York, NY: The Tiresias Press.

Weiss, J. (1984). *Expressive therapy with elders and the disabled: Touching the heart of life*. New York, NY: The Haworth Press.

Weiss, C., & Jamieson, N. (1988). Hidden disabilities: A new enterprise for therapeutic recreation. *Therapeutic Recreation Journal*, 4th Quarter, 9–17.

Wickwire, G. (1955). Activity analysis for rehabilitation. *Archives of Physical Medicine and Rehabilitation*, Vol. 36, 578–586.

C H A P T E R   1 1
•••••••••••••••••••••••••
Marketing and Group Leadership

OBJECTIVES ....

After completing this chapter, you should:

- understand how internal and external marketing techniques help sell your program
- utilize group leadership skills and techniques to succeed with group programming
- plan programs with knowledge of resident behaviors

INTRODUCTION

Marketing, through internal and external means, assists you in drawing attention to your department and programs. Group dynamics and their effective use are instrumental in helping you run successful group activity programs. Leadership techniques, along with successful group activity programs, provide you with the background to manage your programs.

Marketing Your Program Internally ....

Having taken the time to establish your program, you now have the task of marketing your program to all the key players. **Marketing**, defined as the act of selling a particular service or product, is an important component in the success of your program. To sell your program (which is your product), you can utilize both internal and external methods.

Why consider the marketing aspects of your program? You may feel that you have carefully planned your program with the residents' needs in mind, so why should you be concerned about making specific plans to sell what you have developed?

The three main groups in your facility to whom you will market your programs are the residents and their families, the staff, and your administrator or owner. Effectiveness of your program will be lost unless the individuals whom you serve (your residents and indirectly, the facility staff) have a need for your services and see the value in your activity program. Thorn (1984) discussed this issue, and suggests that promotion, which she defines as ". . . that portion of the marketing plan concerning communication," is one of the key factors in marketing. This communication is accomplished by simply informing individuals of the program or using an aggressive effort toward education. In his work, Patterson (1987) discussed how program promotion can be accomplished through personal messages in verbal, written, or visual form.

Internal marketing methods, such as decorations, staff in-service programs, and the use of calendars and newsletters are all important parts of the process.

Newsletters

Using a **newsletter** is an effective way to build a facility community as you market your programs and projects. A newsletter is a written or pictorial publication of a particular business with specific goals and objectives. One of the best things about a facility newsletter is the fact that it can be done on any budget. If you do not have a facility newsletter, start one, but be clear with your administrator concerning the responsibilities of all involved. Even though the newsletter may be initiated by the activity department, it is an example of a team effort that cannot succeed unless all parties are committed to it.

To establish a new newsletter or refine an existing one, Hartmann (1992) offers these benefits of his experience: develop a family atmosphere, improve knowledge, and increase performance. The impact of a newsletter is probably felt the most by the activity department because it is a constant reminder of upcoming programs and their importance, and is a large part of the selling and success of the department. Meals, nursing, and other forms of care follow more of a routine, but the activity department offers changes from month to month, and a newsletter is a perfect way to keep upcoming programs in focus.

Before jumping into the production of a newsletter, there are some things to consider. First, decide how frequently the newsletter will come out. Will it be monthly, bimonthly, or quarterly? Who will be in charge of the newsletter and what mechanisms are in place to see that the final product is of a high caliber? Hartmann feels that internal newsletters have to define goals, mention the departments involved, have an approval process for information in place, be incorporated in the budget, and, of course, have a system of delivery of the newsletter to its intended reader. Is the newsletter really just for the residents' enjoyment or should staff be involved? If the newsletter is to be distributed to family members and friends, will information about staff activities be of interest?

Hartmann (1992) talks about steps in the general production of any newsletter applicable to a facility newsletter that you may be trying to produce. One of the first steps is to decide on a design. Will the newsletter be one page or multiple pages? Will it be produced in color or black and white? Will it contain photos? Will it be serious in intent or be lighthearted? Is a masthead (a list of all the key participants) necessary?

The next two steps involve the personnel who will be involved with the overall production of the newsletter (i.e., the writing and typing). Will you get assistance from other departments for news information, as well as help in handling the production? Can the overall duties be divided among all the departments? Will it be typed and copied in-house or will it be sent out to be produced professionally? The budget allotted for the project, as well as a realistic time frame, will give you the answers to some of your initial questions.

The questions above are meant to help activity professionals starting a newsletter from scratch. Here are some of the ideas to help you begin the process:

1. Meet with your administrator to discuss your ideas for a newsletter. Come prepared to talk about cost, number of copies, who might be involved, and so forth.
2. Conclude your meeting with a "go or no go" as to whether you will produce the newsletter. Use the following outline for newsletter preparation suggested by Lamken (1980), and be sure to answer the questions in each of these key categories concerning your newsletter:
   a. What is its purpose, who will read it, and what will its content be?
   b. What format will the newsletter follow, and will there be a theme for each issue?
   c. How will material be gathered? Who will write and edit the newsletter?
   d. Who will prepare the layout and do the printing and collating?
   e. How will the newsletters be distributed?

Other critical issues on production that should be discussed include the size of the newsletter, production timetable, content, and other editorial issues. A standard 8 1/2" by 11" size paper that can be folded and self-addressed for mailing works well for many facilities. If the size of the newsletter is too small, the ability to read the print (which must also get smaller) could be impaired. The intended readers should dictate the size of the newsletter and the size of the type as well.

A production timetable is important to establish and share with others so they understand the time constraints of their role in the process. If you are planning to distribute finished copies of your newsletter the first of every month, you might set up a production timetable similar to this:

- 5th–10th of each month — collect material for the next issue
- 11th–15th — prepare and do layout for issue
- 16th–20th — fill-ins and first proof reviewed
- 21st–23rd — administrator's review of proof
- 24th–25th — final proof prepared/photos inserted
- 26th–30th — printing, folding, collating
- 1st–4th — distribution
- process begins again

Setting the tone for the newsletter by the information you present may come slowly. At first, it may appear to be a commercial for the activity department because you may not have gathered enough support from other departments or secondary sources for material. If your newsletter's defined purpose is to serve your residents, their families, and the limited community (determined by you through your mailing list), offer material that meets their needs and include all participants. Remember that most people love to see their names in print. The following lists some things you may wish to include in your newsletter to reach each audience:

- *For residents*: activity calendar, highlighted special events, notice of special visits (voter registration, and the like), resident profile, resident birthday list, new admissions
- *For staff*: in-service dates, information about events in each department, special events, employee activities
- *For families and friends*: special events, family functions (milestone birthdays, promotions, and so forth), news about the facility in general (i.e., update on renovations)
- *For the community*: events for the public, community meetings, pictures of the facility

How you present your material each month can be easy if you rough out a "dummy" or template in which you place material for each issue. A sample dummy for page one of a fictitious issue is shown in Figure 11–1. If you prepare a dummy for the size issue you plan to produce, your rough plan will show you where and how much material you need. Plan on including illustrations, drawings, and photographs whenever possible. They will add a great deal of interest to your project.

If you are the editor of the newsletter, you will face some interesting challenges. You may have to trim departmental news or make adjustments to balance your subject matter. You may have to completely (but politely!) reject some material as inappropriate. There will be complaints made no matter what you do, so be prepared. As editor, if you keep your intended audience in mind as you review material, you should be on the right track.

Facility Identifiers and Decorations

Marketing your program visually can be accomplished by using facility identifiers and other decorations. Thorn (1984) discussed "packaging" your program, or allowing your programs to be exposed for the participants to see. Activity professionals have many chances to take advantage of visual marketing opportunities that exist throughout most facilities. Although program space can often be a problem, vertical space needed for wall or other visual presentations are usually underused.

Your lobby or entrance area is the first place that all new (and potential) admissions, families, and the general public see as they enter your facility. A first impression is made by the viewer as to the information and surroundings of the lobby area. In discussing some marketing guidelines for recruiting admissions, Partin (1986) acknowledges that when visitors have to wait for tours or other information, "a comfortable waiting area, with

NEWSLETTER LOGO		
ISSUE #: _____	DATE: _____	
LETTER OF WELCOME	LETTERS TO THE EDITOR	WINNER OF LAST MONTH'S CONTEST
		POEM
BIRTHDAYS		UPCOMING EVENTS
	PHOTO	
QUOTE OF THE MONTH		EDITORIAL INFORMATION

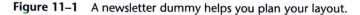

Figure 11–1   A newsletter dummy helps you plan your layout.

reading material or craft displays, makes the time pass more quickly." An easy way to be a part of the first impression in the lobby area is through presentation of an activity calendar mounted colorfully on an easel or special frame. Showcases that lock, but have window access for viewing can be used to display completed projects or draw special attention to upcoming theme programs. Display racks that hold newsletters or other flyers from the activity department also create interest. You may even be lucky enough to have an entrance area that has a corner or a space for seating that you can "take over," and transform each month (or bimonthly) into a special display of your choosing. When you get the attention of every visitor as they first enter the building, you are marketing your "product" effectively.

Around the facility and in your actual program areas, you may find wall space that will accommodate bulletin boards of all sizes. Along with some arts and crafts supplies, these are inexpensive ways to trumpet your programs. Some facilities have found it wise to designate a special bulletin board for resident announcements, such as the telephone number for the ombudsman's office, Department of Health information, and residents' rights guidelines. Residents can also use the space to post their own announcements. The use of other bulletin boards around the facility are limited only by your imagination. You can use them for seasonal themes or change them to correspond with particular special events. Tying the bulletin boards into a facility project, such as fitness month for residents and staff is another use. No matter how you use them, if you gain extra positive attention for your programs, you have achieved much!

Decorating for holidays and seasonal events also helps you sell your programs and makes your residents feel comforted that traditions from home are remembered. Every facility is different in the space it has available for decorating, but the areas that could be used include activity rooms, dayrooms, hallways, nursing stations, closet doors, resident room doors, and dining rooms.

Walls and doors of resident rooms provide spots for small decorations and reaffirmations of resident identity. Doors can be designed with seasonal items for purely decorative purposes, or the areas can be used for resident identification with pictures or other memory-triggering memorabilia. Resident wishes should prevail, and all decorative items should be safe for the inhabitants of a particular area, as well as being tasteful and adult-oriented. Many things can be accomplished inside resident rooms. In addition to traditional bulletin boards with mementos and wall photos, mobiles, suncatchers, memory boxes, and biography boards can help during program implementation. Mobiles can be custom made, using wire and string, tailored to the interests of a particular resident. Suncatchers, used on windows, reflect light and create interesting designs. Preparing memory boxes for mild cognitively impaired residents can be a fun project, especially when the box is mounted in the room as a decoration between program visits. Biography boards give staff and visitors cues about a resident and can be mounted near the bedside in frames or on boards. Memory boxes and biography boards can contain old pictures, information about a resident's hometown or upbringing, or anything that could trigger a memory for the resident or an opportunity for an interaction.

No matter how excited you get in planning your decorations and identifiers, safety issues must be stressed. Wayfinding techniques, discussed in Chapter 6, can be incorporated into your decorating preparation. Oversized signs, wall arrows, footprints, and other helpful identifiers can fit into your overall decorating plan. Facility decorating, which sounds unnecessary and frivolous, can really be a strong marketing focus, as well as a key method for identification for your residents, staff, and families.

Employee Involvement

Marketing may involve staff in two ways: one, by the ability of you and your staff to act as facility advocates to sell the facility through your programs, and two, by offering employee activity programs that sell the facility to all who work there.

Activity programs in progress make a great marketing statement to prospective residents and families touring the facility, as well as to any drop-in visitors. Seeing residents engaged and content in the busy confines of a program dispels the idea that a long-term care facility is an inactive place. Your activity program should be a high point of any tour, with stops made at programs in progress and introductions to activity staff members, when appropriate.

Planning employee activities as a morale booster has other indirect effects. It allows your own long-term care community to grow and markets the services of the activity department to the other departments in the facility. Every facility is different in its approach to staff functions, but most organizations welcome the opportunity to have a department coordinate a bus trip, special event, or other function. Often, these employee programs are offshoots of regular special programming, and affords added benefits. For example, you might schedule a '50s party for your residents and encourage your general staff to attend and give them incentives to assist. You could give a preplanning party for employees who help, then schedule raffles or award special prizes to employee participants.

Forming an employee event council is another good way to help employees bond, as well as ensure support for your regular resident programs. Headed by the activity department, a committee composed of at least one employee from each department can meet on a frequent basis to plan employee functions and improve facility life. As the committee works together on employee projects, it is natural for a rapport to develop that will certainly have beneficial impacts on resident care and relationships.

Marketing Your Program Externally ....

Dealing positively with the public is an important skill to master. Long-term care facilities have the unique characteristic of being open around the clock, but with specific visiting hours: usually 8:00 a.m. to 8:00 p.m. The public comes in for many reasons all day long: tours, visits, performances, deliveries, and so forth. Having the opportunity to interact with the public as they visit, as well as the time to use external channels to make a favorable statement in the outside community, makes sense for activity professionals who are in need of building a quality program. External marketing ideas, such as community involvement, press releases, and a speaker's bureau adds much to draw attention to your growing program.

External Newsletter

The *internal* newsletter you put together for your residents and staff can be useful in external settings that can give you marketing clout. By developing an *external* mailing list that consists of the names of hospital social workers, community based aging groups, residential or assisted living homes (who may need to place clients in your facility), and prominent community members

(mayor, councilman), you will form a written link to advocates of your facility. By using your newsletter to reach these individuals and groups, you have positively positioned your facility as a vital member of the community by informing them of the continued active status of residents.

In addition to mailing out additional copies of an existing newsletter, some facilities have found an opportunity to develop a second professional newsletter to reach particular community members. Tailoring a brief newsletter to give information on regulations, changes in the Medicaid guidelines, coping skills, and so forth, you may be able to perform a community service by reaching out to current caregivers in your area who may eventually need your services. A newsletter with a particular slant can be created for any identified community group who requires specialized information concerning health care services. Some of the groups include physicians, hospital social workers, and informal caregivers. A project of this magnitude may require assistance from other departments such as social services or administration, but the results could be very favorable to the educational and marketing objectives you seek. With increased exposure in the community, your chances for impacting community members with specific information on your activity programming increases.

Community Programs

True community programs take many forms and will be discussed more fully in Chapter 17. Using community programs as a marketing strategy, however, can be a win-win situation for you and outside groups.

Bringing the community "in" for mutual benefit can be accomplished by three methods. First, when you book an outside entertainer or speaker, you provide your residents with a subtle connection to the community. Although you do not look at this as marketing, any time a person visits your facility and leaves with a positive impression of your program, you have provided a form of marketing. A second, more structured way to market occurs when you host large, joint programs with community agencies at the facility. Functions such as a health fair, voter registration drive, craft show, or flea market, bring community members in for an educational and soft selling marketing objective. Take this idea further and you can employ a third marketing strategy by offering the use of facility space for regular meetings or special events sponsored by various community organizations and clubs. When they come into your facility on a regular basis, groups such as the 4H or Lion's Club become the extended community, and are grateful for a place to meet while providing your residents with a connection to the outside world.

Press Releases

Many of your programs may have appeal to individuals outside of your facility, but many may have limited exposure to your programs because of traditional methods. Promoting your specialty and general interest programs to local papers, association newsletters, and professional publications serves to alert people about the special attributes of your program.

Because the busy production schedule of most newspapers and other professional publications, selling your programs through the use of a **press release** is a time-saving method. A press release is a compact version of your program that answers the journalist's questions of who, what, where, when, why and how. Many publications and local newspapers print their own guidelines for submitting press releases by supplying standard forms to complete. Others require that you submit your information in a specific format, or follow a standardized format for press releases or articles, such as the Associated Press. The "who" of the press release should have identifiable people, with their names spelled correctly (James Smith, Ph.D., formerly of Bar Harbor, Maine). The "what" should give a brief sentence about your facility or organization (sponsored by the Jerome Foundation). The "where" should give the location (at the Chauncey Care Center auditorium). The "when" (on January 17th, 20XX at 6:00 pm) gives the date and time. The "why" gives the reason for the event (to celebrate his 75th year of teaching), and the "how" gives information on how to attend (reservations can be made by calling (090)555-1234 before January 1st). Once you answer these questions about your function, you are ready to prepare a release. Press releases should be brief, no more than one or two pages in length and typed double-spaced for easy reading. Write a draft, reread it, and ask a colleague to look at it. Add your name as contact person at the bottom of the release in case any questions arise. The volume of facts does not matter; what does count is concise, clear material. Be sure that all your key information is highlighted and the most important material does not get lost in a sea of information.

What constitutes a good news story? Opinions vary, and some newspapers have an opinion about what makes good copy. A few papers will only cover milestone birthdays (such as 95, 100), whereas other special occasions are not considered important. Other papers want you to go out of your way to establish a rapport with them, to show them that you have many wonderful human interest stories, and follow up by repeat calling and sending releases to get attention.

Photographs speak volumes and can really sell a story. Most newspapers prefer to have their own photographer shoot pictures of a special event. However, because they take a picture does not always mean you will see it in print. Help your press release to be accepted by sending in a good black and white photograph along with it.

If, despite your best efforts, your press releases are not being accepted, contact the editorial staff of the publication. By not following the specific guidelines of the publication or giving confusing or incomplete information may result in repeated rejections. Sometimes the draw of bigger news stories take temporary priority for a particular paper, but with patience and time, your press releases and press coverage should work. A sample press release form is shown in Figure 11–2.

Speaker's Bureau

An ambitious but rewarding project, comes with the formation of a **speaker's bureau**. A speaker's bureau is a compilation of nonprofessional speech-makers brought together to speak on related topics. According to Lovejoy (1988), setting up a speaker's bureau follows some of these steps:

- formulating the idea for the bureau
- defining the intended audience
- securing and training the speakers
- arranging a speaking schedule

Having a group of speakers available to present topics to a group can be a form of community outreach that demonstrates the educational and medical services that your facility can offer. Topics can be based on requests, such as literature searches, talking to community caregivers, and listening to other civic leaders about their needs. As a speaker, you present the topic as an acknowledged expert in the field. You act as a representative of your organization and show further credibility for the goals and objectives of your facility as you do so.

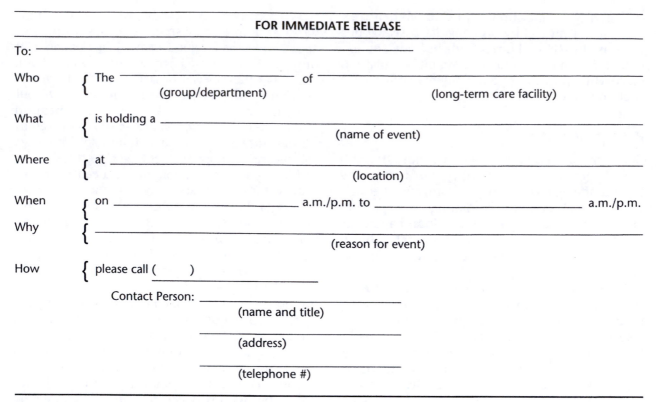

FOR IMMEDIATE RELEASE

To: _____

Who { The _____ of _____
            (group/department)   (long-term care facility)

What { is holding a _____
                    (name of event)

Where { at _____
                  (location)

When { on _____ a.m./p.m. to _____ a.m./p.m.

Why { _____
                  (reason for event)

How { please call (_____) _____

       Contact Person: _____
                 (name and title)

             _____
                 (address)

             _____
                 (telephone #)

Figure 11–2 The elements of a press release.

Group and Leadership Skills ....

Developing competency and self-assurance in the area of leadership and working with groups provides you with the skills you need to run programs, lead groups, and interact effectively with residents, staff, and families. As an activity professional you have the opportunity to act as a leader to host groups and to act as a facilitator (see Figure 11–3). Leading a group requires special skills to manage the needs and behaviors of that group. Acting as a facilitator is a role often used in individual or group work with the cognitively impaired. Instead of leading from a central point, as facilitator you move from individual to individual or table to table to ensure that residents are progressing on their projects. If needed, assist them in starting again or moving on to a different level of programming.

Before you can begin thinking about group dynamics or leadership skills, consider how the experience of aging impacts your ability as a group leader and the dynamics of your group. Toseland (1990) points out that most deliverers of services to the elderly have not personally experienced the changes in development that are felt by older clients. He suggests, therefore, that the negative image of aging be removed, and replaced by a sensitization to the issues of the elderly before

progress can be made. Fortunately, Toseland states that most of the elderly handle their loss of some roles that come as a part of the aging

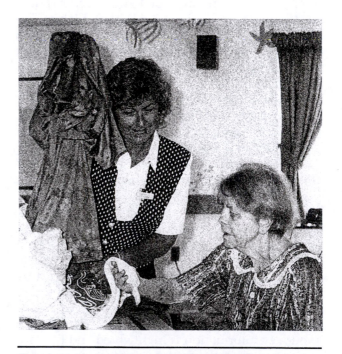

Figure 11–3 In addition to leading groups, activity professionals also function as facilitators.

process in a positive way, and in fact, may be comfortable to relinquish some of the roles from earlier developmental stages.

Leadership Skills

Speaking generally about the leadership abilities that recreation or activity professional should have today, Kraus, Carpenter, and Bates (1981) list twelve principles of successful functioning that professionals should possess. Among them are understanding group dynamics and using approaches that support the group, recognizing and respecting the needs of specific group members, and considering that recreation is ". . . not as an end in itself, but rather as a means to an end."

Skill development is important, but some guidelines have been suggested to aid in the leadership process. Three models of leadership are discussed by Toseland (1990) as reciprocal, remedial, and social goals. A **reciprocal model of leadership** attempts to use the group's concerns as a method for sharing and support. The activity (or other professional) functions as a facilitator or enabler to allow the group to share stressful events and support each other's solutions. An example of the use of the reciprocal model of leadership is a caregivers support group or a grief session for residents. The **remedial model of leadership** acknowledges that group members function at less than their full capacity, and expect to "restore and rehabilitate" elders who are chronically ill or who need social skills to bring them out of isolation. The professional relies less on the group members' input toward approaches and instead guides the members to specific intervention strategies. The remedial model might be the most utilized in long-term care because it has applications in educational and therapy programs such as remotivation or reality orientation. The last aspect of leadership, the **social goals model of leadership**, is designed to assist the elderly in increasing their social consciousness and responsibility through the professional's guidance toward social issues. Often used by civic and other advocacy groups, examples of this model in the long-term care setting include resident's council, current events groups, and resident volunteers.

Selecting the proper leadership model for a program and using skills effectively may not be the only factors to consider. Co-leadership, or administrating a group with two individuals as leaders, has advantages and disadvantages. Although weighed as expensive and impractical because of the use of two staff members, the advantages given by Toseland (1990) include allowing greater participation from challenging groups, such as the frail elderly, and offering support to colleagues during demanding activities.

Looking at the age of the group leader in comparison to those of the participants was done by Maguire (1985), who found that the leadership preferences of the institutionalized aged varies according to the type of program that is being offered. For example, a young man might be the leader of preference for physical activities whereas an older man might be the preferred leader of a group involved in carpentry.

In discussing the basic competencies that a recreation or activity leader must possess in order to run a group effectively, Leitner and Leitner (1985) propose that the group must be planned with the interests and needs of the group in mind, adaptations must be made for the fluctuating levels of participant abilities, group members must be sufficiently motivated to stay in the group through new challenges, and a formal meeting schedule should be established to maintain interest level. Additionally, they discuss offering social development opportunities to group participants and communication techniques such as touch to motivate participants.

Other tips for group leaders come from Burnside (1994) who states that successful group leadership comes from ". . . meticulous communication, careful scheduling, and attention to details."

Group Dynamics

The benefits of group participation for elderly adults are many. Toseland (1990) mentions human relatedness to the group, an outlet for venting, new satisfying roles, information sharing, new learning opportunities, and chances for the resolution of problems as some of the obvious benefits.

Along with benefits of group work comes information on understanding **group dynamics** and the impact that is felt on group work. Although individuals make up a group, a process occurs (group dynamics) during the meeting in which the group as a whole takes on an identity. In his study on group work, Toseland categorizes group dynamics in four areas of interaction and communication patterns: cohesion, social control mechanisms, and group culture.

Group members use verbal and nonverbal communication to express thoughts and feelings. The professional understands the group dynamic of communication and uses skills of repeating and clarification of information to improve the group relationship. Members with special needs, who may not be able to participate as fully as other members, may need extra attention from the group leader to experience the goals of the group.

Monitoring the interaction patterns of groups is another communication challenge for group leaders. Suggestions by Toseland for observing and redirecting inappropriate interaction patterns include making specific seating and group size plans in advance, discouraging subgroups or cliches from continuing, and altering the environment to make the group situation easier for the physically or cognitively impaired to participate.

Cohesion, or the imaginary glue that binds members of a group together, provides higher levels of participation and satisfaction for group members. Increased self-confidence and self-esteem are an additional outgrowth of the cohesive effects of a group. Conversely, cohesive groups tend to be dependent on one another and are more prone toward conformity.

The social control mechanisms of group dynamics, such as norms, roles, and status, are responsible for the behavior of individual members in a group. A mutual belief on the proper way someone should act in a group (called norms) and the feeling about how members relate to their group work (called roles) have implications as to how one group functions with another. Additionally, the status or ranking of group members has a bearing on the interaction patterns.

The last area of the group dynamic process is group culture, outside factors that each individual brings to the group that melds together into a unified culture. This group culture can be positive if it supports different opinions, but it can be destructive if stereotypical behaviors exist.

Other researchers offer these comments on group dynamics and leadership. Johnson, Sandel, and Margolis (1987) suggest that an engaging and interpersonal group atmosphere can be created by leaders offering a protected and stable environment, group members share similar experiences, and leaders use techniques to bring discussions to a "here-and-now" point. Burnside (1994) mentions that a major goal of group work is ". . . to alleviate this general anxiety by helping group members solve immediate problems." In addition to handling the obvious problems of the aged population, a sensitive group leader must offer encouragement and support to increase members' confidence. Burnside also offers that new group leaders need to be aware of potential safety issues, group members who may monopolize the proceedings, and monitor agitated behavior of members.

Participation Factors

Reasons that motivate residents to participate in group and individual programs is often related to a number of factors. The importance of participation was shown in a study by Spector and Takada (1991) that illustrated how low participation in organized activity programs were associated with negative outcomes in residents. Although residents spend only a few hours a day in formal activity programs, Voelkl and Birkel (1988) suggest that recreation professionals should look beyond the traditional programming to the general institutional environment for positive ways to assess and improve their environmental participation.

The early work of researchers, such as DeCarlo (1974), showed that successful aging factors such as the ability to maintain a daily routine, were found to impact recreation participation patterns in a positive manner. Quilitch (1974), and McCormack and Whitehead (1981), in different studies, demonstrated that when activity programs were offered, the residents had a significantly higher engagement level than at times when no programs were available. Other past work, such as the study by Lemmon and Pieper (1980), show that participation in group programs by elderly, institutionalized residents was not as great as their participation in individual activities. Using prompts and reminders when offering a formal program was shown by Burrows, Jason, Quattrochi-Tubin, and Lavelli (1981) to increase the activity and participation of residents in lounge areas.

What are some of the barriers to participation that residents experience that may cause participation levels to vary? The barriers that some residents feel may be physical, cognitive, social, emotional, or environmental. Physical impairments to participation may take the form of decreased bodily functions, inability to stand or walk unaided, or a feeling of not being well. Cognitive problems that may impact participation include memory loss, depression, inaccurate perceptions, or developmental difficulties. Ability to participate may be compromised in the social area because of isolation, language and cultural differences, and sensitivity about condition or appearance. The emotional barriers to participation include inability to control one's behavior, dealing with loss, and feelings of inadequacy or low self-esteem. In the environmental area, barriers may be simply needing to rely on a staff member for transportation to a program or being placed in an awkward spot in a group setting.

Control And Choice. Aspects of choice and control have been found to play a role in the participation level of long-term care of residents. Two studies by Langer and Rodin (1976, 1977) showed that activity participation, overall feelings of well-being, and alert status improved when residents perceived that they took part in their care responsibility. Over time, they also reported that declines in activity and alertness could be slowed or stopped when choice and control factors were made available to them. Iso-Ahola (1980) reported that when resident perceptions of responsibility and choice increased, their interpersonal activities and recreation involvement increased. In talking about freedom and choices, Robertson (1988) advanced the theory of an intervention continuum for allowing a decreasing amount of freedom when the recreation professional interacts with the resident. She defined the intervention continuum as ". . . inform-encourage-coax-coerce-require . . ." and asks colleagues for input on the proper approach that does not reject personal choice, but yields the desired participation.

When choice and control increase morale, the quality of life is also increased. Blair (1994) found that long-term care residents who were told they had more responsibility for themselves felt happier and more active than those who felt they had to rely on the staff for their happiness.

In an important study of the link between certain resident characteristics and activity participation, Voelkl, Fries, and Galecki (1995) found that residents who considered they had impaired functional skills participated in fewer activity programs than those residents with independent functional abilities. Other classifications of residents, associated with lower activity participation, included "high resource use" residents (those who required more nursing care time and costs), those residents receiving rehabilitative services or having greater ADL dependency needs, and those with severe cognitive deficits. The recommendations for activity professionals are to ". . . monitor residents with characteristics related to high resource use, those with few activity preferences, those preferring their own rooms, and those with very severe cognitive limitations."

The work of Gillespie, McLellan, and McGuire (1984) confirms that serving refreshments at activity programs has a greater increase in attendance and participation than not serving refreshments.

Behaviors that Impact Programs

Handling group dynamic issues is most challenging when behavioral problems are present. Behavior, as defined by Dattilo and Murphy (1987), is ". . . any observable and measurable act, response or movement by an individual." With this broad definition, behavior means everything from a smile to a negative response, such as anger. Positive responses are not disruptive to programming; in fact, they are one of the reactions that we seek when we run programs.

We will now look at some of the negative behaviors that you might expect to see during programming and give solutions as to how to manage them.

Causes of Behavioral Problems. A review of some of the research on behaviors by Winger and Schirm (1989) shows that in most skilled nursing facilities, well over fifty percent of the residents in the studies showed some form of behavioral problem including inappropriate language, hazardous conduct, and other nonconforming behaviors. The study demonstrated that aggressive behavior could be a result of causal factors, such as the lack of control or choice that a resident feels he or she has in ADLs (particularly eating and grooming) and his or her ability to perform ADLs.

Another study by Jackson, Drugovich, Fretwell, Spector, Sternberg, and Rosenstein (1989) used the term "disruptive behavior" to describe activities such as verbal or physical abuse of others, noisiness, inappropriate behavior, opposition to care, and wandering. With estimates on the evidence of disruptive behavior ranging from twenty-two percent to sixty-four percent in facilities, they concluded that there are certain resident characteristics that can be correlated to this type of behavior. Their findings indicate that a resident who has ". . . severe cognitive impairment, high dependency in ADL, and incontinence" fits the profile of the candidate who most likely exhibits disruptive behavior. Conclusions are also drawn about residents who may have greater cognitive function, but still exhibit verbal and/or physical abuse and noisiness. The researchers feel that attempts to regain control over loss of some body functions may account for some of their behavior. Interestingly, the study concluded that wandering behavior, which many people feel is related to frustration, may be simply a result of disorientation and confusion.

Although their results were inconclusive, a study was conducted by Rabinovich and Cohen-Mansfield (1992) that used involvement in a formal activity program as an intervention to test the changes that might be seen in agitated behaviors such as verbal and aggressive behavior, pacing, repetitive movements, and touching. Some changes were noted that warrant further investigation by researchers.

Examples of Problem Behaviors. Although each facility may be different in its resident composition, some behaviors are frequently seen. The following sections contain an overview of some commonly experienced behaviors.

Agitation, defined as a disturbed state of restlessness or excitement, and **anxiety**, an overwhelming feeling of nervousness or apprehension, is evidenced in behaviors that include yelling, screaming, crying, rocking, or tapping. Possible causes are confusion about placement or environment, loss of self-esteem, and psychological origins. Approaches and interventions, suggested by Mayers (1994), are distraction, personal attention, and removal of the person from the area. Other methods of handling these situations include reassurance and acknowledgement of feelings.

Catastrophic reaction, as defined by Burnside (1994), is a behavior in a cognitively impaired resident that results when he or she is ". . . overwhelmed by a task or an exercise that he cannot perform." Examples of this behavior are crying, embarrassment, sudden mood change, stubbornness, agitation, anger, and abruptly exiting a situation. Possible causes for the behaviors could be stressful situations that overload the brain, pressure to perform, complicated requests and tasks, and lack of assistance or understanding from caregivers. Approaches and interventions include those suggested by Mace and Rabins (1991): avoidance or limitations of similar situations, simplification of tasks, and reassurance in approach. Other methods include removing the resident from the frustrating environment, slowing down the pace, and lowering your expectations of the resident's ability.

Eloping/exiting are thought to be attempts to leave the secured room, area, unit, or building where a cognitively impaired or psychiatric resident resides. Examples of behavior include increase wandering, agitated or aggressive behavior at exit areas, attempts to push or break down walls or doors, and comments such as "I want to go home." Possible causes for the behaviors are anxiety, confusion, and unfamiliar environment (although noting visual cues at doors and other exits). Approaches and interventions that may work are the redesign of visual cues that both Namazi, Rosner and Calkins (1989) and Dickinson, McLain-Kark, and Marshall-Baker (1995) suggest that include using tape patterns on floors and doors, reworking door knobs and handles, decreasing shiny surfaces on doors, decreasing light, and removing the window portions of doors. Also, allowing freedom of movement through areas with minimal exit cues may help.

Hoarding is the searching and collecting of miscellaneous objects (sugar packets, picture frames, socks) and carrying them away or hiding them in another area. Examples of behavior include reports of missing items, rummaging activity, and agitated searching. Possible causes for the behaviors might be attempts to control the environment, forgetfulness, and confusion about ownership of property. Approaches and interventions that may work are to reduce the number of objects and possessions in the immediate environment, seek compatibility in terms of a roommate, store unsafe items or valuables and other often-used items in specific places, and ask other residents to label their belongings.

Hostility and **anger** are varying degrees of displeasure expressed toward a situation. Examples of behavior include yelling, hitting, screaming, verbal assaults, negative body language, and biting. Possible causes for the behaviors might be frustration at loss of abilities, unhappiness with dependency on caregivers, unhappiness toward family at placement, and fear of the unknown. Approaches and interventions that could work are calm acknowledgment of feelings, individual discussion, and removal of the person from the situation.

Noisemaking is classified as excessive, loud, and disruptive talking or yelling. Ryan, Tainsh, Kolodny, Lendrum, and Fisher (1988) found in their study of long-term care facilities that approximately thirty percent of residents could be considered "disruptively noisy." Examples of behavior include screaming, banging, moaning, requesting attention, continuous singing, or refusal to end conversations. Possible causes for the behaviors are attempts to be a part of, or to control, the environment of others, and deafness. Approaches and interventions suggested by Ryan, Tainsh, Kolodny, Lendrum, and Fisher are changes in caregivers' routine to detect effects on noisemaking, use of conversation-ending techniques, and other modifications of the environment.

Rummaging, similar to hoarding, is the act of repeatedly searching for lost possessions or other items. Examples of this behavior include sorting intently through objects and the resulting anxiety or agitation when the items are not located. Possible causes for the behaviors are confusion, attempts to regain control of environment, and memory loss. Approaches and interventions that may work are providing appropriate rummaging areas, reassurance, and distraction.

Sundowning, defined by Bliwise (1994) as ". . . the phenomenon of agitation seemingly caused by, or at least strongly associated with darkness." Examples of this behavior include increases in noisemaking, pacing, or agitation in the late afternoon or evening. The cause of this behavior is not fully known, but Bliwise speculates that a disruption of the circadian rhythm (a person's internal clock) may cause the behavior. He also mentions that awakening from sleep may also play a role. Thought to involve residents in the mid-range of dementia, Hopkins, Rindlisbacher, and Grant (1992) conclude that sundowning is a sensory deprivation situation in which residents are missing visual cues that usually help them compensate within their environment. However, their research did not support the theory of a relationship between light levels and increased activity. Program interventions for sundowning syndrome include implementing programs during critical time periods and providing appropriate outlets for higher levels of activity.

Suspicion, a feeling of distrust of others, and **delusion**, a belief not based in reality, both have psychological origins. Examples of behavior include doubting of facts, accusatory acts, checking up on others, anger, and hostility. Possible causes for the behaviors are mental illness, confusion about placement or environment, and lack of support from family or others. Approaches and interventions include acknowledgement and validation of feelings, offering of assistance, and distractions.

Wandering and **pacing** are interchangeable terms that mean the act of repeated walking in nonpurposeful ways. Examples of pacing behavior patterns mentioned by Cohen-Mansfield, Werner, Marx, and Freedman (1991) include restless pacing, exit seekers, self-stimulators (turning knobs during pacing), and modelers, who shadow another person while wandering. Possible causes for the behaviors are confusion, restlessness, and, according to the researchers, a higher frequency of stressful situations in previous life experience that release physical energy. Approaches and interventions that may work involve the results that Cohen-Mansfield, Werner, Marx, and Freedman discovered. They concluded that pacing is less apparent during mealtime and has no relevance to a particular day of the week. They suggest that the majority of the pacing occurs in the corridors, with more pacing occurring when no noise is present. Less pacing occurred with darkness, but music or television noise had no significance. Reassurance, redirection, and the provision of safe areas for wandering are other interventions that might work.

Behavior Modification. In addition to strategies for specific behaviors, there is also a methodology for handling or modifying problem behaviors called **behavior modification**. Using the guideline that all humans react to their environment, Dattilo and Murphy (1987) defined behavior modification as ". . . a systematic, performance-based evaluative method for changing behavior." This theory suggests that all behavior is learned, and, therefore, specific behaviors, called target behaviors, can be altered or modified. In activity programming, using behavior modification can be as simple as observing a behavior, describing the behavior, searching for the antecedent (or activity that occurred before the behavior), and then looking at the consequence of the behavior. For example, if a resident was transported to an activity by a nursing assistant (antecedent) and began to cry and scream (behavior), the resident may first be spoken to by the activity professional. If the behavior continued, the resident would be removed from the program (consequence). This procedure of analyzing events for antecedents, behaviors, and consequences is called **sequencing analysis**. After identifying behaviors, change can occur through use of either **positive reinforcement** or **negative reinforcement**. Participation in an activity is an example of a positive reinforcement, and removal after inappropriate behavior is an example of negative reinforcement. These techniques have applications for developing approaches and goal-setting for residents.

SUMMARY

Marketing, both internally and externally, has advantages to showcase your program and invite attendance. Group leadership skills, understanding of group dynamics, and participation factors can assist you in developing appropriate, meaningful programs. Understanding expected behaviors of residents and knowing interventions for modifying these behaviors will help to make your programming plans successful.

R E V I E W   Q U E S T I O N S

1. What are some of the benefits of an internal newsletter?
2. What are the three models for group leadership?
3. Define cohesion, and explain how it relates to group activity.

4. Name three barriers to participation in activity programming.
5. What is a catastrophic reaction, and how can an activity professional intervene?

O N   Y O U R   O W N

1. Using your own facility as an example, what are five additional ways that you can increase the profile of your department?
2. Develop a press release and marketing campaign for a visit to your facility by a famous

Olympic athlete. Funds are limited and the event is three months away.
3. What are some other program methods that can be used to assist in controlling wandering, pacing, and other agitated behaviors?

R E F E R E N C E S

Blair, C. (1994). Residents' who make decisions reveal healthier, happier attitudes. *The Journal of Long-Term Care Administration*, Winter, 32–39.

Bliwise, D. (1994). What is sundowning? *Journal of American Geriatrics Society*, Vol. 42, 1009–1011.

Burnside, I. (1994). Education and preparation for group work. In I. Burnside & M. G. Schmidt (Eds.) *Working with older adults: Group process and techniques*, (65–74). Boston, MA: Jones & Bartlett Publishers.

Burrows, B., Jason, L., Quattrochi-Tubin, S., & Lavelli, M. (1981). Increasing activity of nursing home residents in their lounges using a physical design intervention and a prompting intervention. *Activities, Adaptation and Aging*, Vol. (4), 25–33.

Cohen-Mansfield, J., Werner, P., Marx, M., & Freedman, L. (1991). Two studies of pacing in the nursing home. *Journal of Gerontology*, Vol. 46, No. 3, M77–M83.

Dattilo, J., & Murphy, W. (1987). *Behavior modification in therapeutic recreation: An introductory learning manual*. State College, PA: Venture Publishing.

DeCarlo, T. (1974). Recreation participation patterns and successful aging. *Journal of Gerontology*, 29 (4), 16–22.

Dickinson, J., McLain-Kark, J., & Marshall-Baker, A. (1995). The effects of visual barriers on exiting behavior in a dementia care unit. *The Gerontologist*, Vol. 35, No. 1, 127–130.

Gillespie, K., McLellan, R., & Mcguire, F. (1984). The effect of refreshments on attendance at recreational activities for nursing home activities. *Therapeutic Recreation Journal*, 3rd Quarter, 25–29.

Hartmann, T. (1992). *Producing, designing and writing newsletters*. Marietta, GA: The Newsletter Factory.

Hopkins, R., Rindlisbacher, P., & Grant, N. (1992). An investigation of the sundowning syndrome and ambient light. *The American Journal of Alzheimer's Care & Related Disorders & Research*, March/April, 22–27.

Iso-Ahola, S. (1980). Perceived control and responsibility as mediators of the effect of therapeutic recreation on the institutionalized aged. *Therapeutic Recreation Journal*, 1st Quarter, 36–43.

Jackson, M., Drugovich, M., Fretwell, M., Spector, W., Sternberg, J., & Rosenstein, R. (1989). Prevalence and correlates of disruptive behavior in the nursing home. *Journal of Aging & Health*, Vol. 1, No. 3, 349–369.

Johnson, D., Sandel, S., & Margolis, M. (1982). Waiting at the gate. *Activities, Adaptation and Aging*, Vol. 9, No. 3, 15–24.

Kraus, R., Carpenter, G., & Bates, B. (1981). *Recreation leadership and supervisor: Guidelines for professional development*, 2nd edition. Philadelphia, PA: Saunders College Publishing.

Kubler-Ross, E. (1987). *AIDS: The ultimate challenge*. New York, NY: Macmillan.

Lamken, M. (1980). Editing a newsletter: An activity therapist's perspective. *Activities, Adaptation and Aging*, Vol. 1 (2), 11–25.

Langer, E., & Rodin, J. (1976). The effects of choice and enhanced personal responsibility for the aged: A field experiment in an institutional setting. *Journal of Personality and Social Psychology*, Vol. 34, No. 2., 191–198.

Lemmon, D., & Pieper, H. (1980). Leisure pursuits and their meaning for the institutionalized elderly population. *Journal of Gerontological Nursing*, Vol. 6, No. 2, 74–77.

Leitner, M. J., & Leitner, S. I. (1985). *Leisure in later life: A sourcebook for the provision of recreational services for elders*. Binghamton, NY: Haworth Press.

Lovejoy, M. (1988). *Organizing and operating a speaker's bureau*. Philadelphia, PA: The National Mental Health Consumers' Self-Help Clearinghouse.

Mace, N., & Rabins, P. (1991). *The 36-hour day*. New York, NY: Warner Books.

Maguire, G. (1985). Key issues where intervention can make a difference. In G. H. Maguire (Ed.) *Care of the elderly: A health team approach*. Boston, MA: Little Brown and Co.

Mayers, K. (1994). Calming the agitated demented patient: Use of self-soothing techniques. *The American Journal of Alzheimer's Care and Related Disorders & Research*, July/August, 2–5.

McCormack, D., & Whitehead, A. (1981). The effect of providing recreational activities on the engagement level of long-stay geriatric patients. *Age and Ageing*, 10, 287–291.

Namazi, K., Rosner, T., & Calkins, M. (1989). Visual barriers to prevent ambulatory Alzheimer's patients from exiting through an emergency door. *The Gerontologist*, Vol. 29, No. 5, 699–702.

Partin, R. (1986). The ten most common mistakes in handling inquiries. *Contemporary Long Term Care*, December, 55–56.

Patterson, F. C. (1987). *A systems approach to recreation programming*. Columbus, OH: Publishing Horizons Inc.

Quilitch, H. R. (1974). Purposeful activity increased on a geriatric ward through programmed recreation. *Journal of the American Geriatric Society*, Vol. XXII, No. 5, 226–229.

Rabinovich, B., & Cohen-Mansfield, J. (1992). The impact of participation in structured recreational activ-

ities on the agitated behavior of nursing home residents: An observational study. *Activities, Adaptation and Aging*, Vol. 16 (4), 89–97.

Robertson, R. (1988). Recreation and the institutionalized elderly: Conceptionalization of the free choice and intervention continuums. *Activities, Adaptation and Aging*, Vol. 11 (1), 61–73.

Rodin, J., & Langer, E. (1977). Long-term effects of a control-relevant intervention with the institutionalized aged. *Journal of Personality and Social Psychology*, Vol. 35, No. 12, 897–902.

Ryan, D., Tainsh, S., Kolodny, V., Lendrum, B., & Fisher, R. (1988). Noise-making amongst the elderly in long term care. *The Gerontologist*, Vol. 28, No. 3, 369–371.

Spector, W., & Takada, H. A. (1991). Characteristics of nursing homes that affect resident outcome. *Journal of Aging and Health*, 3 (4), 427–454.

Thorn, B. (1984). Marketing therapeutic recreation services. *Therapeutic Recreation Journal*, 4th Quarter, 42–47.

Toseland, R. (1995). *Group work with the elderly and family caregivers*. New York, NY: Springer Publishing Co.

Voelkl, J., Fries, B., & Galecki, A. (1995). Predictors of nursing home residents' participation in activity programs. *The Gerontologist*, Vol. 35, No. 1, 44–51.

Winger, J., & Schirm, V. (1989). Managing aggressive elderly. *Journal of Gerontological Nursing*, Vol. 15, No. 2, 28–33.

F U R T H E R   R E A D I N G

Abraham, I., Currie, L., & Neundorfer, M. (1992). Effects of cognitive group interventions on depression and cognition among elderly women in long term care. *Journal of Women and Aging*, Vol. 4(1), 5–24.

Backman, S., & Mannell, R. (1986). Removing attitudinal barriers to leisure behavior and satisfaction: A field experiment among the institutionalized elderly. *Therapeutic Recreation Journal*, 3rd Quarter, 46–53.

Curley, J. (1983). Letting the inmates run the asylum: Another point of view. *Activities, Adaptation and Aging*, Vol. 3 (3), 13–15.

Davidhizar, R., & Cosgray, R. (1990). Helping the wanderer. *Geriatric Nursing*, Nov./Dec., 280–281.

Dixon, J. (1978). Expanding individual control in leisure participation while enlarging the concept of normalcy. *Therapeutic Recreation Journal*, 3rd Quarter, 20–24.

Funabiki, D., Edney, C., & Myers, J. (1982). Management of disruptive behaviors in therapeutic recreation setting. *Therapeutic Recreation Journal*, 4th Quarter, 24–25.

Gwyther, L. P. (1985). *Care of Alzheimer's patients: A manual for nursing home staff*. Washington, DC: American Health Care Association & Alzheimer's Disease and Related Disorders Association.

Howe-Murphy, R. (1979). A conceptual basis for mainstreaming recreation and leisure services: Focus on

humanism. *Therapeutic Recreation Journal*, 4th Quarter, 11–18.

McClannahan, L., & Risley, T. (1974). Design of living environments for nursing home residents: Recruiting attendance at activities. *The Gerontologist*, June, 236–240.

McGuire, F. (1985). Recreation leader and co-participant preferences of the institutionalized aged. *Therapeutic Recreation Journal*, 2nd Quarter, 47–54.

Miller, D. (1979). Case studies to challenge the nursing home activity coordinator. *Therapeutic Recreation Journal*, 3rd Quarter, 22–32.

Spector, W., & Jackson, M. (1994). Correlates of disruptive behaviors in nursing homes. *Journal of Aging & Health*, Vol. 6, No. 2, 173–184.

Teaff, J. (1985). *Leisure services with the elderly*. St. Louis, Missouri: Times Mirror/Mosby.

Voelkl, J., & Birkel, R. (1988). Application of the experience sampling method to assess clients' daily experiences. *Therapeutic Recreation Journal*, 3rd Quarter, 23–33.

Vogler, E. W., Fenstermacher, G., & Bishop, P. (1982). Group-oriented behavior management systems to control disruptive behavior in therapeutic recreation settings. *Therapeutic Recreation Journal*, 1st Quarter, 20–24.

C H A P T E R   1 2
Documentation and Medical Records

OBJECTIVES..

After completing this chapter, you should:

- understand your responsibilities, and the formats for documentation for federal programs, including a working knowledge of each section
- understand the Resident Assessment Instrument (RAI) and feel comfortable with the process
- follow standard procedure for other facility documentation, such as policies and procedures, attendance records, and correspondence

INTRODUCTION

Assessing needs, designing programs, and implementing them are all crucial facets of your job. Translating resident needs into workable clinical goals that are appropriate and measurable is part of the role of documentation for the person's medical record. Federal programs, such as Medicare and Medicaid, have standard methods for data collection, addressing needs, and resolving clinical issues. Other recordkeeping procedures, such as the use of policies and procedures, reports, and attendance records are also part of your documentation responsibilities.

Medical Records and Documentation ....

Your role as a member of the interdisciplinary and clinical team begins with knowledge of the aging residents, their needs, and your assessment of them. The **medical record** is a written compilation of all the treatment efforts, interventions, orders, and reports that are conducted by all members of the interdisciplinary team. The team includes physicians, nurses, dietician, activity or recreation professional, social worker, rehabilitative team members (occupational therapy, speech therapy and physical therapy), pharmacist, and other consultants (psychologist, psychiatrist, podiatrist, and so forth). **Documentation** is the physical act by an interdisciplinary team member of writing an assessment, evaluation, order, or update and logging it into a particular resident's medical record. Documentation may be supported by record keeping materials not maintained in the formal medical record, such as attendance records, interest forms, and risk assessment sheets.

Purpose and Benefits of Documentation

There are three main reasons for medical record documentation. First, there must be a central location for all resident information from the various interdisciplinary team members that reflect a person's needs and care. Second, documentation is used as a means to support proper reimbursement for federal programs, such as Medicaid and

Medicare. The actual amount that a facility is reimbursed for on a daily basis is impacted by the documentation efforts that support the actual care and services that were rendered. The third, and most recently evolving reason for documentation, is to assist in "data driven" surveys by state and federal regulatory agencies.

In addition to serving important functions in the facility, documentation has numerous benefits, according to Miller (1989). She suggests that increased communication and cooperation among staff members and evaluation and explanation of services and progress are some of the key reasons for keeping accurate records.

Understanding Your Responsibilities

In all phases of documentation, some crucial factors must be considered to ensure professionalism. **Confidentiality** is the *expected practice* of all interdisciplinary team members. This is not a suggestion; it is a mandated protocol based on resident rights. The only discussions or written information that should occur are those that have a direct bearing on a resident issue. Gossip, unprofessional comments, and off-hand remarks about residents are not part of any professional conduct. Rough drafts of notes used to prepare your documentation should be destroyed to protect them from the public sector. Check with your medical records designee in the facility to determine the medical records policies that apply to all interdisciplinary team members in the areas of confidentiality and proper destruction of records.

Activity professionals and all interdisciplinary team members should provide documentation information that is accurate and simple. Other general tips come from Miller (1989), who mentions that clarity and comprehensiveness of information are important in any effort. She also suggests that labeling or personal judgement of a resident situation not be conducted. Straightforward, factual information should be reported in any documentation instead of any personal commentary. Crepeau (1989) proposes that to be useful, documentation should have four qualities of addressing all pertinent issues: meeting the time frames set up by regulatory agencies, making sense from an organizational standpoint, and writing simply and in an understandable manner.

General procedures usually apply to the handling of medical records. Uniack (1994) suggests that since a medical record is considered "evidence of care," it is a legal document that may be required as proof of care in another setting and should be legible enough to be photocopied. Documentation entries on the medical record are done in ink or by computer and signatures may be required, depending on facility policy. In addition to keeping your notes brief and without judgemental opinion, your documentation should reflect information of which you have personal knowledge. Medical and other abbreviations are acceptable as long as they conform to your facility's approved list. (Chapter 3 gives some examples of medical terminology and abbreviations to which you may wish to refer.) Errors made in charting are usually handled by placing a single, solid line through the incorrect information, writing the word "error," signing the correction with your initials, and the date. Medical records or parts of the records usually are not to be removed from the facility. At times, you may need to make an addendum to an existing episodic or progress note or perhaps you have forgotten a key detail in your first note. Correct that situation by making an addendum note or late entry to your original note. Label the new note "addendum to (date)" or "late entry to (date)." Your facility may have a policy for removing records temporarily from the nurses' station. Be sure to check with your administrator or medical records designee if you are unsure of the policy in your facility. Access to medical records by nonprofessional personnel (families, outside agencies) follows strict policies of state laws and the facility. Your medical records designee can help you in learning about access requirements.

Some documentation will be conducted individually by you or your staff members, such as initial assessment information or episodic progress notes. The bulk of your documentation work, however, will be based on the interdisciplinary team approach. Although an interdisciplinary team is not a mandated requirement, presenting coordinated care in an organized fashion is the goal of every facility. The interdisciplinary team approach works well because many professional and clinical members bring a special understanding of resident needs and work together to resolve problems. With responsibilities for documentation spelled out clearly in policies, each member of the interdisciplinary team has major input to the RAI process. (The RAI process will be discussed later in this chapter.) Meeting weekly or on some other schedule that fits the needs of your facility, a group of professionals, such as the RN coordinator, nurses, dietician, activity professional, resident, resident's family member, certified nurses' aide, occupational therapist, speech therapist and physical therapist, review specific resident care based on the MDS full assessment form or the MDS quarterly, based on the requirements of the resident. Usually, a registered nurse is designated as the person responsible for coordinating all the information contained on an MDS. Some facilities, however, may charge a social worker or other staff member with managing the schedule of resident cases up for initial review or quarterly review during on a particular week. The designated "scheduler" often has the additional responsibility of sending notices out to all interdisciplinary staff members to remind them of the upcoming case reviews. This person sends out invitations to residents and family members, requesting their attendance and participation. Family members may be invited to attend these sessions if the resident is unable to participate in issues concerning his or her care. Identifying problems and formulating team approaches and interventions to solving them is the purpose of the interdisciplinary team meeting. It serves no purpose if each member comes to the meeting with "tunnel-vision" and is not open to developing approaches together. Team members often may note behavioral changes in residents or small indicators overlooked by others. By pooling information and working together, innovative plans for meeting resident needs can emerge.

Required Documentation for Federal Programs

Having a method for handling resident data collection and assessment grew from two sources. The enactment of the Omnibus Budget Reconciliation Act (OBRA) of 1987 that contained a section on Nursing Home Reform required that a resident assessment method be implemented to monitor and support the new quality of life focus. Other researchers, such as the Committee On Nursing Home Reform (1986) (discussed in Chapter 1) also supported the idea of using collected resident information to design and implement a better survey process. The Resident Assessment Instrument (RAI) in use today is a direct result of these groundbreaking regulatory changes.

Resident Assessment Instrument (RAI)

The **Resident Assessment Instrument (RAI)** is defined by the Health Care Financing Administration (HCFA) (1995) as "an instrument which requires for completion the performance of a standardized assessment system, comprised of the MDS and utilization guidelines (including RAPs and triggers)." The system was designed to be a standardized instrument for measuring the functional capabilities and medical concerns of all res-

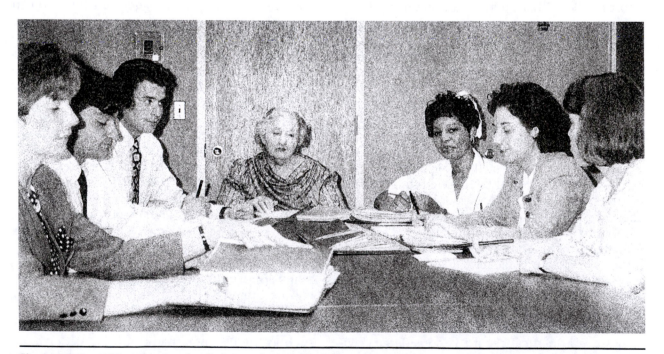

Figure 12–1   With resident or family input, the interdisciplinary team develops a coordinated and individualized plan of care.

idents residing in a facility that participates in the Medicare or Medicaid program. Figure 12–2 illustrates the components of the RAI process.

Before discussing the specifics of the RAI, the concept of **assessment** should be reviewed. Crepeau (1989) suggests "activity assessment is the process by which data is collected to identify the activity-related resources, strengths, and limitations of the patient." She outlines the assessment process as data collection, interpretation, validation, and documentation. Crepeau adds that "clinical reasoning," defined as ". . . a narrative process in which initial assumptions are formed. . . ," begins as interdisciplinary professionals consider how to assist residents in bringing about change. In handling assessment, Budge (1989) mentions that there are many purposes for assessment, including ways to determine the level of confusion of a resident, placement options within a program, and overall planning for programs. She suggests that an "observational assessment" process view the resident's abilities to participate in terms of social interactions, levels of participation, orientation and memory, initiative, mobility, and cognitive skills. Gallo, Reichel, and Anderson (1988) discuss the use of a multidimensional assessment process that incorporates physical, social, and functional observations to complete a total assessment picture of an individual. Referring to a "holistic" assessment process, Perschbacher (1993) suggests that the beginning stages of assessment involve areas such as functioning, distinct resident characteristics, and current patterns. Resident functioning in all areas (physical, social, cognitive, and emotional) are examined on an individual basis and for interrelationships. Identifying resident characteristics, such as their interests, typical routines, and viewing of past and present habits offers a great deal of information to the activity professional, according to Perschbacher. Using a data collection form (discussed in Chapter 4) will help you to learn about your resident and prepare the initial phases of the data collection for the MDS together with your interdisciplinary team.

The RAI was developed to assist interdisciplinary care team members standardize a method to assess and make care planning decisions for residents. The American Health Care Association (1995) suggests that the RAI offers benefits to facility staff in such areas as helping to gather specific information on resident abilities and methods to look at residents holistically. They also state that staff communication is improved and individualized care has increased.

Subgroups within the Resident Assessment Instrument include the MDS 2.0, the **triggers** and **Resident Assessment Protocol (RAPs)**, and the **utilization guidelines**. The MDS 2.0 is a set of forms that comprises the assessment process. The triggers are resident responses noted for particular MDS elements with resident assessment protocols (RAPs) set up to handle each trigger. The utilization guidelines are the instructional directions as to how to use the parts of the RAI. Each of these components of the RAI will be discussed in the following section, but it is important to understand the framework of the problem identification model and how it relates to the RAI. In Figure 12–2, a problem identification model is shown, that consists of a pathway beginning with the assessment process (consisting of the MDS 2.0) to the decision-making section (that involves triggers and RAPs) into care plan development, implementation, and evaluation.

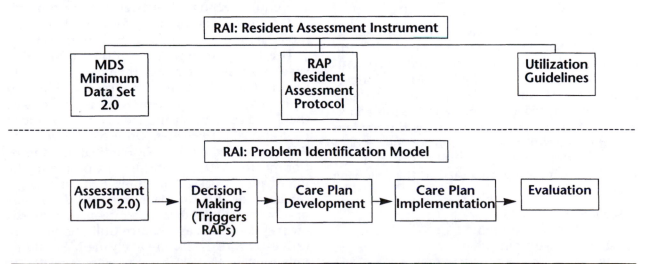

Figure 12–2 An overview of the steps in the Resident Assessment Instrument (RAI).

Minimum Data Set (MDS)2.0

The **Minimum Data Set (MDS) 2.0** is defined by HCFA (1995) as "A core set of screening and assessment elements, including common definitions and coding categories, that forms the foundation of the comprehensive assessment for all residents of long term care facilities certified to participate in Medicare and Medicaid." At first glance, the Minimum Data Set 2.0 looks like a confusing set of documents. The simple layout of fill-in-the-boxes with limited choices for each box, however, are designed to make the assessment instrument as user-friendly as possible. There are three major MDS forms that require review: the basic assessment tracking form, the full assessment form, and the quarterly assessment form. We will discuss other related forms as well.

The basic assessment tracking form is a brief background face sheet completed at the time of admission. The full assessment form is the total assessment conducted within fourteen days of admission and contains the input of the interdisciplinary team members. Section N is an area devoted exclusively to activity pursuit patterns. All the other full assessment sections have been broken out into separate areas to highlight important information. The entire set of MDS forms are available in Appendix F for you to review and use.

Basic Assessment Tracking Form. The **Basic Assessment Tracking Form** contains vital information and must be completed after every full assessment, quarterly assessment, or any other assessment required in a particular state. The Basic Assessment Tracking Form shown in Figure 12–3 consists of information such as birth date, race, social security number, and reasons for assessment.

Full Assessment Form. The MDS 2.0 **Full Assessment Form** is used in conjunction with the **Background (Face Sheet) Information At Admission Form**. The Background (Face Sheet) Information At Admission Form, shown in Figure 12–4, is completed at the time a resident is admitted to a facility. The sheet contains information on patterns and living conditions of the resident prior to admission. An activity professional should be particularly interested in the following section of the form:

- Sections AB
  —box 2: Admitted from
  —box 3: Lived alone prior
  —box 4: Zip code, primary residence
  —box 6: Lifetime occupations

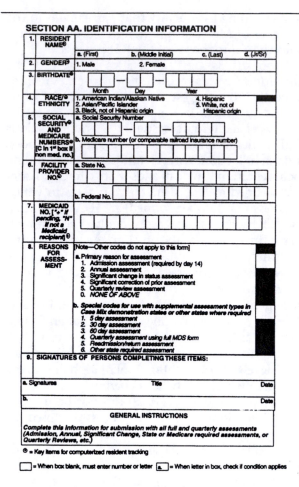

Figure 12–3 MDS 2.0 Basic Assessment Tracking Form.

—box 7: Education
—box 8: Language

The entire Section AC lists customary routines and is a good starting point for the activity professional to conduct in the assessment process.

The Full Assessment Form of the MDS 2.0 spans six pages or more, including the Background (Face Sheet) Information at Admission Form. The Full Assessment Form is prepared at the time a resident is admitted to a facility, and at least annually thereafter. Once completed, verified, and signed by the RN Coordinator, information on the MDS is considered closed and the information "locked," meaning that no changes can be made after that date. Some states are using or plan to use MDS data for a case-mix reimbursement system, such as Resource Utilization Groups (RUGs-II or RUGs-III), in which the Medicaid reimbursement that a facility receives is related to the type of medical cases being handled. It should

SECTION AB. DEMOGRAPHIC INFORMATION

1.	DATE OF ENTRY	Date the stay began. Note — Does not include readmission if record was closed at time of temporary discharge to hospital, etc. In such cases, use prior admission date

Month — Day — Year

2.	ADMITTED FROM (AT ENTRY)	1. Private home/apt. with no home health services 2. Private home/apt. with home health services 3. Board and care/assisted living/group home 4. Nursing home 5. Acute care hospital 6. Psychiatric hospital, MR/DD facility 7. Rehabilitation hospital 8. Other
3.	LIVED ALONE (PRIOR TO ENTRY)	0. No 1. Yes 2. In other facility
4.	ZIP CODE OF PRIOR PRIMARY RESIDENCE	
5.	RESIDEN-TIAL HISTORY 5 YEARS PRIOR TO ENTRY	(Check all settings resident lived in during 5 years prior to date of entry given in item AB1 above) Prior stay at this nursing home ... a. Stay in other nursing home ... b. Other residential facility—board and care home, assisted living, group home ... c. MH/psychiatric setting ... d. MR/DD setting ... e. NONE OF ABOVE ... f.
6.	LIFETIME OCCUPA-TION(S) [Put "/" between two occupations]	
7.	EDUCATION (Highest Level Completed)	1. No schooling 5. Technical or trade school 2. 8th grade/less 6. Some college 3. 9-11 grades 7. Bachelor's degree 4. High school 8. Graduate degree
8.	LANGUAGE	(Code for correct response) a. Primary Language 0. English 1. Spanish 2. French 3. Other b. If other, specify
9.	MENTAL HEALTH HISTORY	Does resident's RECORD indicate any history of mental retardation, mental illness, or developmental disability problem? 0. No 1. Yes
10.	CONDITIONS RELATED TO MR/DD STATUS	(Check all conditions that are related to MR/DD status that were manifested before age 22, and are likely to continue indefinitely) Not applicable—no MR/DD (Skip to AB11) ... a. MR/DD with organic condition Down's syndrome ... b. Autism ... c. Epilepsy ... d. Other organic condition related to MR/DD ... e. MR/DD with no organic condition ... f.
11.	DATE BACK-GROUND INFORMA-TION COMPLETED	Month — Day — Year

SECTION AC. CUSTOMARY ROUTINE

1.	CUSTOMARY ROUTINE (In year prior to DATE OF ENTRY to this nursing home, or year last in community if now being admitted from another nursing home)	(Check all that apply. If all information UNKNOWN, check last box only.)

CYCLE OF DAILY EVENTS

Stays up late at night (e.g., after 9 pm)	a.
Naps regularly during day (at least 1 hour)	b.
Goes out 1+ days a week	c.
Stays busy with hobbies, reading, or fixed daily routine	d.
Spends most of time alone or watching TV	e.
Moves independently indoors (with appliances, if used)	f.
Use of tobacco products at least daily	g.
NONE OF ABOVE	h.

EATING PATTERNS

Distinct food preferences	i.
Eats between meals all or most days	j.
Use of alcoholic beverage(s) at least weekly	k.
NONE OF ABOVE	l.

ADL PATTERNS

In bedclothes much of day	m.
Wakens to toilet all or most nights	n.
Has irregular bowel movement pattern	o.
Showers for bathing	p.
Bathing in PM	q.
NONE OF ABOVE	r.

INVOLVEMENT PATTERNS

Daily contact with relatives/close friends	s.
Usually attends church, temple, synagogue (etc.)	t.
Finds strength in faith	u.
Daily animal companion/presence	v.
Involved in group activities	w.
NONE OF ABOVE	x.
UNKNOWN—Resident/family unable to provide information	y.

END

SECTION AD. FACE SHEET SIGNATURES

SIGNATURES OF PERSONS COMPLETING FACE SHEET:

a. Signature of RN Assessment Coordinator			Date
b. Signatures	Title	Sections	Date
c.			Date
d.			Date
e.			Date
f.			Date
g.			Date

□ = When box blank, must enter number or letter   [a.] = When letter in box, check if condition applies

October, 1995   MDS 2.0 10/18/94n

Figure 12–4 MDS 2.0 Background (Face Sheet) Information At Admission, Sections AB–AD.

also be mentioned that some states require additional, specific MDS sections for meeting their own documentation requirements. Check with your MDS coordinator to ensure that all the required sections are properly completed.

Some **significant changes** that occur in resident's status may require that a full assessment be completed sooner than planned. For states using case-mix and quality demonstrations, a seventh page is added in Section T. To have an understanding of important elements of the MDS as they relate to the activity department, we have broken the MDS into the following segments for discussion purposes in this text:

Section A—Identification and Background Information of the Full Assessment Form. The highlights of this section are :

—box 2: Room number
—box 5: Marital status
—box 8: Reason for assessment
—box 9: Responsibility/legal guardian
—box 10: Advanced directives (see Figure 12–5)

Section B—Cognitive Patterns. Contains information on cognitive patterns. All of the information in this section, such as memory, recall, and cognitive skills, should be of interest to the activity professional in program planning (see Figure 12–6).

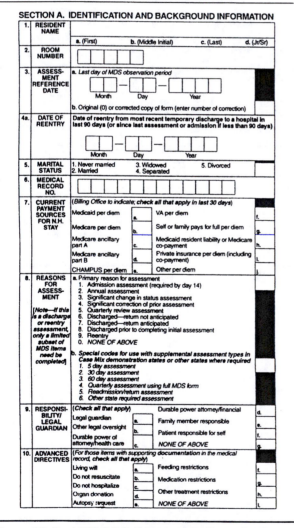

Figure 12–5 MDS 2.0 Full Assessment Form, Section A.

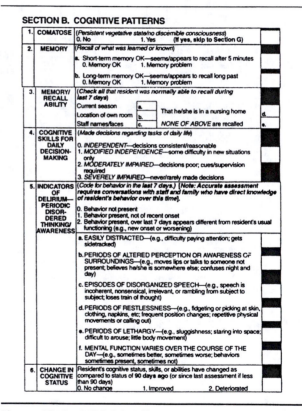

Figure 12–6 MDS 2.0 Full Assessment Form, Section B.

Section C—Communication/Hearing Patterns and *Section D—Vision Patterns.* These sections are important in order to gain an understanding of the level of participation that can be expected for a particular resident based on his or her abilities (see Figure 12–7).

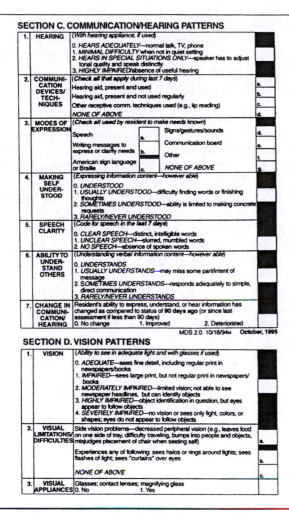

Figure 12–7 MDS 2.0 Full Assessment Form, Section C and D.

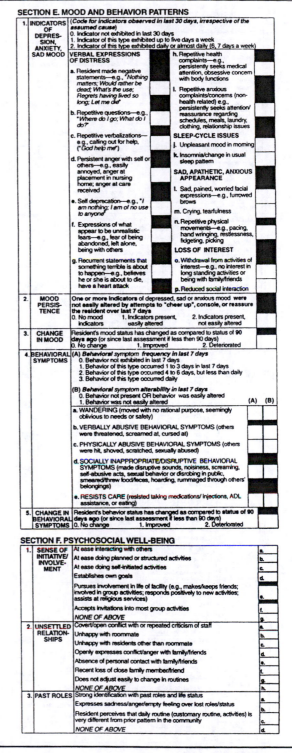

Figure 12–8 MDS 2.0 Full Assessment Form, Section E and F.

Section E—Mood and Behavior Patterns and *Section F—Psychosocial Well-Being.* These sections show areas crucially linked to the level of information you need in order to effectively plan programs. Evidence of depression, mood, relationships, and behavioral symptoms such as wandering definitely will have a bearing on your planning aspects (see Figure 12–8).

Section G—Physical Functioning and Structural Problems. Box 1 is important to note because it deals with a resident's ability to be independent and has impacts on the person's skill level for attending programs without intervention. Box 4 would be useful for planning exercise or other movement programs. Boxes 5, 6, 7, 8, and 9 have

to do with ambulation, locomotion, and a resident's ability in activities of daily living skills (see Figure 12–9).

SECTION G. PHYSICAL FUNCTIONING AND STRUCTURAL PROBLEMS

1. (A) ADL SELF-PERFORMANCE—*(Code for resident's PERFORMANCE OVER ALL SHIFTS during last 7 days—Not including setup)*

0. **INDEPENDENT**—No help or oversight —OR— Help/oversight provided only 1 or 2 times during last 7 days
1. **SUPERVISION**—Oversight, encouragement or cueing provided 3 or more times during last 7 days —OR— Supervision (3 or more times) plus physical assistance provided only 1 or 2 times during last 7 days
2. **LIMITED ASSISTANCE**—Resident highly involved in activity; received physical help in guided maneuvering of limbs or other nonweight bearing assistance 3 or more times —OR— More help provided only 1 or 2 times during last 7 days
3. **EXTENSIVE ASSISTANCE**—While resident performed part of activity, over last 7-day period, help of following type(s) provided 3 or more times:
   — Weight-bearing support
   — Full staff performance during part (but not all) of last 7 days
4. **TOTAL DEPENDENCE**—Full staff performance of activity during entire 7 days
8. **ACTIVITY DID NOT OCCUR** during entire 7 days

(B) ADL SUPPORT PROVIDED—*(Code for MOST SUPPORT PROVIDED OVER ALL SHIFTS during last 7 days; code regardless of resident's self-performance classification)*

0. No setup or physical help from staff
1. Setup help only
2. One person physical assist
3. Two+ persons physical assist
8. ADL activity itself did not occur during entire 7 days

			(A) SELF-PERF	(B) SUPPORT
a.	BED MOBILITY	How resident moves to and from lying position, turns side to side, and positions body while in bed		
b.	TRANSFER	How resident moves between surfaces—to/from: bed, chair, wheelchair, standing position (EXCLUDE to/from bath/toilet)		
c.	WALK IN ROOM	How resident walks between locations in his/her room		
d.	WALK IN CORRIDOR	How resident walks in corridor on unit		
e.	LOCOMO-TION ON UNIT	How resident moves between locations in his/her room and adjacent corridor on same floor. If in wheelchair, self-sufficiency once in chair		
f.	LOCOMO-TION OFF UNIT	How resident moves to and returns from off unit locations (e.g., areas set aside for dining, activities, or treatments). If facility has only one floor, how resident moves to and from distant areas on the floor. If in wheelchair, self-sufficiency once in chair		
g.	DRESSING	How resident puts on, fastens, and takes off all items of street clothing, including donning/removing prosthesis		
h.	EATING	How resident eats and drinks (regardless of skill). Includes intake of nourishment by other means (e.g., tube feeding, total parenteral nutrition)		
I.	TOILET USE	How resident uses the toilet room (or commode, bedpan, urinal); transfer on/off toilet, cleanses, changes pad, manages ostomy or catheter, adjusts clothes		
J.	PERSONAL HYGIENE	How resident maintains personal hygiene, including combing hair, brushing teeth, shaving, applying makeup, washing/drying face, hands, and perineum (EXCLUDE baths and showers)		

2. BATHING—How resident takes full-body bath/shower, sponge bath, and transfers in/out of tub/shower (EXCLUDE washing of back and hair.) *Code for most dependent in self-performance and support.*
(A) BATHING SELF-PERFORMANCE codes appear below

0. Independent—No help provided
1. Supervision—Oversight help only
2. Physical help limited to transfer only
3. Physical help in part of bathing activity
4. Total dependence
8. Activity itself did not occur during entire 7 days
(Bathing support codes are as defined in Item 1, code B above)

(A) ___ (B) ___

3. TEST FOR BALANCE (see training manual)—*(Code for ability during test in the last 7 days)*
0. Maintained position as required in test
1. Unsteady, but able to rebalance self without physical support
2. Partial physical support during test; or stands (sits) but does not follow directions for test
3. Not able to attempt test without physical help

a. Balance while standing
b. Balance while sitting—position, trunk control

4. FUNCTIONAL LIMITATION IN RANGE OF MOTION (see training manual)—*(Code for limitations during last 7 days that interfered with daily functions or placed resident at risk of injury)*

(A) RANGE OF MOTION	(B) VOLUNTARY MOVEMENT
0. No limitation	0. No loss
1. Limitation on one side	1. Partial loss
2. Limitation on both sides	2. Full loss

(A) ___ (B) ___

a. Neck
b. Arm—Including shoulder or elbow
c. Hand—Including wrist or fingers
d. Leg—Including hip or knee
e. Foot—Including ankle or toes
f. Other limitation or loss

5. MODES OF LOCOMO-TION *(Check all that apply during last 7 days)*

Cane/walker/crutch	a.	Wheelchair primary mode of locomotion	d.
Wheeled self	b.		
Other person wheeled	c.	NONE OF ABOVE	e.

6. MODES OF TRANSFER *(Check all that apply during last 7 days)*

Bedfast all or most of time	a.	Lifted mechanically	d.
Bed rails used for bed mobility or transfer	b.	Transfer aid (e.g., slide board, trapeze, cane, walker, brace)	e.
Lifted manually	c.	NONE OF ABOVE	f.

7. TASK SEGMENTA-TION—Some or all ADL activities were broken into subtasks during last 7 days so that resident could perform them
0. No   1. Yes

8. ADL FUNCTIONAL REHABILITA-TION POTENTIAL
a. Resident believes he/she is capable of increased independence in at least some ADLs
b. Direct care staff believe resident is capable of increased independence in at least some ADLs
c. Resident able to perform tasks/activity but is very slow
d. Difference in ADL Self-Performance or ADL Support, comparing mornings to evenings
e. NONE OF ABOVE

9. CHANGE IN ADL FUNCTION—Resident's ADL self-performance status has changed as compared to status of 90 days ago (or since last assessment if less than 90 days)
0. No change   1. Improved   2. Deteriorated

Figure 12–9 MDS 2.0 Full Assessment Form, Section G.

Section H—Continence in Last 14 Days, Section I—Disease Diagnoses, and *Section J—Health Conditions.* In Section H, box 1, the continence pattern should be noted to understand a resident's potential needs during programming. Box 3 lets you know if a specialized program or appliance (i.e., catheter) is being used by the resident. If a resident is on a bladder training program, you should be familiar with his or her schedule to ensure that your programs and the training programs do not conflict. Section I gives you insight into the disease process, acute infection, or chronic condition that has brought your resident into the long-term care facility. By refamiliarizing yourself with the disease processes discussed in previous chapters, you will learn the specific needs of your resident. In Section J, all the boxes are important. Box 1 relates to problem conditions, and boxes 2 and 3 relate to pain symptoms and areas where pain is present (see Figure 12–10).

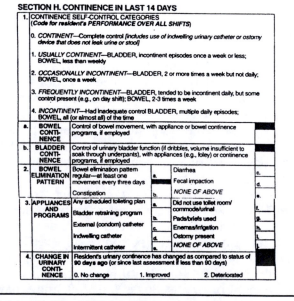

SECTION H. CONTINENCE IN LAST 14 DAYS

1. CONTINENCE SELF-CONTROL CATEGORIES *(Code for resident's PERFORMANCE OVER ALL SHIFTS)*

0. **CONTINENT**—Complete control *[includes use of indwelling urinary catheter or ostomy device that does not leak urine or stool]*
1. **USUALLY CONTINENT**—BLADDER, incontinent episodes once a week or less; BOWEL, less than weekly
2. **OCCASIONALLY INCONTINENT**—BLADDER, 2 or more times a week but not daily; BOWEL, once a week
3. **FREQUENTLY INCONTINENT**—BLADDER, tended to be incontinent daily, but some control present (e.g., on day shift); BOWEL, 2-3 times a week
4. **INCONTINENT**—Had inadequate control BLADDER, multiple daily episodes; BOWEL, all (or almost all) of the time

| a. | BOWEL CONTI-NENCE | Control of bowel movement, with appliance or bowel continence programs, if employed | |
| b. | BLADDER CONTI-NENCE | Control of urinary bladder function (if dribbles, volume insufficient to soak through underpants), with appliances (e.g., foley) or continence programs, if employed | |

2. BOWEL ELIMINATION PATTERN

Bowel elimination pattern regular—at least one movement every three days	a.	Diarrhea	c.
		Fecal impaction	d.
Constipation	b.	NONE OF ABOVE	e.

3. APPLIANCES AND PROGRAMS

Any scheduled toileting plan	a.	Did not use toilet room/commode/urinal	f.
Bladder retraining program	b.	Pads/briefs used	g.
External (condom) catheter	c.	Enemas/irrigation	h.
Indwelling catheter	d.	Ostomy present	i.
Intermittent catheter	e.	NONE OF ABOVE	j.

4. CHANGE IN URINARY CONTI-NENCE—Resident's urinary continence has changed as compared to status of 90 days ago (or since last assessment if less than 90 days)
0. No change   1. Improved   2. Deteriorated

Figure 12–10 MDS 2.0 Full Assessment Form, Sections H, I, and J *(continued on next page).*

Section K—Oral/Nutritional Status and Section L—Oral/Dental Status. In Section K, boxes 4 (nutritional problems) and 5 (nutritional approaches) provide the activity professional with information as to how nutritional goals can be supported in activity programming. Section L provides information about the resident's ability to chew and digest foods (see Figure 12–11).

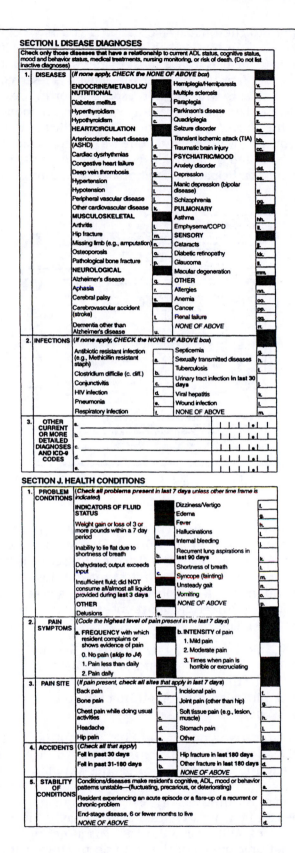

Figure 12–10 MDS 2.0 Full Assessment Form, Sections H, I, and J (continued).

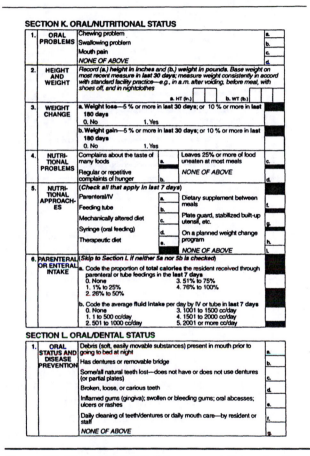

Figure 12–11 MDS 2.0 Full Assessment Form, Sections K and L.

Section M—Skin Condition. The activity professional should know if serious skin conditions exist that may limit a resident's participation outside the room, or if a treatment or turning schedule impacts programming times (see Figure 12–12).

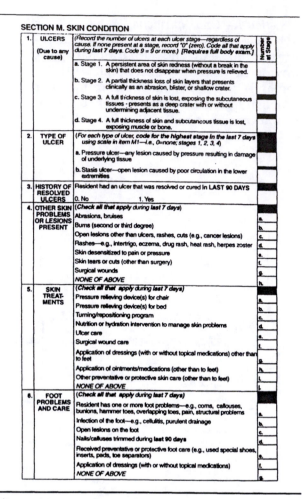

Figure 12–12 MDS 2.0 Full Assessment Form, Section M.

Section N—Activity Pursuit Patterns. Review with the team the other MDS items before jumping into Section N in order to understand the framework for activity department information in the total assessment picture. The intent of Section N (see Figure 12–13), according to AHCA (1995), is to "record the amount and types of interests and activities that the resident currently pursues, as well as activities the resident would like to pursue that are not currently available at the facility." Five boxes require completion in Section N. Using your pre-assessment or data collection forms, and observations you have made of the resident, complete this section. Area 1 refers to the amount of time a resident is currently awake, on average. This section remains the same from the older version of the MDS. Your observations and data collection will tell you to check A. morning, B. afternoon, C. evening, or D. none of the above. Simply check off all the boxes that

apply to the time-awake patterns you have observed. You may check more than one area if your resident is awake most of the day. The last category (area D., none of the above), is reserved for residents who are nonresponsive or in a comatose state for the majority of the day. If "none of the above" is your choice for a particular resident, you will not be required to complete areas 2, 3, 4, and 5 of Section N because the resident cannot participate in traditional programming.

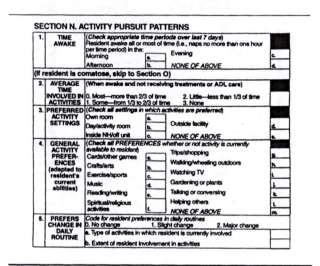

Figure 12–13 MDS 2.0 Full Assessment Form, Section N.

Another area in Section N deals with the average time spent in activities. A number is chosen from the four categories listed and placed in the empty box in Area 2. Choices for this area (that mention that the resident should be awake and not receiving treatment in calculating time frames) include:

- 0. most–more than two-thirds of the time
- 1. some–from one-third to two-thirds of the time
- 2. little–less than one-third of the time
- 3. none

The older versions of the MDS did not have explanations for "most," "some," and "little," and made the choosing of categories variable from one person to the next. To calculate the time frames for this category as accurately as possible, determine what a typical length of day is for this resident. What time did the person get up and what time did he or she go to sleep? Once that is determined, subtract time for bathing, dressing, treatments, and so forth, to arrive at the time a resident has to participate in activity programming. Look to see what portion of this available time the resident actually uses for activity pursuits. Is it two-thirds of the time, one-third to two-thirds of the time, less than a third of the time, or none of the time? Your answers should be placed in the box in Area 2.

Area 3 refers to the resident's preference of a setting for attending activities. The choices are: A. own room, B. day/activity room, C. inside nursing home/off unit, D. outside facility, and E. none of the above. More than one box may be checked if they apply to the resident. This area has remained unchanged from the older version of the MDS.

The fourth area in Section N concerns the general pattern of activities preferred by residents or "adapted to the resident's current abilities." In the new MDS 2.0, this section contains three new categories of activity choices, Areas J., K., and L. The sections are as follows: A. cards/other games, B. crafts/arts, C. exercise/sports, D. music, E. reading/writing, F. spiritual/religious activities, G. trips/shopping, H. walking/wheeling outdoors, I. watching TV, J. gardening or plants, K. talking or conversing, L. helping others, and M. none of the above. Using the assessment information you have gathered by observations and interviews with the resident and family members, check all the preferences, even if the program or activity is not available to the resident at this time.

The last area of the activity pursuit patterns in Section N has been changed in the new MDS 2.0 to elaborate on the preferences that a resident has in changes to the daily routine. AHCA (1995) defines the intent of this area as "determining if the resident has an interest in pursuing activities not offered at the facility (or on the nursing unit), or not made available to the resident. This included situations in which an activity is provided but the resident would like to have other choices in carrying out the activity." The choices for this category are: 0. no change (resident is satisfied with current situation), 1. slight change (resident may want to see minor changes, but is satisfied overall) and 2. major change (resident is not content for a specific reason and would like to see a change in routine). The choices for residents are applied to two separate categories in Area 5: A. the type of activities in which the resident is currently involved, and B. the extent of involvement in activities. This information must be gained from discussions with the resident, observations, and discussions with family members. Other than your signature on the last page of the MDS, this is the only area that requires your specific input and completion. Activity professionals who work in states using MDS+ or in case-mix states may have additional items to complete concerning isolation and sensory stimulation.

Section O—Medications and *Section P—Special Treatments and Procedures.* These sections are of interest to activity professionals because of expected behaviors and changes that may occur with medications changes and special treatments that may cause participation issues. Key areas in Section O are: 1. number of medications, 2. new medications, and 4. days received the following medications: antipsychotic, antianxiety, antidepressant, hypnotic, and diuretic. Residents on a high overall level of medications may experience drug interactions or may not function at full capacity. Additionally, the type and number of days on new medications is important information to have as well. Often, when a new medication is introduced, especially psychotropic drugs, it takes a period of time before a stabilization or other desired effect occurs. That is why the number of days on a new medication should be of interest to other caregivers. In Section P, Areas 1, 2, and 4 are important to the activity professional. Area 1 gives information about specific treatment programs in which the resident may be participating that takes time away from other facility programs. Additionally, these programs are related to a disease or chronic condition and gives insights into moods, feelings, and behaviors. Interventions that can be listed in Area 2 relate to programs you may be initiating to help your residents change behaviors, moods, or compensate for cognitive loss. This includes Item D., resident specific deliberate changes in the environment to address mood/behavior patterns (i.e., providing a bureau in which to rummage) and Item E., reorientation (i.e., cueing) related to specific team interventions to assist in modifying moods or behaviors. Become involved in the discussion and formation of these interventions in Area 2. Area 4 gives the activity professional insight into types of restraints or other devices used in resident care. It is crucial to understand the safety issues, other interventions that are being tried, and the release schedule for restraints in use. Sections O and P are shown in Figure 12–14.

Section Q—Discharge Potential And Overall Status and *Section R—Assessment Information.* These sections contain information of use in programming. Section Q, Item 1, relates to the possibility of discharge. Knowing the status of a resident's expected stay and overall changes in care that have occured since the last assessment are key items to note for planning. Section R notes if family and resident attended the planning session and provides space for

SECTION O. MEDICATIONS

1.	NUMBER OF MEDICATIONS	(Record the number of different medications used in the last 7 days; enter "0" if none used)
2.	NEW MEDICATIONS	(Resident currently receiving medications that were initiated during the last 90 days) 0. No 1. Yes
3.	INJECTIONS	(Record the number of DAYS injections of any type received during the last 7 days; enter "0" if none used)
4.	DAYS RECEIVED THE FOLLOWING MEDICATION	(Record the number of DAYS during last 7 days; enter "0" if not used. Note—enter "1" for long-acting meds used less than weekly) a. Antipsychotic b. Antianxiety c. Antidepressant d. Hypnotic e. Diuretic

SECTION P. SPECIAL TREATMENTS AND PROCEDURES

1. SPECIAL TREATMENTS, PROCEDURES, AND PROGRAMS

a. SPECIAL CARE—Check treatments or programs received during the last 14 days

TREATMENTS
- Chemotherapy a.
- Dialysis b.
- IV medication c.
- Intake/output d.
- Monitoring acute medical condition e.
- Ostomy care f.
- Oxygen therapy g.
- Radiation h.
- Suctioning i.
- Tracheostomy care j.
- Transfusions k.

Ventilator or respirator l.

PROGRAMS
- Alcohol/drug treatment program m.
- Alzheimer's/dementia special care unit n.
- Hospice care o.
- Pediatric unit p.
- Respite care q.
- Training in skills required to return to the community (e.g., taking medications, house work, shopping, transportation, ADLs) r.
- NONE OF ABOVE s.

b. THERAPIES - Record the number of days and total minutes each of the following therapies was administered (for at least 15 minutes a day) in the last 7 calendar days (Enter 0 if none or less than 15 min. daily) [Note—count only post admission therapies]
(A) = # of days administered for 15 minutes or more
(B) = total # of minutes provided in last 7 days

	DAYS (A)	MIN (B)
a. Speech - language pathology and audiology services		
b. Occupational therapy		
c. Physical therapy		
d. Respiratory therapy		
e. Psychological therapy (by any licensed mental health professional)		

2. INTERVENTION PROGRAMS FOR MOOD, BEHAVIOR, COGNITIVE LOSS

(Check all interventions or strategies used in last 7 days—no matter where received)
- Special behavior symptom evaluation program a.
- Evaluation by a licensed mental health specialist in last 90 days b.
- Group therapy c.
- Resident-specific deliberate changes in the environment to address mood/behavior patterns—e.g., providing bureau in which to rummage d.
- Reorientation—e.g., cueing e.
- NONE OF ABOVE f.

3. NURSING REHABILITATION/RESTORATIVE CARE

Record the NUMBER OF DAYS each of the following rehabilitation or restorative techniques or practices was provided to the resident for more than or equal to 15 minutes per day in the last 7 days (Enter 0 if none or less than 15 min. daily)
- a. Range of motion (passive)
- b. Range of motion (active)
- c. Splint or brace assistance

TRAINING AND SKILL PRACTICE IN:
- d. Bed mobility
- e. Transfer
- f. Walking
- g. Dressing or grooming
- h. Eating or swallowing
- i. Amputation/prosthesis care
- j. Communication
- k. Other

4. DEVICES AND RESTRAINTS

(Use the following codes for last 7 days:)
0. Not used
1. Used less than daily
2. Used daily

Bed rails
- a. — Full bed rails on all open sides of bed
- b. — Other types of side rails used (e.g., half rail, one side)
- c. Trunk restraint
- d. Limb restraint
- e. Chair prevents rising

5. HOSPITAL STAY(S) — Record number of times resident was admitted to hospital with an overnight stay in last 90 days (or since last assessment if less than 90 days). (Enter 0 if no hospital admissions)

6. EMERGENCY ROOM (ER) VISIT(S) — Record number of times resident visited ER without an overnight stay in last 90 days (or since last assessment if less than 90 days). (Enter 0 if no ER visits)

7. PHYSICIAN VISITS — In the LAST 14 DAYS (or since admission if less than 14 days in facility) how many days has the physician (or authorized assistant or practitioner) examined the resident? (Enter 0 if none)

8. PHYSICIAN ORDERS — In the LAST 14 DAYS (or since admission if less than 14 days in facility) how many days has the physician (or authorized assistant or practitioner) changed the resident's orders? Do not include order renewals without change. (Enter 0 if none)

9. ABNORMAL LAB VALUES — Has the resident had any abnormal lab values during the last 90 days (or since admission)?
0. No 1. Yes

Figure 12–14 MDS 2.0 Full Assessment Form, Sections O and P.

---

the team members' signatures, titles, which sections have been completed, and the date. The RN Coordinator verifies that the full assessment document is complete and accurate and signs to that effect. Figure 12–15 shows Sections Q and R.

SECTION Q. DISCHARGE POTENTIAL AND OVERALL STATUS

1.	DISCHARGE POTENTIAL	a. Resident expresses/indicates preference to return to the community 0. No 1. Yes b. Resident has a support person who is positive towards discharge 0. No 1. Yes c. Stay projected to be of a short duration— discharge projected within 90 days (do not include expected discharge due to death) 0. No 2. Within 31-90 days 1. Within 30 days 3. Discharge status uncertain
2.	OVERALL CHANGE IN CARE NEEDS	Resident's overall self sufficiency has changed significantly as compared to status of 90 days ago (or since last assessment if less than 90 days) 0. No change 1. Improved—receives fewer supports, needs less restrictive level of care 2. Deteriorated—receives more support

SECTION R. ASSESSMENT INFORMATION

1.	PARTICIPATION IN ASSESSMENT	a. Resident: 0. No 1. Yes b. Family: 0. No 1. Yes 2. No family c. Significant other: 0. No 1. Yes 2. None
2.	SIGNATURES OF PERSONS COMPLETING THE ASSESSMENT:	

a. Signature of RN Assessment Coordinator (sign on above line)

b. Date RN Assessment Coordinator signed as complete

	Month	Day	Year

c. Other Signatures	Title	Sections	Date
d.			Date
e.			Date
f.			Date
g.			Date
h.			Date

Figure 12–15 MDS 2.0 Full Assessment Form, Sections Q and R.

Quarterly Minimum Data Set

Called a "subset" of the MDS items by HCFA (1995), the quarterly review of an MDS is completed every three months at minimum to "assure the continued accuracy of the care plan." The **Quarterly Minimum Data Set 2.0** helps to monitor resident changes between the full assessments (required at least annually). The quarterly minimum data set contains a sampling of mandated items from the full assessment form that must be addressed for each resident three months after their first full assessment. Variations may exist from state to state on the components required in the quarterly assessment. Check with your MDS Coordinator. Within the first year of admission, a new resident should have at least one full assessment and three quarterly reviews. At the end of a twelve-month period, another full assessment should be conducted.

All items on the quarterly form are of importance because it highlights the status of a resident's condition. Activity professionals are responsible for completing Section N, which has only two areas in the quarterly review: 1. time awake, and 2. average time involved in activities. Completion of these items should be handled in the same manner as those on the full assessment form. In Area 1, "time awake," refers to the behavior of the resident in the last seven days, not a composite of their time awake over the last three months. If you check off "none of the above" in this section, you do not need to complete the N2 Area. Signatures, titles, sections completed, and dates are required at the bottom of the second page of this two-page document by all interdisciplinary team members who contributed information. The RN Coordinator for the MDS signs and verifies that the quarterly document is complete. The Quarterly MDS 2.0 Assessment Form is shown in Figure 12–16.

MDS QUARTERLY ASSESSMENT FORM

A1. RESIDENT NAME
a. (First) b. (Middle Initial) c. (Last) d. (Jr/Sr)

A2. ROOM NUMBER

A3. ASSESSMENT REFERENCE DATE
A. Last day of MDS observation period
Month — Day — Year
b. Original (0) or corrected copy of form (enter number of correction)

A4a. DATE OF REENTRY
Date of reentry from most recent temporary discharge to a hospital in last 90 days (or since last assessment or admission if less than 90 days)
Month — Day — Year

A6. MEDICAL RECORD NO.

B1. COMATOSE (Persistent vegetative state/no discernible consciousness)
0. No 1. Yes *(Skip to Section G)*

B2. MEMORY (Recall of what was learned or known)
a. Short-term memory OK—seems/appears to recall after 5 minutes
0. Memory OK 1. Memory problem
b. Long-term memory OK—seems/appears to recall long past
0. Memory OK 1. Memory problem

B4. COGNITIVE SKILLS FOR DAILY DECISION-MAKING (Made decisions regarding tasks of daily life)
0. INDEPENDENT—decisions consistent/reasonable
1. MODIFIED INDEPENDENCE—some difficulty in new situations only
2. MODERATELY IMPAIRED—decisions poor; cues/supervision required
3. SEVERELY IMPAIRED—never/rarely made decisions

B5. INDICATORS OF DELIRIUM—PERIODIC DISORDERED THINKING/AWARENESS (Code for behavior in the last 7 days.) [Note: Accurate assessment requires conversations with staff and family who have direct knowledge of resident's behavior over this time.]
0. Behavior not present
1. Behavior present, not of recent onset
2. Behavior present, over last 7 days appears different from resident's usual functioning (e.g., new onset or worsening)
a. EASILY DISTRACTED—(e.g., difficulty paying attention; gets sidetracked)
b. PERIODS OF ALTERED PERCEPTION OR AWARENESS OF SURROUNDINGS—(e.g., moves lips or talks to someone not present; believes he/she is somewhere else; confuses night and day)
c. EPISODES OF DISORGANIZED SPEECH—(e.g., speech is incoherent, nonsensical, irrelevant, or rambling from subject to subject; loses train of thought)
d. PERIODS OF RESTLESSNESS—(e.g., fidgeting or picking at skin, clothing, napkins, etc; frequent position changes; repetitive physical movements or calling out)
e. PERIODS OF LETHARGY—(e.g., sluggishness; staring into space; difficult to arouse; little body movement)
f. MENTAL FUNCTION VARIES OVER THE COURSE OF THE DAY—(e.g., sometimes better, sometimes worse; behaviors sometimes present, sometimes not)

C4. MAKING SELF UNDERSTOOD (Expressing information content—however able)
0. UNDERSTOOD
1. USUALLY UNDERSTOOD—difficulty finding words or finishing thoughts
2. SOMETIMES UNDERSTOOD—ability is limited to making concrete requests
3. RARELY/NEVER UNDERSTOOD

C6. ABILITY TO UNDERSTAND OTHERS (Understanding verbal information content—however able)
0. UNDERSTANDS
1. USUALLY UNDERSTANDS—may miss some part/intent of message
2. SOMETIMES UNDERSTANDS—responds adequately to simple, direct communication
3. RARELY/NEVER UNDERSTANDS

E1. INDICATORS OF DEPRESSION, ANXIETY, SAD MOOD (Code for indicators observed in last 30 days, irrespective of the assumed cause)
0. Indicator not exhibited in last 30 days
1. Indicator of this type exhibited up to five days a week
2. Indicator of this type exhibited daily or almost daily (6, 7 days a week)
VERBAL EXPRESSIONS OF DISTRESS
a. Resident made negative statements—e.g.,"Nothing matters; Would rather be dead; What's the use; Regrets having lived so long; Let me die"
b. Repetitive questions—e.g.,"Where do I go; What do I do?"
c. Repetitive verbalizations—e.g., calling out for help, ("God help me")
d. Persistent anger with self or others—e.g., easily annoyed, anger at placement in nursing home; anger at care received
e. Self deprecation—e.g., "I am nothing; I am of no use to anyone"

E1. INDICATORS OF DEPRESSION, ANXIETY, SAD MOOD (cont.)
VERBAL EXPRESSIONS OF DISTRESS
f. Expressions of what appear to be unrealistic fears—e.g., fear of being abandoned, left alone, being with others
g. Recurrent statements that something terrible is about to happen—e.g., believes he or she is about to die, have a heart attack
h. Repetitive health complaints—e.g., persistently seeks medical attention, obsessive concern with body functions
i. Repetitive anxious complaints/concerns (non-health related) e.g., persistently seeks attention/reassurance regarding schedules, meals, laundry, clothing, relationship issues
SLEEP-CYCLE ISSUES
j. Unpleasant mood in morning
k. Insomnia/change in usual sleep pattern
SAD, APATHETIC, ANXIOUS APPEARANCE
l. Sad, pained, worried facial expressions—e.g., furrowed brows
m. Crying, tearfulness
n. Repetitive physical movements—e.g., pacing, hand wringing, restlessness, fidgeting, picking
LOSS OF INTEREST
o. Withdrawal from activities of interest—e.g., no interest in long standing activities or being with family/friends
p. Reduced social interaction

E2. MOOD PERSISTENCE One or more indicators of depressed, sad or anxious mood were not easily altered by attempts to "cheer up", console, or reassure the resident over last 7 days
0. No mood indicators 1. Indicators present, easily altered 2. Indicators present, not easily altered

E4. BEHAVIORAL SYMPTOMS (A) Behavioral symptom frequency in last 7 days
0. Behavior not exhibited in last 7 days
1. Behavior of this type occurred 1 to 3 days in last 7 days
2. Behavior of this type occurred 4 to 6 days, but less than daily
3. Behavior of this type occurred daily
(B) Behavioral symptom alterability in last 7 days
0. Behavior not present OR behavior was easily altered
1. Behavior was not easily altered (A) (B)
a. WANDERING (moving with no rational purpose, seemingly oblivious to needs or safety)
b. VERBALLY ABUSIVE BEHAVIORAL SYMPTOMS (others were threatened, screamed at, cursed at)
c. PHYSICALLY ABUSIVE BEHAVIORAL SYMPTOMS (others were hit, shoved, scratched, sexually abused)
d. SOCIALLY INAPPROPRIATE/DISRUPTIVE BEHAVIORAL SYMPTOMS (made disruptive sounds, noisiness, screaming, self-abusive acts, sexual behavior or disrobing in public, smeared/threw food/hoarding, rummaged through others' belongings)
e. RESISTS CARE (resisted taking medications/injections, ADL assistance, or eating)

G1. (A) ADL SELF-PERFORMANCE—(Code for resident's PERFORMANCE OVER ALL SHIFTS during last 7 days— Not including setup)
0. INDEPENDENT—No help or oversight—OR—Help/oversight provided only 1 or 2 times during last 7 days
1. SUPERVISION—Oversight, encouragement or cueing provided 3 or more times during last 7 days—OR—Supervision (3 or more times) plus physical assistance provided only 1 or 2 times during last 7 days
2. LIMITED ASSISTANCE—Resident highly involved in activity; received physical help in guided maneuvering of limbs or other nonweight bearing assistance 3 or more times—OR—More help provided only 1 or 2 times during last 7 days
3. EXTENSIVE ASSISTANCE—While resident performed part of activity, over last 7-day period, help of the following type(s) provided 3 or more times:
— Weight-bearing support
— Full staff performance during part (but not all) of last 7 days
4. TOTAL DEPENDENCE—Full staff performance of activity during entire 7 days
8. ACTIVITY DID NOT OCCUR during entire 7 days (A)

a. **BED MOBILITY** How resident moves to and from lying position, turns side to side, and positions body while in bed.
b. **TRANSFER** How resident moves between surfaces—to/from: bed, chair, wheelchair, standing position (EXCLUDE to/from bath/toilet).
c. **WALK IN ROOM** How resident walks between locations in his/her room.
d. **WALK IN CORRIDOR** How resident walks in corridor on unit.
e. **LOCOMOTION ON UNIT** How resident moves between locations in his/her room and adjacent corridor on same floor. If in wheelchair, self-sufficiency once in chair.
f. **LOCOMOTION OFF UNIT** How resident moves to and returns from off unit locations (e.g., areas set aside for dining, activities, or treatments). If facility has only one floor, how resident moves to and from distant areas on the floor. If in wheelchair, self-sufficiency once in chair.
g. **DRESSING** How resident puts on, fastens, and takes off all items of street clothing, including donning/removing prosthesis.
h. **EATING** How resident eats and drinks (regardless of skill). Includes intake of nourishment by other means (e.g., tube feeding, total parenteral nutrition).

Figure 12–16 MDS 2.0 Quarterly Assessment Form (*continued on next page*).

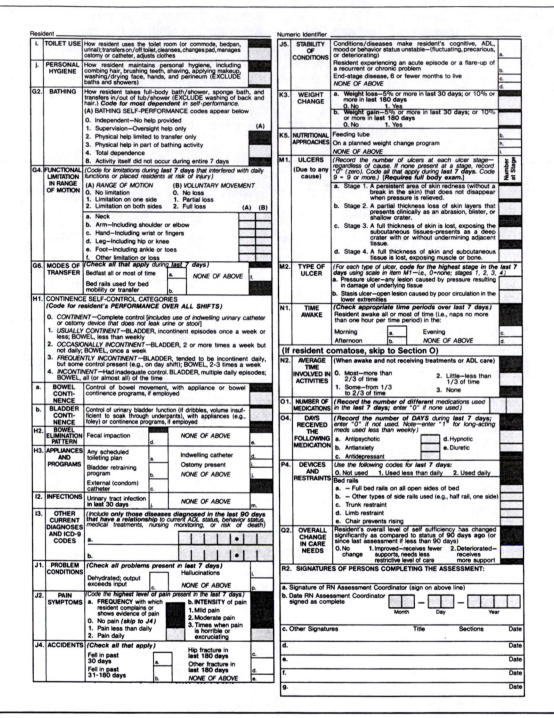

Figure 12–16 MDS 2.0 Quarterly Assessment Form (*continued*).

Significant changes refer to changes in resident status that require a new Full Assessment Form be completed. A significant change is defined by HCFA (1995) as " . . . a major change in the resident's status that is not self-limiting, impacts on more than one area of the resident's health status and requires interdisciplinary review or revision of the care plan." Self-limiting refers to a condition that resolves itself without intervention. Declining conditions, such as changes in unplanned weight loss of certain percentages, a negative change in an ADL physical functioning area, and positive improvements such as changes in incontinence patterns are all examples of significant changes.

A timetable that spells out the type of assessment document and the expected timing of each is summarized in Figure 12–17.

Resident Assessment Protocols (RAPs)

As part of the utilization guidelines, Resident Assessment Protocols (RAPs) are defined by HCFA (1995) as ". . . structured, problem-oriented frameworks for organizing MDS information and additional clinically relevant information about an individual that identifies medical problems and forms the basis for individualized care planning." The MDS is the first screening step to identify problems and residents' preferences. The triggers and the RAP process use the collected MDS information to develop solutions and determine types of interventions. The RAP process expects interdisciplinary team members to look for causes and risk factors involved in declines, poor improvement, limited abilities, or lack of participation. RAP starts the actual decision-making process whereas the MDS was simply the data collection stage. Following the development of the MDS, the interdisciplinary team reviews the document to see if certain conditions require intervention, if improvement of function is possible, if a predicted decline can be slowed or reduced, and if negative symptoms and pain are controlled as

much as possible. Using the RAP process helps address these team concerns and forms the necessary structure for the development of care plans.

There are four components to each RAP that must be understood before the sequence of steps in the RAP process are discussed. Each RAP contains a problem statement, triggers that illustrate an MDS response to one or more assessment items, guidelines for evaluation of triggered conditions (looking at causes and contributing factors), and a RAP key that provides a summarized list of triggered items. Eighteen RAPs have been identified for the MDS 2.0, including one in the area of activities. The full resident assessment protocol developed by HCFA for use in activities is shown in Figure 12–18. Reviewing this figure before we begin the discussion of each point will help you to better understand the process.

The general guidelines for using the RAP process start with the interdisciplinary staff completing the MDS and identifying "triggered" items. The HCFA (1995) defines triggers as "specific resident responses for one or a combination of MDS elements. These triggers identify residents who require further evaluation using resident assessment protocols designated within the State specified RAI." In reviewing the summary of Section One, the area of the RAP protocol for activities shown in Figure 12–18, the third paragraph informs us that certain assessment responses on the MDS should "trigger" our attention to review ". . . certain cases where the system may have failed the resident or where the resident has distressing conditions that warrant review of the activity care plan." The types of situations that should trigger an activity professional's attention include those residents who wish additional activity choices, those who have full cognitive skills, but are distressed and need activity interventions, those with cognitive problems who may also be distressed and in need of evaluated activity levels, and those whose high level of involvement may be causing health risks. The second page of the Trigger Legend Form that references the activity sections of the MDS is a tool to identify triggered items quickly during the RAP process, and is shown in Figure 12–19 on page 190. Locating triggered items begins by referencing the left hand column of Figure 12–19 to locate the four activity MDS items that have the capacity to generate triggers. Once located, the activity professional checks the responses on a particular resident's MDS to see if any automatic triggers have occurred. A solid circle indicates an automatic trigger and a circle with the number "2" inside indicates that a second

TYPE OF ASSESSMENT	TIMING OF ASSESSMENT
Admission (Initial) Assessment	Must be completed by 14th day of resident's stay.
Annual Reassessment	Must be completed within 12 months of most recent full assessment.
Significant Change in Status Reassessment	Must be completed by the end of the 14th calendar day following determination that a significant change has occurred.
Quarterly Assessment	Set of MDS items, mandated by state (contains at least HCFA established subset of MDS items). Must be completed no less frequently than once every 3 months.

Figure 12–17 Documentation timetable.

item is required to trigger. To evaluate the problems in the activity section that have been triggered, the activity professional begins asking himself or herself questions similiar to those in paragraph four in the problem section of Figure 12–18.

HCFA's RAI Version 2.0 Manual
RESIDENT ASSESSMENT PROTOCOL: ACTIVITIES

I. PROBLEM

The Activities RAP targets residents for whom a revised activity care plan may be required to identify those residents whose inactivity may be a major complication in their lives. Resident capabilities may not be fully recognized: the resident may have recently moved into the facility or staff may have focused too heavily on the instrumental needs of the resident and may have lost sight of complications in the institutional environment.

Resident involvement in passive as well as active activities can be as important in the nursing home as it was in the community. The capacities of the average resident have obviously been altered as abilities and expectations change, disease intervenes, situational opportunities become less frequent, and extended social relationships less common. But something that should never be overlooked is the great variability within the resident population: many will have ADL deficits, but few will be totally dependent; impaired cognition will be widespread, but so will the ability to apply old skills and learn new ones; and sense may be impaired, but some type of two-way communication is almost always possible.

For the nursing home, activity planning is a universal need. For this RAP, the focus is on cases where the system may have failed the resident, or where the resident has distressing conditions that warrant review of the activity care plan. The types of cases that will be triggered are: (1) residents who have indicated a desire for additional activity choices; (2) cognitively intact, distressed residents who may benefit from an enriched activity program; (3) cognitively deficient, distressed residents whose activity levels should be evaluated; and (4) highly involved residents whose health may be in jeopardy because of their failure to "slow down."

In evaluating triggered cases, the following general questions may be helpful:

- Is inactivity disproportionate for the resident's physical/cognitive abilities or limitations?
- Have decreased demands of nursing home life removed the need to make decisions, to set schedules, or meet challenges? Have these changes contributed to resident apathy?
- What is the nature of the naturally occurring physical and mental challenges the resident experiences in everyday life?
- In what activities is the resident involved? is he/she normally an active participant in the life of the unit? Is the resident reserved, but actively aware of what is going on around him/her? Or is he/she unaware of surroundings and activities that take place?
- Are these proven ways to extend the resident's inquisitive/active engagement in activities?
- Might simple staff actions expedite resident involvement in activities? For example: Can equipment be modified to permit greater resident access of the unit? Can the resident's location or position be changed to permit greater access to people, views, or programs? Can time and/or distance limitations for activities be made less demanding without destroying the challenge? Can staff modes of interacting with the resident be more accommodating, possibly less threatening, to resident deficits?

II. Triggers

ACTIVITIES TRIGGER A (Revise)
Consider revising activity plan if one or more of following present:
- Involved in activities little or none of time
  (N2 = 2, 3)
- Prefers change in daily routine
  (N5a = 1, 2)
  (N5b = 1, 2)

ACTIVITIES TRIGGERS B (Review)
Review of activity plan suggested if both of following present:
- Awake all or most of time in morning
  (N1a = checked)
- Involved in activities most of time
  (N2 = 0)

III. Guidelines

The followup review looks for factors that may impede resident involvement in activities. Although many factors can play a role, age as a valid impediment to participation can normally be ruled out. If age continues to be linked as a major cause of lack of participation, a staff education program may prove effective in remedying what may be overprotective staff behavior.

Issues to be Considered as Activity Plan is Developed.

Is Resident Suitably Challenged, Overstimulated? To some extent, competence depends on environmental demands. When the challenge is not sufficiently demanding, a resident can become bored., perhaps withdrawn, may resort to fault-finding and perhaps even behave mischievously to relieve the boredom. Eventually, such a resident may become less competent because of the lack of challenge. In contrast, when the resident lacks the competence to meet challenges presented by the surroundings, he or she may react with anger and aggressiveness.

- Do available activities correspond to resident lifetime values, attitudes, and expectations?
- Does resident consider "leisure activities" a waste of time - he/she never really learned to play or to do things just for enjoyment?
- Have the resident's wishes and prior activity patterns been considered by activity and nursing professionals?
- Have staff considered how activities requiring lower energy levels may be of interest to the resident - e.g., reading a book, talking with family and friends, watching the world go by, knitting?
- Does the resident have cognitive/functional deficits that either reduce options or preclude involvement in all/most activities that would otherwise have been of interest to him/her?

Confounding Problems to be Considered

Health-related factors that may affect participation in activities. Diminished cardiac output, an acute illness, reduced energy reserves, and impaired respiratory function are some of the many reasons that activity level may decline. Most of these conditions need not necessarily incapacitate the resident. All too often, disease-induced reduction of activity may lead to progressive decline through disuse, and further decrease in activity

---

Figure 12–18 RAP for Activities (*continued on next page*).

levels. However, this pattern can be broken: many activities can be continued if they are adapted to require less exertion of if the resident is helped in adapting to a lost limb, decreased communication skills, new appliances, and so forth.

- Is resident suffering from an acute health problem?
- Is resident hindered because of embarrassment/unease due to presence of health-related equipment (tubes, oxygen tank, colostomy bag, wheelchair)?
- Has the resident recovered from an illness? Is the capacity for participation in activities greater?
- Has an illness left the resident with some disability (e.g., slurred speech, necessity for use of cane/walker/wheelchair, limited use of hands)?
- Does resident's treatment regimen allow little time or energy for participation in preferred activities?

Other Issues to be Considered.
Recent decline, in resident status — cognition, communication, function, mood, or behavior. When pathologic changes occur in any aspect of the resident's competence, the pleasurable challenge of activities may narrow. Of special interest are problematic changes that may be related to the use of psychoactive medication. When residents or staff overract to such losses, compensatory strategies may be helpful - e.g., impaired residents may benefit from periods of both activity and rest; task segmentation can be considered; or available resident energies can be reserved for pleasurable activities (e.g., using usual stamina reserves to walk to the card room, rather than to the bathroom) or activities that have individual significance (e.g., sitting unattended at a daily prayer service rather than at a group activity program).

- Has staff or the resident been overprotective? Or have they misread the seriousness of resident cognitive/functional decline? In what ways?
- Has the resident retained skills, or the capacity to learn new skills, sufficient to permit greater activity involvement?
- Does staff know what the resident was like prior to the most recent decline? Has the physical/other staff offered a prognosis for the resident's future recovery, or change of continued decline?
- Is there any substantial reason to believe the the resident cannot tolerate or would be harmed by increased activity levels? What reasons support a counter opinion?
- Does resident retain any desire to learn or master a specific new activity? Is this realistic?
- Has there been a lack of participation in the majority of activities which he/she stated as preferences even though these types of activities are provided?

Environmental factors.
Environmental factors include recent changes in resident location, facility rules, season of the year, and physical space limitations that hinder effective resident involvement.

- Does the interplay of personal, social, and physical aspects of the facility's environment hamper involvement in activities? How might this be addressed?
- Are current activity levels affected by the season of the year or the nature of the weather during the MDS assessment period?
- Can the resident choose to participate in or create an activity? How is this influenced by facility rules?
- Does resident prefer to be with others, but the physical layout of the unit gets in the way? Do other features in the physical plan frustrate the resident's desire to be involved in the life of the facility? What correction actions are possible? Have any been taken?

Changes in availability of family/friends/staff support.

Many residents will experience not only a change in residence but also a loss of relationships. When this occurs, staff may wish to consider ways for resident to develop a supportive relationship with another resident, staff member or volunteer that may increase the resident to socialize with others and/or to participate in activities with this new friend.

- Has a staff person who has been instrumental in involving a resident in activities left the facility/been reassigned?
- Is a new member in a group activity viewed by a resident as taking over?
- Has another resident who was a leader on the unit died or left the unit?
- Is resident shy, unable to make new friends?
- Does resident's expression of dissatisfaction with fellow residents indicate he/she does not want to be a part of an activities group?

Possible Confounding Problems to be Considered for Those Now Actively Involved in Activities.

Of special interest are cardiac and other diseases that might suggest a need to slow down.

Figure 12–18   RAP for Activities (*continued*).

Following evaluation of the triggered issues, the activity professional and care planning team makes a decision as to whether or not a triggered condition warrants care planning intervention. The triggers shown in Figure 12–18, Section II, show activity care plan review and revision suggestions for particular triggers. The Activities RAP guidelines, section III, in Figure 12–18 offer questions to consider before developing or reviewing an activity plan for a resident. Is a resident understimulated or overstimulated? Are related health factors present that could impact enjoyment or participation? Have any declines occurred in resident status, such as communication, or changes in the environment or the family support network? To reduce the RAP items into a manageable format, the RAP key was developed for activities and summarizes the triggers and guidelines that should be used in care planning. The **RAP Key for Activities** is shown in Figure 12–20.

When using a **Resident Assessment Protocol Summary Form**, each area where problems were triggered or the need of an intervention appeared must be indicated on this form. The Resident

RESIDENT ASSESSMENT PROTOCOL TRIGGER LEGEND FOR REVISED RAPS (FOR MDS VERSION 2.0)

Key:
- ● = One item required to trigger
- ❷ = Two items required to trigger
- ✱ = One of these three items, plus at least one other item required to trigger
- @ = When both ADL triggers present, maintenance takes precedence

Proceed to RAP Review once triggered

MDS ITEM	CODE	Delirium	Cognitive Loss/Dementia	Visual Function	Communication	ADL-Rehabilitation Trigger A @	ADL-Maintenance Trigger B @	Urinary Incontinence and Indwelling Catheter	Psychosocial Well-Being	Mood State	Behavioral Symptoms	Activities Trigger A	Activities Trigger B	Falls	Nutritional Status	Feeding Tubes	Dehydration/Fluid Maintenance	Dental Care	Pressure Ulcers	Psychotropic Drug Use	Physical Restraints	MDS ITEM
J1n	Unsteady gait	✓																			●	J1n
J4a,b	Fell	✓												●							●	J4a,b
J4c	Hip fracture	✓																			●	J4c
K1b	Swallowing problem	✓																			●	K1b
K1c	Mouth pain	✓																●				K1c
K3a	Weight loss	1														●							K3a
K4a	Taste alteration	✓														●							K4a
K4c	Leave 25% food	✓														●							K4c
K5a	Parenteral/IV feeding	✓														●		●					K5a
K5b	Feeding tube	✓															●	●					K5b
K5c	Mechanically altered	✓														●							K5c
K5d	Syringe feeding	✓														●							K5d
K5e	Therapeutic diet	✓														●							K5e
L1a,c,d,e	Dental	✓																	●				L1a,c,d,e
L1f	Daily cleaning teeth	Not ✓																	●				L1f
M2a	Pressure ulcer	2,3,4														●							M2a
M2a	Pressure ulcer	1,2,3,4																		●			M2a
M3	Previous pressure ulcer	1																		●			M3
M4a	Impaired tactile sense	✓																		●			M4a
N1a	Awake morning												❷										N1a
N2	Involved in activities	0											❷										N2
N2	Involved in activities	2,3											●										N2
N5a,b	Prefers change in daily routine	1,2											●										N5a,b
O4a	Antipsychotics	1-7																			✱		O4a
O4b	Antianxiety	1-7													●						✱		O4b
O4c	Antidepressants	1-7													●						✱		O4c
O4e	Diuretic	1-7																●					O4e
P4c	Trunk restraint	1,2													●							●	P4c
P4c	Trunk restraint	2																		●			P4c
P4d	Limb restraint	1,2																				●	P4d
P4e	Chair prevents rising	1,2																				●	P4e

MDS 2.0 10/18/94N   October, 1995

Figure 12–19 Partial Trigger Legend Form.

TRIGGER — REVISION	GUIDELINES

ACTIVITIES TRIGGER A (Revise)
Consider revising activity plan if one or more of the following present:
• Involved in activities little or none of time
    [N2 = 2, 3]
• Prefers change in daily routine
    [N5 = 1, 2]
    [N5a = 1, 2]
    [N5b = 1, 2]
 	
ACTIVITIES TRIGGERS B (Review)
Review of activity plan suggested if both of following present:
• Awake all or most of time in morning
    [N1a = checked]
• Involved in activities most of time
    [N2 = 0]
	Issues to be considered as activity plan is developed:
	• Time in facility [AB1]
	• Cognitive status [B2, B4]
	• Walking/locomotion pattern [G1c,d,e,f]
	• Unstable/acute health conditions [J5a,b]
	• Number of treatments received [P1]
	• Use of Psychoactive medications [O4a,b,c,d]
	Confounding problems to be considered:
	• Performs tasks slowly and at different levels (reduced energy reserves) [G8c,d]
	• Cardiac dysrhythmias [I1e]
	• Hypertension[I1h]
	• CVA [I1t]
	• Respiratory diseases [I1hh, I1ii]
	• Pain [J2]
	Other issues to be considered:
	• Customary routines [AC]
	• Mood [E1, E2] and Behavioral Symptoms [E4]
	• Recent loss of close family member/friend or staff [F2f; from record]
	• Whether daily routine is very different from prior pattern in the community [F3c]

Figure 12–20 Activities RAP Key for MDS 2.0.

Assessment Protocol Summary Form, shown in Figure 12–21, illustrates RAP problem area #10. This section shows activities triggers that have been identified or other activity problems that need to be addressed. Often, problems come to light that have not actively triggered a RAP, but they must be handled as well. Column A on the form should be checked if the item referred to was triggered. A notation in the next column is made to indicate where this issue will be addressed in the medical record, and when, so that other care team members or the survey team can reference your handling of this matter The actual documentation of RAP decisions and results can be placed in the progress notes for activities or in care plan summary notes. A decision must be made within seven days of completing the RAI as to whether or not to address the specific triggered item in the care plan. A check must be made in the B column on the Resident Assessment Protocol Summary Form if the issue will be addressed in the care plan.

Care Planning

Following the RAP process, the development of a care plan begins. In the case of existing care plans, revisions can be made to care plans at this stage. HCFA (1995) refers to the care plan as "the blueprint for meeting the needs of individual resi-

dents." The RAI manual proposes that assessment and care planning should flow into a "seamless" process that looks holistically at residents, views separate functional areas of each resident, uses information to identify problems through triggers, looks at causes and risks for problems, and formulates and puts into effect an interdisciplinary care plan. The care planning decisions are actually based on the RAI process. Decisions of the interdisciplinary team may indicate at the time of their meeting that certain triggered items do not have impacts on a resident's functioning and may not need to be addressed in the care plan. The RAP review should generate the need for any care planning by suggesting specific issues at which to look. Identified problems, conditions, and so forth, should be reduced to functional or behavorial terminology, then, translated into **goals** that have measurable objectives with specific time frames for completion. Goals should include improvement, maintenance, or prevention. HCFA suggests a goal-writing formula as the subject + the verb + modifiers + time frame = goal. For example, Mrs. Smith (the subject) will choose and attend (the verb) two morning activities (the modifiers) each week (the time frame). **Approaches** or interventions are also mentioned in detail as the methodology of how to achieve the goals specific to a particular resident. An approach to the example above might be "review

SECTION V. RESIDENT ASSESSMENT PROTOCOL SUMMARY   Numeric Identifier _____

Resident's Name: Medical Record No.:

1. Check if RAP is triggered.

2. For each triggered RAP, use the RAP guidelines to identify areas needing further assessment. Document relevant assessment information regarding the resident's status.

- Describe:
  — Nature of the condition (may include presence or lack of objective data and subjective complaints).
  — Complications and risk factors that affect your decision to proceed to care planning.
  — Factors that must be considered in developing individualized care plan interventions.
  — Need for referrals/further evaluation by appropriate health professionals.

- Documentation should support your decision-making regarding whether to proceed with a care plan for a triggered RAP and the type(s) of care plan interventions that are appropriate for a particular resident.

- Documentation may appear anywhere in the clinical record (e.g., progress notes, consults, flowsheets, etc.).

3. Indicate under the Location of RAP Assessment Documentation column where information related to the RAP assessment can be found.

4. For each triggered RAP, indicate whether a new care plan, care plan revision, or continuation of current care plan is necessary to address the problem(s) identified in your assessment. The Care Planning Decision column must be completed within 7 days of completing the RAI (MDS and RAPs).

A. RAP PROBLEM AREA	(a) Check if triggered	Location and Date of RAP Assessment Documentation	(b) Care Planning Decision—check if addressed in care plan
1. DELIRIUM	☐		☐
2. COGNITIVE LOSS	☐		☐
3. VISUAL FUNCTION	☐		☐
4. COMMUNICATION	☐		☐
5. ADL FUNCTIONAL/ REHABILITATION POTENTIAL	☐		☐
6. URINARY INCONTINENCE AND INDWELLING CATHETER	☐		☐
7. PSYCHOSOCIAL WELL-BEING	☐		☐
8. MOOD STATE	☐		☐
9. BEHAVIORAL SYMPTOMS	☐		☐
10. ACTIVITIES	☐		☐
11. FALLS	☐		☐
12. NUTRITIONAL STATUS	☐		☐
13. FEEDING TUBES	☐		☐
14. DEHYDRATION/FLUID MAINTENANCE	☐		☐
15. DENTAL CARE	☐		☐
16. PRESSURE ULCERS	☐		☐
17. PSYCHOTROPIC DRUG USE	☐		☐
18. PHYSICAL RESTRAINTS	☐		☐

B. _____

   1. Signature of RN Coordinator for RAP Assessment Process   2. ☐☐ – ☐☐ – ☐☐☐☐   Month Day Year

_____

   3. Signature of Person Completing Care Planning Decision   4. ☐☐ – ☐☐ – ☐☐☐☐   Month Day Year

Figure 12–21   RAP Summary Form.

activity calendar with resident at the beginning of each week and encourage resident to attend programs that resident has selected." There are many activity care planning books that give you specific examples of sample goals and approaches to help you in your care planning endeavors.

Progress Notes or Episodic Notes

Documenting responses to goals, approaches, and interventions is the purpose of progress or episodic notes. **Progress notes** list the progress a resident has made toward particular goals. These notes used to be required on a regularly scheduled basis for each resident. Traditional charting allows each discipline to write progress notes in their own tabbed section of the chart. The advantage of this system is that all the information concerning a particular discipline, such as activities, can be found easily in one section. The disadvantage is that many of the notes are not read and shared by other disciplines because of the time involved. **Episodic notes** are becoming an accepted form of documenting changes in resident status, noting "episodes" of changes in behavior or moods and charting brief segments of information that relate directly to changes noted, as well as any responses to specific approaches to goals. **Integrated progress notes** or **focused charting**, described by DePaul Healthcare Corporation (1993), are used by all disciplines to document or describe ". . . all findings, focuses, or progress that requires communication to other disciplines." This style of charting, used by many facilities around the country, suggests that all disciplines document their interventions and other notes collectively in one area of the chart instead of segregated into separate discipline sections in the medical record. The advantages of this system is that members of all disciplines have only one area to look at for updates on resident status, and, at the same time, know that their documentation on progress will be read by the other team members. As more and more facilities become comfortable with the true value of the RAI process and meaningful care planning, we may see this type of focused charting replacing the traditional progress note methods.

Using Computers

Computers are already part of the information management system of many long-term care facilities and will gain further popularity because of the requirements of MDS 2.0 to be fully computerized. The standardized assessment procedure brought about by the Omnibus Budget Reconciliation Act (OBRA) regulations (1987) and the Institute of Medicine's 1986 report, suggested that one of the purposes of standardized assessment was to gain essential information to develop more efficient regulatory polices for long-term care facilities. HCFA has determined that an automated system, such as computers for data collection and transmission, results in more immediately available data for use in planning survey group samples, tracking data, and developing key long-term care policies based on the needs of facilities. For example, the MDS 2.0 data for a particular facility would be collected by the interdisciplinary team

and the information would be entered into the facility computer by a designated individual. Guidelines have been established by HCFA for the type of system and software specifications required for each facility. Once systems are set up in each state regulatory agency (such as the Department of Health), facilities would be informed as to how to send the MDS 2.0 information to the state regulatory office by means of computer transmission. The state office would then be able to review the information, and in the case of survey visits to your facility, the state agency would be able to select a resident sample from the MDS records or plan to check particular residents, based on the facility's computer records. In addition to using the MDS 2.0 records for use in selecting survey samples, the state agency will eventually be able to use the data to tabulate information about the scope of long-term care in that particular state. The MDS 2.0 data from state facilities can then be transmitted to the HCFA on a routine basis for federal review and tabulation. At this level, regulations, policies, and survey processes can hopefully be guided by the compiled information contained in the MDS 2.0 from each state. Variations by geographic area, trends in diseases or age groups, and an overall direction for policy development will be the biggest benefits of the MDS 2.0 computerization. These changes, although initially intimidating, should be welcomed by all professionals in the field because the problems they experience (i.e., high levels of cognitively impaired residents in the facility population) will force policies to address these critical care issues. Although you may not have to type your own MDS information into the computer, become familiar with your facility's computer system so you can "call-up" any MDS for review at a computer terminal. Most facilities use code numbers or passwords in their computer systems to limit access to those professionals with "a need to know."

Record keeping for the RAI requires a hard copy be maintained at the time of admission, after significant change in resident status, for quarterly assessments, and at the time of the annual assessment. This amounts to the last fifteen months of records for each resident. In facilities that maintain electronic records, it is not required to maintain hard copies if the last fifteen months can be printed out upon request, have a full back-up system to prevent damage, follow all guidelines for safekeeping and maintaining confidentiality of records, and have readily accessible electronic records.

Record Keeping to Assist With Documentation ....

To assist in justifying the goals and approaches used in resident care planning, record keeping of activity participation, resident interests, and other information should be collected and maintained. These records are not housed in the formal medical record, but are kept in a secure location (such as the activity office) and are considered supplementary to the medical record information. The kinds of records maintained varies from facility to facility, but many keep records of daily, weekly, and monthly attendance at group programs, as well as individual logs of participation for bedside and other individualized programs. Attendance records simply record the date of a particular program and list (or require check-offs for) the attendees. A master list of all residents can be kept for each month or quarterly period to record daily activity participation. Maintaining these attendance records can be time-consuming and are sometimes viewed negatively because probably, you would prefer to use the time with your residents instead. You may find it easier to keep journals or communication books for particular programs in which all activity department staff could write daily, use a single sheet for each resident to make weekly notes of their participation, or devise a system of your own that works for you.

When you initially planned programs and updated them, you used another record keeping system to help you to calculate information about the overall resident interests in your facility. These records show how you built and modified your program calendar to meet resident needs. Revising your programming rationale was part of the program planning process covered in earlier chapters. You should maintain your notes and tally sheets to show how and why you added or subtracted new programs from your calendar. Although the survey process may be less geared to viewing piles of records, some aspects of the survey process require that you explain your reasons for a particular plan or approach based on your determined resident interests. With proper record keeping, you will easily be able to produce the written rationale for your choices. Figure 12–22 shows two examples of traditional attendance record keeping that you may wish to adapt.

Policies and Procedures ....

Important documentation that supports the purpose and function of your entire department, as well as the methods of implementation, are **policies and procedures**. A **policy** is a written statement of the standard practice in a particular area in your department. For example, "It is the policy of the Activity Department of Chauncey Care Center to permit volunteers to work with residents only after completing two hours of orientation and training." A **procedure** outlines the step-by-step process of meeting the objectives of

NAME OF RESIDENT	1	2	3	4	5	6	7	8	9	10	11	12	13	14	15	16	17	18	19	20	21	22	23	24	25	26	27	28	29	30	31

NAME OF RESIDENT: _____

DATE	PROGRAM PARTICIPATED IN	COMMENTS/RECOMMENDATIONS

Figure 12–22 Examples of attendance record keeping.

the policy statement. A procedure for the example above might be "Step 1—After the volunteer application and interview process has been completed, the activity director will schedule the volunteer for a training session. Step 2—After successfully completing the training session, the activity director will arrange for the first day of volunteering at the facility, with an activity staff person to be present to arrange for introductions and assistance."

Policies and procedures are vital documents because they outline the objectives and goals of the department and translate every key area into a step-by-step procedure for all employees to understand and follow. The formation of policies and procedures, similar to the resident assessment instrument, provides a standardized format for delivery of services in your department. With a clear policy, you have a quality approach to special events planning or bedside programming. In every area, you can set departmental standards of practice on which to judge performance and delivery of services.

The starting place for developing policies and procedures is through the use of a standard form for your department. Your facility may have a form for policy writing or you may have the opportunity to develop your own. The major elements that need to be included are facility name, title of policy section, department name, space for the actual policy statement, a large section for the procedural steps, a signature and date space for the person preparing the policy, and a signature and date space for the supervisor who approves the policy. An optional area might be a space for dates of revision. A sample of a policy and procedure form is shown in Figure 12–23.

Each of the policy and procedural elements contained on the policy and procedure form must be understood in order for you to write an entire policy book for your department or revise an existing one. The title of your policy should be chosen carefully for two reasons: first, policies are usually filed alphabetically. You will want key words present in order to make the locating of policies easy for everyone. (i.e., a policy called "Volunteer Application Process" may be quicker to find than "The Application Process For Volunteers"). The second reason is that you want the policy to be as descriptive in title as possible to avoid confusion. You may have a number of policies that sound alike; therefore, specifying the title is important. The department name listed is meant for the dominant user of the policy. For all policies specific to the activity department, list "Activity Department" in the "Department" slot. For other policies, such as one on universal precautions, nursing or administration might be the originating department. In the section marked "policy," outline, in one or two sentences, the purpose or general meaning of your policy. Some examples of policy statements include: "A written schedule of the monthly activity programs is available to residents and staff by the first day of each month," "Use of facility space by outside community groups must be requested and approved in writing," or "Activity department staff meetings are held on the first Friday of every month." The procedure section requires a brief but detailed methodology to explain the usual steps in accomplishing the policy statement. All of the steps should be listed in detail, no matter how trivial a step may seem. The person responsible for completing a certain step should also be listed such as "office manager." Having specific accountability for each step helps ensure that all stages in the process will be properly completed.

Writing Guidelines

Writing policies and procedures is easy when you use a standard format and keep a few guidelines in mind. When writing the steps of a procedure, the information should be given in specific enough detail to be clear, but in the simplest terms possible. As you write policies, imagine that a new co-worker will be reading them who has little or no understanding of the workings of your department. If the policy and procedure works under that scenario, it will probably be an operational policy. As a double check, ask one of your colleagues to read the completed policy for accuracy and clarity. Remember that policy development has an approval stage where your administrator, another member of administration, or your owner needs to review, approve, and sign that a policy is approved and in effect as of a certain date. Some policies involve more than one department and could take weeks before they are agreed upon by all participants. Larger policies that have more than one page should also have spaces to indicate page numbers with reference to the total number of pages for the entire policy. For example, on a three-page policy, number the first page "Page 1 of 3," the second page "Page 2 of 3," and so on. Policies should be reviewed annually by you and your administrator. If necessary, revisions should be made, the new version dated with the revision date, and distributed to any departments or individuals who require a copy. After your policy book is reviewed by you

FACILITY NAME

Department:	Policy Name:

Policy:

Procedure:

Original Date of Policy: **Policy Revision Dates:**

Policy Developed By:

Policy Approved by: Page ___ of ___

Figure 12–23   Blank Policy and Procedure Form.

and your administrator, indicate in writing that a review has taken place and sign and date the sheet together. A partial list of policies and procedures that you should have for your department is included in Figure 12–24.

Other Facility Documentation ....

In addition to required medical record participation, and writing and revising policies and procedures, you may also be required to submit reports and send memos or letters. There are many specialty books that help to develop sharper writing or organizational skills, but a few guidelines when discussing reports and other written communication is necessary.

Monthly or Quarterly Reports

Many facilities, especially those with corporate ties, may require that a written report be submitted monthly, quarterly, or on another schedule to the administrator, owner, or board of directors.

SUGGESTED POLICIES AND PROCEDURES

Administrative Rounds
Assessment
Attendance At Meetings
Attendance Records
Bloodborne Pathogens
Budget Preparation
Community Use of Space
Documentation Schedules
Employee Appraisal
Employee Orientation
Employee Work Schedules
Function Request Form
Handling Groups
Handling Resident Precautions
Incident Reports
In-service Attendance
Maintaining Storage Areas
Meal Breaks
MDS
MSDS
Preparing for Programs
Professional Departmental Standards
Program Guidelines
Resident Council
Total Quality Management
Volunteer Applications
Volunteer Orientations

Figure 12–24 A list of sample policies and procedures to develop for your department.

This should not be viewed as another chore. Look at it as an opportunity to demonstrate in writing what you have accomplished over the period of time in question. Determine if a format exists for all reports or if you can devise your own. Some administrators may want reports filled with numbers: How many people did you reach through programs? How many activities were attended? Unfortunately, numbers may look good on paper, but do not indicate the full picture of the interventions that you have made in your department. A quality-based report (using a quarterly format for this example) includes a few key elements: overall review of the last three months, personnel changes (hirings, firings, or resignations), new programs added or subtracted and why, problems and how they were solved, number of volunteers added or subtracted and why, adherence to budget, current issues without resolution, and upcoming programs. When this report is submitted to your administrator, there will be no item of surprise if you have been using good communication techniques. As with any item that you submit, take care to ensure that it is neat (typing would be preferred) and legible. Keep a copy for your records, and review against your next report to ensure that all outstanding items were rectified and not moved forward from the last report.

Memos and Letters

Committing your thoughts to paper and sending correspondence to staff or the outside world may seem intimidating to some people, but it is an effective way of connecting professionally with your peers and the public.

Memos should be sent to other department heads and/or your administrator to notify them of schedule changes, upcoming events, reminders, special assistance you may need, or simple "thank yous." All memos should indicate clearly to whom they are being sent (i.e., To: All Third Floor 3–11 Staff), who is sending them (i.e., From: Stephen Chu, Activity Director), and what the subject of the memo is (i.e., Subject: New Evening Programs). It is important to include the date of your memo, and in the body of the written information, be sure to state clearly what you expect from the people who will receive your memo. Is it information only (i.e., please be aware that beginning on August 2nd, evening programs will be start at 6:15)? Or are you expecting a specific response (i.e., please submit your ideas for the next fund raiser by June 13th)? All expected responses should be explained clearly and a definite time for the response given. Leaving an open-ended response allows the recipient to use his or her own judgement as to when you need the information! Again, keep copies of all memos for future reference.

Letters sent to the public should follow standard letter format used by your business office manager or other reference books. When you send a letter out as an employee, you act as a representative of your facility and should conduct yourself as professionally as if you appeared in person. Letters, in proper format, should be typed, with no spelling or grammatical errors. The point of the letter should be clear and expressed in a friendly, business-like manner. Similiar to the memos, indicate what response you are looking for or what action you will be taking. Are you sending letters for recruitment of volunteers? In that case, close the letter by saying that you will contact the person by telephone next week. Are you sending a press release? Ask the person to consider using your information. This may sound elementary, but many people forget to include the basics in letters and memos

and are disturbed when they do not get the expected responses. Always include your full name, title, the address of the facility, and your telephone number. Proper courtesy dictates that you thank the recipient for his or her time and consideration. Copies of letters should go into your administrative files for reference.

SUMMARY

Learning about your specific documentation responsibilities and the overall need for accurate assessment is a large part of programming for resident needs. Developing a clear understanding of the Resident Assessment Instrument (RAI) and the role of the activity professional in the interdisciplinary care team process is a vital link to full assessment and delivery of care based on needs. Knowing the other documentation areas, such as record keeping, policies and procedures, and correspondence will also assist you in providing a professional and high level of service to your residents.

R E V I E W   Q U E S T I O N S

1. What are the components of the RAI?
2. What are the benefits of the RAI?
3. Why is care planning done after the MDS and RAPs?
4. What is the difference between a policy and a procedure?
5. Why is integrated or focused charting important?

O N   Y O U R   O W N

1. How can the interdisciplinary team use information in the MDS for quality assurance and improvement projects?
2. Write three new policies that addresses quality maintenance. Plan a schedule for implementation and for appropriate in-service staff.
3. Using a fictitious resident, complete the MDS and the RAP Summary sheet. Write a care plan to address various issues and make recommendations for program planning.

R E F E R E N C E S

American Health Care Association (1995). *The long term care survey*. Washington, DC: author.

Budge, M. (1989). *A wealth of experience: A guide to activities for older people*. Melbourne, Australia: MacLennan & Petty.

Committee on Nursing Home Regulation-Institute of Medicine. (1986). *Improving the quality of care in nursing homes*. Washington, DC: National Academy Press.

Crepeau, E. (1989). The process of activity assessment in geriatrics. *Topics in Geriatric Rehabilitation*, 4(4), 31–44.

The DePaul Healthcare Corporation (1993). *The interdisciplinary care planning process*. [training materials] Philadelphia, PA: author.

Federal Register (1991). Vol. 56., No. 187. Omnibus budget reconciliation Act.

Gallo, J., Reichel, W., & Anderson, L. (1988). *Handbook of geriatrics assessment*. Rockville, MD: Aspen Publishers.

Health Care Financing Administration (1995). *Long term care resident assessment instrument: User's manual for version 2.0*. Baltimore, MD: author.

Miller, M. (1989). *Documentation in long term care facilities*. Silver Spring, MD: Manor Healthcare Inc.

Perschbacher, R. (1993). *Assessment: The cornerstone of activity programs*. State College, PA: Venture Publishing Inc.

Uniack, A. (1994). *Documentation in a SNAP for activity programs*, 2nd edition. San Anselmo, CA: Skilled Nursing Assessment Program.

FURTHER READING

American Association of Homes and Services for the Aging (1995). *Preparing for your next survey: Understanding the new survey, certification & enforcement regulations.* (videotape). Washington, DC: author.

American Health Care Association (1993). *Health care decisionmaking in long-term care facilities.* Washington, DC: author.

Brasile, F., Conway-Callahan, M., Dager, D., & Kleckner, D. (1986). Computer applications in therapeutic recreation. *Therapeutic Recreation Journal*, 2nd Quarter, 8–18.

Beddall, T., & Kennedy, D. (1985). Attitude of therapeutic recreation toward evaluation and client assessment. *Therapeutic Recreation Journal*, 1st Quarter, 62–70.

Cunninghis, R. (1988). *The new art of documentation.* Holmes Beach, FL: Geriatric Educational Consultants.

Davis, E., & Greenwald, S. (1996). *The care-plan answer book for activity psychosocial and social service programs: A partner in definitive OBRA care plan compliance*, 2nd printing. Skokie, IL: SCG Consulting.

Fain, G., & Shank, J. (1980). Individual assessment through leisure profile construction. *Therapeutic Recreation Journal*, 4th Quarter, 46–53.

Ferguson, D. (1983). Assessment interviewing techniques: A useful tool in developing individual plans. *Therapeutic Recreation Journal*, 2nd Quarter, 16–22.

Hall, B., Hotelling, C.,& Nolta, M. (1995). *The album of activity policies and procedures.* San Diego, CA: Recreation Therapy Consultants.

Hall, B., & Nolta, N. (1992). *The activity care planning cookbook.* San Diego, CA: Recreation Therapy Consultants.

Howe, C. (1984). Leisure assessment/ instrumentation in therapeutic recreation. *Therapeutic Recreation Journal*, 2nd Quarter, 14–24.

Kane, R. A., & Kane, R. L. (1981). *Assessing the elderly: A practical guide to measurement.* Lexington, MA: Lexington Books.

Moore, E. A. (1987). *Directions for ICD-9-CM coding: Exclusively for long term care facilities.* Dryden, NY: Health Record Consultant.

Morris, J., Hawes, C., Fries, B., Phillips, C., Mor, V., Katz, S., Murphy, K., Drugovich, M., & Friedlob, A. (1990). Designing the national resident assessment instrument for nursing homes. *The Gerontologist*, Vol. 30(3), 293–302.

Morris, J., Hawes, C., Murphy, K., & Nonemaker, S. (1994). *Resident assessment instrument training manual and resource guide.* Natick, MA: Eliot Press

Rogers, J., Weinstein, J., & Figone, J. (1978). The interest check list: An empirical assessment. *The American Journal of Occupational Therapy*, Vol. 32(10), 628–630.

Sander, P. (1993). *Activity care plans for long term care facilities*, 4th edition. LaGrange, TX: M & H Publishing Co.

Sander, P. (1993). *Activity and volunteer service policies and procedures*, 3rd edition. LaGrange, TX: M & H Publishing Co.

Touchstone, W. (1984). A personalized approach to good planning and evaluation in clinical settings. *Therapeutic Recreation Journal*, 2nd Quarter, 25–31.

U.S. Department of Labor—Occupational Safety and Health Administration (1989). *Access to medical and exposure records.* (U.S. Government Printing Office-241-406/06626) Washington, DC: author.

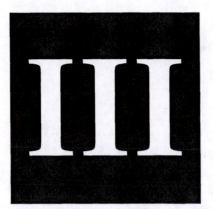

S E C T I O N   I I I

Program Evaluation and Enhancement

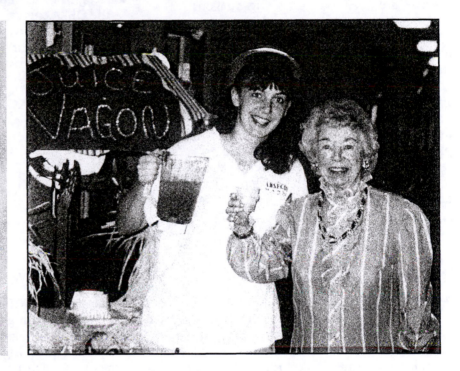

CHAPTER 13
Regulatory Compliance

OBJECTIVES..

After completing this chapter, you should:

- understand and interpret the regulations that apply to activity programming
- recognize the new enforcement guidelines for the OBRA survey
- handle the survey process and prepare a plan of correction for deficiencies.

INTRODUCTION

Providing activity programming to your residents does not occur in a vacuum. You are part of a larger health care team in your facility and a segment of the core of facilities that receive funding for servicing residents according to certain standards. Performance guidelines are set for your job responsibilities by your administrator and professional organizations, including regulatory mandates that govern the performance of staff members who work in a long-term care facility and the level of services they deliver. Learning about the regulatory system will help you to place your activity performance at the top.

Regulations and Accreditation ....

Whether you are in a privately funded facility or in an organization that participates in the Medicare or Medicaid program, there are guidelines called **regulations** monitored by an agency (such as the state or federal government) at particular intervals to determine if certain conditions are being met. Regulations are written standards of practice for all parts of the operation of a facility.

Determining Your Regulatory Agencies

As discussed in Chapter 1, the first step in the process of learning about the regulatory system comes from understanding which specific agencies have governing authority over your facility. Does your facility participate in the Medicare and/or Medicaid program? A facility that acts as a provider of services for either program (or both) is subject to a survey based on federal regulations. The same facility is also judged by all state regulations that apply. The survey in a facility that participates in the Medicare or Medicaid program is administered by the designated state agency (usually the Department of Health). This agency will view facility compliance with federal and state regulations, as applicable.

If your facility does not participate in the Medicare or Medicaid program, the same state agency will conduct the survey, but your facility will only be expected to comply with the regulations at the state level.

Omnibus Budget Reconciliation Act

The nursing home reform section of the **Omnibus Budget Reconciliation Act (OBRA)** of 1987 created a substantial change in the way that facilities have been surveyed and ultimately in the manner in which facilities deliver care. Focusing on resident needs, the OBRA standards underwent amendment changes in 1988, 1989, and 1990 at which time they arrived at today's version. The **Health Care Financing Administration (HCFA)**, a federal agency that determines financing and participation in federal and state programs such as Medicaid, responded to the new reforms by retailoring the survey process to be more interested in resident outcomes instead of strict compliance to written regulations. Friedlob, Steinfort, Santoro, and Luten (1990) reviewed and commented on the four areas of the revised OBRA survey process that include quality of care assessment, review of residents rights/quality of life, environmental quality assessment, and dietary services system assessment.

The quality of care assessment component of the OBRA survey looks at the resident's care over a period of time. Questions about participation in ADLs, if a resident's condition is improving or declining, and what interventions were made to improve or slow the declining process are asked to determine this review. Along with quality of care assessment came the mandate to begin using a minimum data set (MDS), considered a uniform method to measure and assess residents over a period of time. When conducting a survey, the interdisciplinary team members use the MDS, care planning materials, and resident observations to ascertain if quality care has been rendered.

To view the residents' rights component of the OBRA mandate, surveyors must determine the amount of control that residents have over decision-making and control of their lives. Resident rights are a written standard, but the facility must individualize them and allow a resident freedom enough to meet needs. Chemical or physical restraints, a method of restricting or changing resident movement or behavior, fall into this category and are reviewed in detail by the survey team. A review of quality of life issues in all departments are included with particular focus on activity services.

The physical scope of the building is included in the environmental quality assessment portion of the OBRA survey. Surveyors evaluate the sanitation and safety of the environment, as well as the ways in which the facility staff has made use of space and services to assist residents in their needs.

The tasks of the dietary assessment portion of the OBRA survey include a review of sanitation, food preparation and distribution, dining room environments, and individual nutritional status.

OBRA Survey and Enforcement Guidelines

A new set of OBRA rulings have been introduced into the Federal Register (1994) and stipulate guidelines for enforcement for the OBRA regulations, effective July 1, 1995. The new information enhances the focus on quality of life for residents. The two major changes come in the survey process and in the enforcement procedures when **negative outcomes** are found.

In terms of survey types, the revised OBRA guidelines describe four: **standard survey, extended survey, special survey** and **validation survey**. A survey is an observational review of facility procedures and practices by an outside regulatory agency and how these practices impact the life of the residents in the facility. Standard surveys are to be conducted by the state agency sometime between twelve and fifteen months from the date of the last survey. A survey team can conduct an extended survey (adding days to the original survey) if there are indications of "substandard quality of care" during the regular survey. A special survey can occur as a result of change of ownership or key staff (such as administrator) or because of a complaint. A validation survey is normally conducted by a federal team from HCFA a few months after the standard survey to monitor the performance of the state agency.

All the surveys are conducted by a multidisciplinary survey team composed of nurses, physicians, dieticians, and so forth, who are trained in the survey process. As of this writing, there may be at least one state that has survey teams with activity professionals as members.

Major changes in OBRA have come in the area of enforcement. The decision of the surveyors noting deficiencies through a group judgement process of the survey team remains unchanged. What alters radically is the **remedy** imposed for deficiencies. Some of the remedies for documented deficiencies include termination of the provider agreement with Medicare, Medicaid, or both, assignment of temporary management, denial of payments, civil monetary penalties, request for a specific **plan of correction**, and facility closure.

In order for the survey team to recommend a remedy, they must make a survey determination based on these three factors:

■ How serious is the deficiency or group of deficiencies? Is there an immediate threat to resident health and safety?

- What is the **severity** of the deficiency? What is the impact of this deficiency on the residents? Is there no harm to residents but potential for minimal harm (level 1), no harm but potential for more than minimal harm but no immediate jeopardy (level 2), actual harm but no immediate jeopardy (level 3), or immediate jeopardy to resident health or safety (level 4)?
- What is the **scope** of the deficiency? Are the deficiencies isolated, occasional, part of a pattern, or widespread?

The survey team may also consider a facility's past history of compliance as well as factors concerning clustering of deficiencies.

Based on the combined findings of the survey team in the areas of scope and severity, a series of remedies will be recommended in three categories:

- *Category 1:* the survey team will direct a required plan of correction, state monitoring, and directed (mandatory) in-service training.
- *Category 2:* denial of payment for new admissions, denial of payment for all residents (only can be imposed by HCFA), and civil monetary penalties of $50.00 to $3,000.00 per day.
- *Category 3:* temporary management assigned, immediate termination of provider agreement, and civil monetary penalties of $3,050.00 to $10,000.00 per day.

The surveyors use a scale with severity on one side and scope on the other to determine the category of remedy. Designations of letters A through L have also been included for each box to make referencing easier. They can select one or more remedies from each category, depending on the deficiency. Figure 13–1 illustrates the Scope and Severity Scale.

OBRA and Activity Services

The overview of OBRA surveys and the new enforcement guidelines are meant to give you a broad understanding of the entire view of regulatory compliance. Your part in the process begins with complete knowledge of the federal regulations that are within your jurisdiction. Each federal regulation contains a **tag number**, proceeded by the letter "F," which designates a federal guideline. The following are some highlights of the federal regulations from the American Health Care Association (1995) with which you and your staff must become familiar:

Direct Activity Federal Regulations

- *F 248 (1):* The facility must provide for an ongoing program of activities designed to meet, in accordance with the comprehensive assessment, the interests and the physical, mental, and psychosocial well-being of each resident
- *F 249 (2):* Staffing requirements covered in Chapter 1 of this text.

Indirect Activity Federal Regulations

- *F 151 (a) (1):* The resident has the right to exercise his or her rights as a resident of the facility and as a citizen or resident of the United States.
- *F 155 (4):* The resident has the right to refuse treatment, to refuse to participate in experimental research, and to formulate an advance directive as specified in paragraph (8) of this section.
- *F 240:* A facility must care for its residents in a manner and in an environment that promotes maintenance or enhancement of each resident's quality of life.
- *F 241 (a):* The facility must promote care for residents in a manner and in an environment that maintains or enhances each resident's dignity and respect in full recognition of his or her individuality.
- *F 242 (b):* Self-determination and participation. The resident has a right to:
- *F 242 (b) (1):* Choose activities, schedules, and health care consistent with his or her interests, assessments, and plans of care,
- *F 242 (b) (2):* Interact with members of the community inside and outside the facility.
- *F 242 (b) (3):* Make choices about aspects of his or her life in the facility that are significant to the resident.
- *F 245 (d):* Participation in other activities. A resident has the right to participate in social, religious, and community activities that do not interfere with the rights of other residents in the facility.
- *F 245 (e):* Accommodation of needs. A resident has the right to:
- *F 246 (1):* Reside and receive services in the facility with reasonable accommodations of individual needs and preferences, except when the health or safety of the individual or other residents would be endangered.

Within the AHCA book, each tag number corresponds to a listing called **interpretive guidelines**, the surveyor's method of determining if compliance has taken place. The interpretive guidelines give the surveyor a list of questions to ask and observations

	Isolated	Pattern	Widespread
Immediate Jeopardy to Resident Health or Safety	**PoC** Required: Cat. 3 Optional: Cat. 1 Optional: Cat. 2 **J**	**PoC** Required: Cat. 3 Optional: Cat. 1 Optional: Cat. 2 **K**	**PoC** Required: Cat. 3 Optional: Cat. 2 Optional: Cat .1 **L**
Actual Harm that is not Immediate Jeopardy	**PoC** Required* Cat. 2 Optional: Cat. 1 **G**	**PoC** Required* Cat. 2 Optional: Cat. 1 **H**	**PoC** Required* Cat. 2 Optional: Cat. 1 Optional: Temporary Mgmt. **I**
No Actual Harm with Potential for More than Minimal Harm that is not Immediate Jeopardy	**PoC** Required* Cat. 1 Optional: Cat. 2 **D**	**PoC** Required* Cat. 1 Optional: Cat .2 **E**	**PoC** Required* Cat. 2 Optional: Cat. 1 **F**
No Actual Harm with Potential for Minimal Harm	No Remedies Commitment to Correct Not on HCFA-2567 **A**	**PoC** **B**	**PoC** **C**

Substandard quality of care: any deficiency in §483.13 Resident Behavior and Facility Practices, §483.15 Quality of Life, or in §483.25, Quality of Care that constitutes: immediate jeopardy to resident health or safety; or, a pattern of or widespread actual harm that is not immediate jeopardy; or, a widespread potential for more than minimal harm that is not immediate jeopardy, with no actual harm.

Substantial compliance

Remedy Categories

Category 1 (Cat. 1)	Category 2 (Cat. 2)	Category 3 (Cat. 3)
Directed Plan of Correction State Monitor; and/or Directed In-service Training	Denial of Payment for New Admissions; Denial of Payment for All Individuals, Imposed by HCFA; and/or Civil Money Penalties: $50 - $3,000 per day	Temporary Management Termination **Optional:** Civil Money Penalties: $3,050 - $10,000 per day

DENIAL OF PAYMENT FOR NEW ADMISSIONS must be imposed when a facility is not in substantial compliance within three months after being found out of compliance.

DENIAL OF PAYMENT AND STATE MONITORING must be imposed when a facility has been found to have provided substandard quality of care on three consecutive standard surveys.

Note: Termination may be imposed by the State or HCFA at any time when appropriate.

*Required only when decision is made to impose alternate remedies instead of or in addition to termination.

Figure 13–1 The Scope and Severity Scale.

to make in order to gauge a facility's adherence to the regulations in a particular area. Because the guidelines are interpreted by this series of observations and questions, differences are possible in the way that survey teams assess what they observe.

To understand the impact of the severity and scope requirements along with the corresponding remedies, Figure 13–2 illustrates some examples of activity services issues that could cause a deficiency in each of the key areas A through L.

Complying with Regulations

Knowing the regulations is one thing; complying with them is another. Your focus with any rule or regulation is to act in the interests of the resident.

You need to stay in a middle ground in the area of compliance. Be aware of and follow the necessary steps that provide proper activity services, but balance your enthusiasm so that you are not swamped with new forms you have created and unnecessary jobs you may have given yourself. The old survey process that OBRA replaced relied heavily on "paper compliance." Everything looked great on paper, but the resident care observed may not have been the same as what was documented on paper.

Take the time to learn the regulations and survey process until you are comfortable with it. Look beyond the actual written regulation to the meaning and interpretation of the guideline. All of your staff must be aware of how the regulations set the framework for the work we do. Use your quality assurance program to help you determine compliance with the regulations.

Accreditation Surveys

In addition to OBRA surveys which are mandated, some facilities have sought accreditation through special surveys offered by the **Joint Commission on Accreditation of Healthcare Organizations (JCAHO)** and the **Commission on Accreditation of Rehabilitation Facilities (CARF)**.

JCAHO, founded in Illinois in 1967, promotes quality care in long-term care facilities that operate independently or as part of a hospital setting. Using strict survey procedures in key operational areas, a facility undergoes a voluntary and scheduled survey by the JCAHO team. If a facility meets the JCAHO standards, accreditation status is achieved. To evaluate activity services, JCAHO (1995) looks at staffing, policies and procedures, quality improvement, and activities in progress for groups and bed-bound residents.

CARF, based in Arizona since 1966, offers specific accreditation to facilities that offer inpatient rehabilitation programs. The CARF process looks at indicators of quality in the rights and participation of the disabled.

Both the CARF and JCAHO accreditation differ from the federal OBRA survey process in three main areas. First, facilities are judged on standards that CARF and JCAHO have determined are important, not on mandated regulations. Second, participation is voluntary with notice of the survey date given in advance. Third is the cost factor. The accreditation process of both organizations costs a few thousand dollars for facilities who opt for accreditation. And, after paying the survey fees, there is no guarantee that a facility will meet the necessary accreditation guidelines and be granted accreditation.

SCOPE AND SEVERITY SCALE APPLIED TO THE ACTIVITY DEPARTMENT

	Isolated	Pattern	Widespread
Immediate jeopardy to resident health and safety	**J** Residents noted in unsafe activity; activity not adapted to needs.	**K** More than 25% of residents noted in unsafe activities; programs not adapted to needs.	**L** More than 50% of residents noted in unsafe activities; programs not adapted to needs.
Actual harm; no immediate jeopardy	**G** Resident expressed desire for more activities; none were offered.	**H** More than 25% of residents expressed desire for more activities; none were offered.	**I** More than 50% of residents expressed desire for more activities; none were offered.
No actual harm, but potential for more than minimal harm	**D** Resident wishes to attend an activity, but care schedule conflicts.	**E** More than 25% of residents are prevented from attending programs due to care schedules.	**F** More than 50% of residents are prevented from attending programs due to care schedules.
No actual harm, with potential for minimal harm	**A** Resident is left in an activity for 15 minutes after a program concludes.	**B** More than 25% of residents are left in an activity for 15 minutes after a program concludes.	**C** More than 50% of residents are left in an activity for 15 minutes after a program concludes.

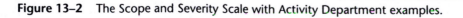

Figure 13–2 The Scope and Severity Scale with Activity Department examples.

Dealing with a Survey Visit ....

Most staff members shake in fear when the survey team comes in for its annual visit. They are trained professionals and they have a job to do. They are verifying that your facility and staff continue to meet the conditions of participation for certification for Medicaid or Medicare. Or, if you are in an all-private facility, the team will be checking its adherence to regulations on the state level. During the survey, the team observes, interviews, and reviews the records.

Meeting the Team

The survey teams always come unannounced, and their visit will be a surprise. Teams usually visit a facility every nine to fifteen months from their last visit. With careful attention to the regulations guiding care throughout the year, you will be prepared. Normally, team members meet briefly with the administrator and then go on a short facility tour. One of the first orders of business for the survey team is to select an anonymous resident sample for their observations and interviews. A **resident sample** is a target representation of a resident population and includes residents of varying medical and cognitive levels. With the computerization of the MDS, the selection of the resident sample for your facility began in the survey team's office. You may be asked to accompany a survey member on an extended tour or to assist in locating residents for interviews.

Questions You may be Asked

The survey team will be busy conducting their survey over the next few days (facility size determines the length of stay) and will have many opportunities to interact with you and your staff. Advanced preparation of all necessary documentation is a given. You could, however, be asked about policies and procedures of your department, the general operation of the facility, or interventions you have tried in an attempt to assist in identified resident problems or needs. The bulk of your intervention attempts (along with those of other team members), should be on the care plan or in your interdisciplinary progress notes. Additionally, you may have information in your "hot file" about special programs or intervention methods that are too detailed to write on the medical record. This information should be available in case a discussion comes up with a surveyor and it is needed for supporting documentation.

The survey team may also question you about participation levels and particular program offerings you have made. You may be asked to assemble your residents' council for a special meeting. The survey team uses a closed session of the resident council forum to gain insight into resident concerns. Attendance records may be requested, but because the focus is on the positive outcome of the resident, few surveyors want to look at twelve months' worth of attendance sheets. As far as your choice of programs, you may have to produce justification for a particular program. Your quality assurance records will be valuable to show you are monitoring your program and to reaffirm that your selected programs are meeting the goals you established.

Attending the Exit Conference

When the survey is finally complete, you and fellow department heads, along with the extended health care team of consultants and others, will probably be invited to attend the **exit conference**. With all the designated staff in attendance that your administrator has deemed appropriate, the surveyors will use their findings in their resident samples to illustrate whether or not care objectives for the facility have been met. If they have encountered major problems early in the survey process, they would have requested an extended survey to further investigate the problems. Each member of the survey team usually reports on the items they found and will state whether or not a deficiency has been found. Using the enforcement guidelines, they will also make a recommendation for remedies. It is helpful to take notes during the conference. All functions of the facility should be of interest to you. You will have a fairly good "feel" for how the survey went by the time the team is ready to leave. Often, final determinations on deficiencies and corresponding remedies are made at the office after the team returns, and your administrator can expect a written report in a few weeks.

Responding to Deficiencies ....

Deficiencies can occur, even in the best facilities. If your department has received a **deficiency**, you probably had some indication of it during the exit conference. The time to begin formulating a plan for correcting the problem is immediately after the exit conference. You may have already been aware of the issue before the survey and begun steps to correct the problem. If the problem is relatively

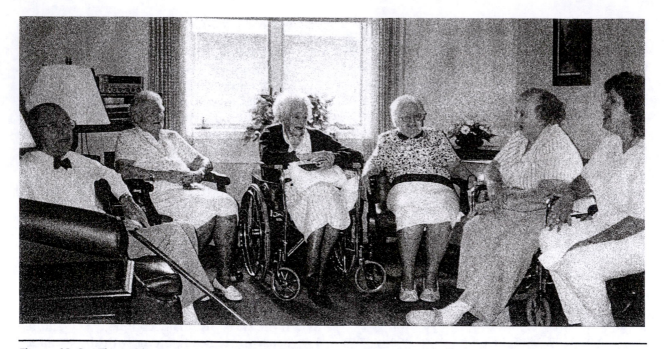

Figure 13–3 The resident council meeting is an important group for survey teams to visit, and listen to any concerns.

minor, make a plan to present to your administrator and begin to tackle the problem. If the issue is more serious, meet with your administrator as soon as possible to get input on how the problem should be handled. He or she may suggest a detailed plan that involves other departments and the quality assurance team. Once the plan is underway, monitor the situation closely, and report progress often to your administrator.

Writing A Plan Of Correction

When the deficiency package arrives from the state agency, your administrator will write a plan of correction for the more minor issues and formulate a game plan for anything larger. Depending on your administrator's style, you may be asked to submit a written plan of correction or discuss your plans in person. The written plan has to be global in nature; it should address the problem and provide a new situation so that similar problems will not recur. As you saw from the scope and severity grid, some of the problems that could be found are so serious that they all require a plan of correction, and involve interdepartmental relationships or a critical "relook" at the overall way in which the department is delivering services. The correction plan must have clear target dates for completion and should include a notation on who will monitor the compliance of the plan of correction. Your administrator will have the whole plan prepared and mailed back to the state agency in the time frame

allowed. If there is any disagreement in interpretation or receipt of particular deficiencies by either you or your administrator, your administrator may participate in a conflict resolution procedure with the regulatory agency, as outlined by the AHCA (1995).

Using OSCAR Data

As the data obtained during a survey process is compiled in state and federal agencies, some continuous historical information is being compiled on each facility's survey records called **Online Survey Certification And Reporting Data (OSCAR)**. An OSCAR 3 report is a compilation of a particular facility's record of past deficiencies whereas an OSCAR 4 report is a comparison of a particular facility's results against national, state, and regional reporting averages.

Why is the OSCAR information useful? These reports are part of the public record and consumers have access to them. More important, facilities should monitor the information on past performance to dictate needed quality assurance programs and other changes in facility practices. Become aware of the contents of these reports forwarded periodically to your administrator.

Using Quality Assurance and Supervision to Make Corrections

Having a plan of correction that involves your quality assurance team makes sense. If there are areas that have been unintentionally neglected or have the potential to become bigger problems, structure a quality assurance monitoring system to keep track of these issues.

Assignments of direct supervision to vulnerable areas is another way to make new progress in areas of concern. Additionally, you should form ad hoc committees with other departmental staff to solve problems with overlapping issues.

In every case, the dialogue you have with your administrator on the progress you are making is critical.

SUMMARY

The regulatory system imposes structure and rules for the way you and your staff render activity services. The OBRA survey process, with its focus on the resident's quality of life, measures resident outcomes through observations and interviews. Your participation in the survey process and exit conference is important for your growth as a health care team member.

R E V I E W   Q U E S T I O N S

1. What is OBRA, and why is this survey different from other procedures?
2. What are scope and severity in relation to the survey process?
3. What are some of the questions that you may be asked by surveyors?
4. What is a resident sample?
5. Define OSCAR data.

O N   Y O U R   O W N

1. Using the full list of all the federal regulations, what other tag numbers can you find that would have applications to the activity program?
2. How would you handle the issue in your programming raised in F 245 and F 246 about a resident's accommodation of needs?
3. Design and present an in-service program to your residents explaining the OBRA survey process.

R E F E R E N C E S

American Health Care Association (1995). *The long term care survey*. Washington, DC: American Health Care Association.

American Health Care Association (1995). *Proposal for conflict resolution.* (16–18). Washington, DC: author.

Committee on Nursing Home Regulation-Institute of Medicine (1986). *Improving the quality of care in nurs-*ing homes. Washington, DC: National Academy Press.

Federal Register (1994). Vol. 59, No. 217. *Medicare and Medicaid Programs; Survey, Certification and Enforcement of Skilled Nursing Facilities and Nursing Facilities.*

F U R T H E R   R E A D I N G

Friedlob, A., Steinfort, L., Santoro, V., & Luten, E. (1990). Moving ahead with the challenge: Meeting the OBRA mandate. *Provider*, April 1992.

Martin, S., & Smith, R. (1993). OBRA legislation and recreational activities: Enhancing personal control in nursing homes. *Activities, Adaptation & Aging*, Vol. 17(3), 1–14.

U.S. Department of Health and Human Services (1995). *Survey, certification and enforcement of skilled nursing facilities and nursing facilities.* (Health Care Financing Administration, HSQ-156-F) Baltimore, MD: author.

C H A P T E R   1 4
- -
Quality Assurance and Total Quality Management

OBJECTIVES ....

After completing this chapter, you should:

- master the differences between evaluation, quality assurance, and total quality management
- understand the variations in creating workable measurement procedures
- design and implement quality improvement teams to assist in resolving departmental issues

....

INTRODUCTION

Evaluating resident needs and offering programs to meet those needs is the main function of your department. But what methodology is in place to ensure that departmental objectives and programming efforts reach the needs of your residents? How will acknowledged problem areas in your department be resolved in an efficient manner? Learning about quality, evaluation, quality assurance, and quality improvement will ensure that your top-notch program continues successfully for many years.

What is Quality? ....

The American Health Care Association (1994) mentioned the importance of quality initiatives in their view of the future, and acknowledged that "quality may be the single most important issue facing long-term care providers." The definition of **quality** is hard for researchers to agree on, but one that summarizes the current thinking is offered by Leebov and Ersoz (1991): "Quality in health care means doing the right things right and making continuous improvements." According to Organizational Dynamics (1987), the "father" of quality, W. Edwards Deming (who pioneered the quality prin-

ciples in Japan that we use today) makes this statement about our view of quality: "Americans still care about quality. The country is full of intelligent, courageous people who would change if they only knew how." Other random quotes about quality, collected by McAlindon (1992), give a flavor of the varied meanings of quality in management and service-driven environments such as long-term care. "Quality is not a department responsibility. Quality is everyone and everything within an organization," "Quality is essentially attention to detail," "Quality improvement is a never ending process," "A commitment to quality must start at the top," and "Quality is never an accident; it is always the result of high intention, sincere effort, intelligent direction and skillful execution; it represents the wise choice of many alternatives."

Gaining an understanding of key quality terminology will help you as you proceed through this chapter. Some of the commonly used terms sound the same but have different meanings. **Quality assurance (QA)**, as defined by Riley (1987), is "... a process that enables the health professional to identify areas of improvement, detect potential problem areas, and design strategies for overcoming deficient areas in patient care." **Total quality management (TQM)** (also called **continuous quality improvement [CQI]** or quality improvement) is defined by Raimondo (1994) as ". . . a management philosophy and practice that establishes quality as an organization's highest priority. . . ."

The Relationship of Quality to Evaluation

Striving for quality begins as a function of the process and need for **evaluation**. The concept of evaluation is defined by Edginton, Compton, and Hanson (1980) as ". . . the process whereby information is obtained in order to assess the efficiency and effectiveness of an organization. . . ." They also state that the reason evaluation takes place is to guide professionals in making efficient decisions about meeting residents' needs and desires. Farrell and Lundegren (1991) mention that evaluation involves determining the value of something and assessing whether or not program objectives have been met. As discussed in Chapter 8, the process of providing activity services to residents follows a sequence of steps. One of the most widely accepted systems approach to the delivery of recreation services was proposed by Gunn and Peterson (1984). A process occurs that includes setting objectives, designing a program based on goals, planning a method for delivery of services, implementing the program, and finally evaluating and, if necessary, revising the program. Evaluation is part of the effort to make improvements to existing programs as well as to set up a system for **accountability** or responsibility.

Farrell and Lundegren (1991) suggest that an evaluation process to determine a program's effectiveness should contain three steps: measurement, judging the value of the measurement against a standard, and making a decision based on the data and options available. What kinds of activity related items could be evaluated? Edginton, Compton, and Hanson (1980) discuss evaluation categories such as personnel, programs and operations, policies, participation, and resources. Farrell and Lundegren (1991) offer other areas such as administration, leadership, programs, or facility spaces. Evaluation occurs against a set of objectives or standards using any number of measurement tools, such as observation, checklists, interviews, rating scales, questionnaires, and research studies.

Benefits of Quality Efforts

Researchers like Graves and MacDowell (1994) cite that poor quality efforts result in costs to long term care facilities of between twenty-five and forty per-

cent of their total costs. It is, therefore, easy to see why making an effort to control quality is so important in the long-term care environment. Additionally, Leebov and Ersoz (1991) list numerous benefits of exploring quality efforts, such as assisting patients in achieving high outcomes, reducing costs, eliminating frustration, and giving employees positive feelings. Another obvious benefit is remembering that "quality is the right and ethical thing—we are in the business of caring."

Quality efforts among a number of facilities can also be pooled to look at the prevalence of **quality indicators**, defined as warning signs or flags that quality improvement efforts may be needed when certain items are present. The AHCA (1995) mentions quality indicators such as weight loss and pressure ulcers and those identified through assessment information on the MDS in test facilities as being ranked as ". . . the most useful quality indicators for facility quality improvement efforts." Interesting to activity professionals, one of the top ten quality indicators they identified was "the prevalence of bedfast residents" as a area for quality intervention.

Quality Methodologies and Theories ....

Quality, as a management concept and tool, has evolved over the last few decades. Originally thought of in narrow terms as the end product of a process, quality first surfaced as "quality control" in service industries and factories to ensure that products and services met standards. The next phase of quality development occurred when quality assurance was instituted. Considered an intermediate stage in the overall quality developmental picture, quality assurance looked at measuring performance against specified objectives. The last and current phase of quality is the total quality management area where continuous quality improvement in all management systems is the operational key to success. Raimondo (1994) states that total quality management was introduced to the health care industry by the mid-1980s, was first accepted in hospitals, and more recently in long-term care facilities. The Joint Commission of Accreditation Of Healthcare Organizations amended their manual in 1992 to reflect the shift from quality assurance to total quality management.

Quality Assurance (QA)

The focus of a quality assurance program is to set standards for performance, then measure the per-

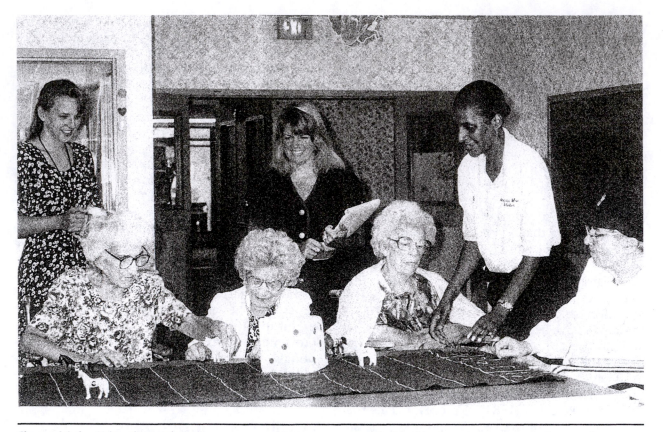

Figure 14–1   Using the total quality management process ensures that resident programs are meeting needs.

formance to determine if standards are met. Huston (1987) mentions that the primary goal of quality assurance is ". . . the monitoring and evaluation of clinical performance and quality of care." She suggests that a quality assurance program must be "comprehensive" in scope, but deal with problems related to increasing the level of patient care and raising clinical performance. Huston outlines the process of monitoring and evaluating activities through quality assurance. They include noting key aspects of care vital in professional and quality services, identifying problem areas, determining criteria with which to judge outcomes, collecting data, and evaluating the data. Riley (1987) listed basic steps involved in the quality assurance process as program planning, setting of standards, systematic monitoring, evaluation of recognized deficiencies, recommendations for alternative methods, and establishment of methods to utilize recommendations. **Quality monitoring** is the term Riley uses to describe ". . . the data-collection phase of quality assessment. . . ." Another term, **performance objectives**, mentioned by Edginton and Hayes (1976), refers to ". . . statements which are observable, measurable, and have some dimension of time" and are also applicable in the quality

assurance process. The systems approach of the quality assurance process has a goal of measuring performances in order to make informed decisions in the future.

Total Quality Management (TQM)

"Quality must be active rather than re-active" said McAlindon (1992), and is an appropriate way of describing the total quality management or continuous quality improvement process. The concept of total quality management was noticed in the United States in 1980 by Kim and Johnson (1994) when W. Edwards Deming discussed some of the highly successful quality efforts he encountered in Japanese management during a television documentary. Total quality management is a long-range change in organizational culture, a process for seeking continuous quality improvement.

Raimondo (1994) claims that three key factors are essential to total quality management: customer focus, use of quality improvement tools, and employee involvement. Customer focus begins by achieving and exceeding the expectations of customers and "delighting them." A "customer" in a long-term care facility is the resident and his or her family. Other secondary external customers are community members, volunteers, employees, vendors, and others who have contact with the facility. Raimondo mentions another level of internal customers who are the "supplier relationships" that exist between departments, such as dietary and nursing or nursing and housekeeping. These internal customers rely on the quality services of the supplier so that their work can be be achieved properly. The needs of all customers have to be identified first, then translated into a level of service that can be ensured and maintained. Leebov and Ersoz (1991) suggest four strategies for total quality management or continuous quality improvement: identifying customers, raising performance standards for improvement, developing a process to improve performance, and having a supportive organizational climate to support the process. Along with the strategies, they mention four easy managerial steps to carry out the strategy: plan, do, check, and act. The strategies and managerial steps are shown in Figure 14–2.

To achieve continuous quality improvement, Raimondo (1994) cites the work of Deming who suggests using quality improvement tools such as checklists, flowcharts, and diagrams. Using these mechanisms produce factual information instead of basing quality efforts on guesswork.

Quality improvement can only occur in a total quality management system when all employees are involved in the process. Raimondo mentions Deming's assumption that employees are willing to do their best and will seek opportunities to participate in quality efforts. The key to involving employees is not to delegate work responsibilities for quality improvement but rather to find ways to help employees to enhance their work performance, as well as showing them how they can participate in decisions that effect their work. Teams, formed by employees who have similar needs in work functions, can follow a step-by-step approach to solve problems by using the quality improvement tools.

Differences Between Quality Assurance and Total Quality Management

There are distinct differences between quality assurance and total quality management practices that explain why the total quality management concept is gaining more acceptance as the primary mode of quality programming in most facilities today. Leebov and Ersoz (1991) summarize some of the key differences in the two major theories. In quality assurance, the focus has been on whether or not things are done properly; if problems are found, specific or individual improvements should be made. The emphasis in total quality management is on "doing right things right," but attention is directed to the process of the problem and focusing on the root cause. Quality assurance programs often have been designed with regulations in mind, whereas total quality management programs have regulatory issues in mind, as well as the important needs of the customers. The focus in quality assurance is to measure performance against standards, but in total quality management, prevention rather than inspection is the driving force. Quality assurance also differs by zeroing in on poor performances or inadequate performers instead of the

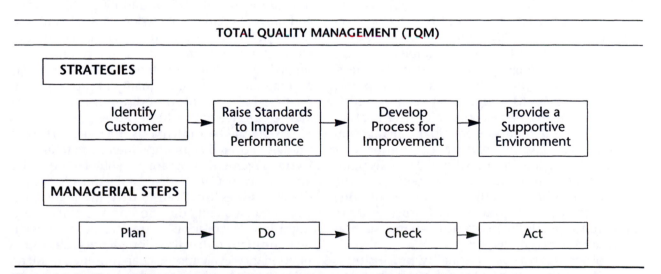

Figure 14–2 Total quality management (TQM) strategies and managerial steps.

total quality management initiative of locating the reasons for substandard performance. Finally, quality assurance has traditionally looked at certain areas of certain departments, whereas total quality management views organizational issues to create a "seamless organization" for residents and staff. Use of the total quality management method with continuous quality improvement as a focus is the preferred method in the evolution of quality programs.

Tools and Measurement Procedures

Using the TQM techniques, the process of measurement and data collection requires the use of various tools to ensure that the data obtained is factual and not merely opinion.

Organizational Dynamics (1987) presents an easy summary of quality improvement steps that also correspond to particular measurement tools. The **FADE process** stands for "Focus, Analyze, Develop and Execute." During the focus stage of quality improvement, problems are generated using tools such as **brainstorming** and a **selection grid**. A selection grid is a method of selecting one option from many possibilities. During the "analyze" stage, **checklists, surveys, flowcharts**, and other tools such as the **fishbone diagram** or **Pareto analysis** are used to decide how to find and determine the most influential factors. Checklists are simply a list of things to be done or items to be obtained. Surveys and lists of gathered information are compiled by asking individuals for knowledge or opinions. Flowcharts are sequential drawings of the stages in a process. A fishbone diagram illustrates the largest number of potential causes for a problem and a Pareto analysis is a bar chart that visually illustrates the layout of the events being studied. As part of the "develop" section, looking at possible solutions and narrowing a choice to one solution with an implementation plan is done through tools such as **cost-benefit analysis, force-field analysis**, and **action plans**. Cost-benefit analysis is a method to compare costs to actual benefits whereas the force-field analysis lists the forces that impede or help the change you wish to make. Action plans are a summary of what will be done and by whom. The execution stage involves receiving commitment from the participants, starting up the plan, and monitoring the results. Tools are **presentations**, such as a formal group meeting, and measurements, such as charts and trend graphs.

Another way to look at quality processing is through a technique called **benchmarking**. As de-

fined by Gift and Mosel (1994), benchmarking in health care means ". . . the continual and collaborative discipline of measuring and comparing the results of key work processes with those of the best performers." Simply put, benchmarking requires that standards of your department be placed against the best activity department of which you are aware as a basis of comparison. Benchmarking as a process is usually used by large companies to judge their performance against industry leaders. It is a technique that has merit when used properly in the long-term care setting.

To utilize the above approaches, many researchers suggest forming quality teams or groups to focus on particular issues. Teams that are formed should have similar work processes in order to understand the identified issue. A quality resource person or coordinator should act as a focal point for the teams to ensure they remain on track. An agenda should be set annually with quarterly updates on the progress of quality teams.

Using the Results

The results or the evaluation stage noted in the FADE process requires that a change be made based on the study by the quality team. New systems are put in place that require periodic monitoring whereas the quality team goes on to identify other new areas for study and resolution. The cycle repeats as the processes and systems continually improve.

An area of study that may be impacted during the measurement and results phase of total quality management is **risk management**. Pozgar (1992) defined risk management as ". . . the identification of potential accidents with an emphasis on claims prevention." A viable risk management program is established to identify problem areas and prevent accidents to residents, staff, and visitors. Quality improvement tools can be used as feedback mechanisms to the safety committee to supply information on potential risks. Darr (1991) also mentions the use of quality improvement in relationship to clinical and administrative services connected with ethical issues.

Despite the best intentions, there will be some hurdles to overcome in implementing a total quality management program in your facility. Kim and Johnson (1994) discuss Deming's "seven deadly diseases" that can impact an organization working in a quality direction. In summary, Deming lists problem areas as unclear purpose, focus on short-term rather than long-term goals, use of performance evaluations, changing management, using fiscal numbers only to drive management decisions, high medical costs, and costs of insurance. Kim and Johnson also discuss the problem of total quality management implementation in the long-term care industry as one of difficulty in defining the customer. The complexity of health organizations, with some departments functioning as both supplier and customer, it is often easy to lose sight of the true customer. Raimondo (1994) also mentions that varying educational levels of employees in organizations also pose problems for the quality process as well as of members of the facility who partially participate in group work instead of fully involving themselves.

Quality Implementation Within the Activity Department

Quality implementation throughout the total quality management process can be useful to monitor the functioning of your department and work on improving processes. Monitoring certain functions, such as the participation levels of residents, the numbers of attendees at programs, the status of charting requirements (discovered through a chart audit), or how your programs are directly meeting needs can be done through checklists, surveys, and charts that you develop specifically for your facility. You should have certain monitoring checkpoints in place to ensure that normal standards of practice are being conducted. The total quality management process takes this one step further by setting up teams to continually look for ways to improve services to the customer, the resident, and his or her family. Other areas you may look at during quality intervention will be determined by using the FADE process or other total quality management technique. For example, your quality team which is studying the activity services in your building may have determined that an area for improvement is the level of participation at your resident council meetings or the initial contact with the resident after admission. Following the outlined TQM process, your team will come up with workable solutions that will allow new systems to be put in place. Although each facility is unique in its needs, Figure 14–3 shows some possible areas for quality intervention.

Critical Pathways

Another area in the literature that has a relationship to quality is the concept of **critical pathways**. Defined by Thompson (1994), a critical pathway ". . . outlines the crucial incidents that normally take place on a given day and the appro-

priate interventions to achieve standardized results." The pathway approach, normally used as a technique in acute care settings, uses an interdisciplinary approach to determine expected outcomes of certain commonly seen situations. For example, a resident may return to your facility following a fall that resulted in a fractured hip. The critical pathways approach suggest that a time frame has already been established for each department (nursing, dietary, and so forth), and that guidelines are available to allow the clinical team to repeat quality standards of practice. On the first day of our example above, the critical pathway indicates specific tests to be performed by the medical team and consultants to be contacted. The activity department may be expected to visit briefly.

Although the benefits of having a specific plan for certain circumstances is a way of ensuring similar quality care for every resident, critical pathways should be individualized for a particular resident (adding steps, reducing days, and so forth). Thompson (1994) states that another benefit of critical pathways is giving staff an interdisciplinary approach to viewing the routines of each department, but cautions that critical pathways are neither "cookbook medicine" nor a cost-saving replacement for good care. Kane and Kane (1995) mention that critical pathways may be seen in the future as a part of the quality improvement process

---

**ACTIVITY DEPARTMENT
POSSIBLE AREAS FOR QUALITY INTERVENTION**

Activity Administration
  Policy Development
  Staff Training
  Time Management
  Interdepartmental Relations
  Volunteer Training

Service Delivery to Residents
  Resident Satisfaction
  Needs Assessment
  Program Offerings vs. Needs
  Family Programs
  Community Projects

Documentation
  Resident Patterns Based on MDS
  Attendance/Interest Surveys
  Interdisciplinary Meetings

Other
  Employee Programs
  Team Building

Figure 14–3 Examples of some activity areas to explore in quality interventions.

in such areas as the MDS to formulate expected outcomes from certain circumstances.

SUMMARY

Through the use of the evaluation methods, quality assurance, and quality improvement techniques, the offerings of your department can remain at the highest level of service for your residents. Integrating the results of total quality management efforts into your department completes the cycle of service delivery.

R E V I E W   Q U E S T I O N S

1. What is the difference between quality assurance and quality improvement?
2. To what process is evaluation more related?
3. What is risk management?
4. Describe the steps in the FADE process.
5. What are some of the barriers to implementing quality programs?

O N   Y O U R   O W N

1. Using your facility as an example, plan out a monitoring program for key functions, as well as two areas of quality improvement that you feel need attention.
2. What are three interdepartmental quality issues that impact your resident, and because of the departmental crossovers, may need administrative intervention?
3. A multipurpose room that had been used exclusively for the activity department is now to be utilized as a dining area during the lunch and supper meal. Many of the residents are upset to hear that their activity space is being taken. How would you use the total quality management techniques and form a quality team to resolve this issue?

R E F E R E N C E S

American Health Care Association (1994). *Vision 2000: The American health care association blue print for the future.* Washington, DC: author.

American Health Care Association (1995). *Data developments, QUIIX-ed quality indicator list,* pg. 13, Washington, DC: author.

Darr, K. (1991). *Ethics in health services management,* 2nd edition. Baltimore, MD: Health Professions Press.

Edginton, C., Compton, D., & Hanson, C. (1980). *Recreation and leisure programming: A guide for the professional.* Philadelphia, PA: Saunders College.

Edginton, C., & Hayes, G. (1976). Using performance objectives in the delivery of therapeutic recreation services. *Leisurability,* Vol. 3(4), 20–26.

Gift, R., & Mosel, D. (1994). *Benchmarking in health care: A collaborative approach.* Chicago, IL: American Hospital Publishing.

Graves, J., & MacDowell, N. M. (1994). Mapping out the road to quality. *The Journal of Long-Term Care Administration,* Winter, 12–17.

Huston, A. (1987). Clinical application of quality assurance in the therapeutic recreation setting. In B. Riley (Ed.). *Evaluation of therapeutic recreation through quality assurance,* (67–75). State College, PA: Venture Publishing Inc.

Kane, R., & Kane, R. (1995). Long-term care. *Journal of The American Medical Association,* Vol. 273, No. 21, 1690–1691.

Kim, P., & Johnson, D. (1994). Implementing total quality management in the health care industry.

Health Care Supervisor, 12(3), 51–57.

Leebov, W., & Ersoz, C. (1991). *The health care manager's guide to continuous quality improvement.* Chicago, IL: American Hospital Publishing Inc.

Lunegren, H., & Farrell, P. (1985). *Evaluation for leisure service managers: A dynamic approach.* Philadelphia, PA: Sanders College Publishing.

McAlindon, H. R. (1992). *Commitment to quality.* Chattanooga, TN: Celebrating Excellence Inc.

Organizational Dynamics, Inc. (1987). *Total quality improvement system: Quality action teams.* Burlington, MA: author.

Peterson, C. A., & Gunn, S. L. (1984). *Therapeutic recreation program design.* Englewood Cliffs, NJ: Prentice Hall Inc.

Pozgar, G. D. (1992). *Long-term care and the law: A legal guide for health care professionals.* Gaithersburg, MD: Aspen Publishers Inc.

Raimondo, M. (1994). Total quality management. In S. B. Goldsmith (Ed.). *Essentials of long-term care administration,* (186–209). Gaithersburg, MD: Aspen Publishers Inc.

Riley, R. (1987). Conceptual basis of quality assurance: Application to therapeutic recreation service. In B. Riley (Ed.). *Evaluation of therapeutic recreation through quality assurance.* (7–24). State College, PA: Venture Publishing Inc.

Thompson, D. G. (1994). Critical pathways: Good idea, right reason? *Critical Care Nurse,* December, 112.

F U R T H E R   R E A D I N G

Annand, V. (1977). A review of evaluation in therapeutic recreation. *Therapeutic Recreation Journal*, 11(2), 42–47.

Bronson, S., Nelson, A., Bronksen, S., & Woos, S. (1993). *Patient satisfaction pays: Quality service for practice success*. Gaithersburg, MD: Aspen Publication.

Coyne, P., & Turpel, L. (1984). Peer program review: A model for implementation of standards. *Therapeutic Recreation Journal*, 2nd Quarter, 7–13.

Fox, N. (1986). *You, your parent, and the nursing home: A family's guide to long-term care*. Buffalo, NY: Prometheus Books.

Goodman, A. (1990). *The quality freeway*. Quality Progress, July, 39–42.

Greenblatt, F. (1993). From custodial care to quality care: Implications for the therapeutic recreation professional. In M. P. Lahey, R. Kunstler, A. H. Grossman, F. Daly, S. Waldman, and F. Schwartz (Eds.). *Recreation, leisure and chronic illness: Therapeutic rehabilitation as intervention in health care*, (87–98). New York, NY: The Haworth Press.

Johnson-Dawlson, J. (1991). *Quest for quality: A continuous quality improvement program for long term care facilities*. Washington, DC: American Health Care Association.

Joint Commission of Accreditation of Hospitals (1986). Quality assurance in long term care. Chicago, IL: author.

Houston, P. (1990). Quality awards: Dubious achievement? *Business Month*, July, 40–44.

King, R. D. (1995). Starting up a quality improvement program. *Provider*, July, 87–88.

Miller, D. (1975). Suggested methodologies for auditing activity programs in long term care facilities. *Therapeutic Recreation Journal*, 3rd Quarter, 99–105.

Miller, T. (1995). Castle manor: The nursing home that surveyed itself. *Nursing Homes*, April, 12–28.

Mobily, K. (1983). Quality analysis in therapeutic recreation curricula. *Therapeutic Recreation Journal*, 1st Quarter, 18–25.

Mosher, C., Cronk, P., Kidd, A., McCormick, P., Stockton, S., & Sulla, C. (1922). Upgrading practice with critical pathways. *American Journal of Nursing*, January, 41–44.

Navar, N., & Dunn, J. (1981). Quality assurance: Concerns for therapeutic recreation. Champaign, IL: University of Illinois.

Navar, N. (1987). Therapeutic recreation's written plan of operation: The step before quality assurance. In B. Riley (Ed.). *Evaluation of therapeutic recreation through quality assurance*, (43–54). State College, PA: Venture Publishing Inc.

Pearlman, R., & Uhlmann, R. (1991). Quality of life in elderly, chronically ill outpatients. *Journal of Gerontology: Medical Sciences*, Vol. 46(2), M31–38.

Rhodes, M. (1991). The use of patient satisfaction data as an outcome monitor in therapeutic recreation quality assurance. In B. Riley (Ed.). *Quality management: Applications for therapeutic recreation*, (83–106). State College, PA: Venture Publishing Inc.

Riley, B. (1991). Quality assessment: The use of outcome indicators. In B. Riley (Ed.). *Quality Management: Applications for therapeutic recreation*, (53–68). State College, PA: Venture Publishing Co.

Roberts, K., LeSage, J., & Ellor, J. (1987). Quality monitoring in nursing homes. *Journal of Gerontological Nursing*, Vol. 13(10), 34–40.

Russoniello, C. (1991). "Vision statements" and "mission statements": Macro indicators of quality performance. In B. Riley (Ed.). *Quality management: Applications for therapeutic recreation*, (21–28). State College, PA: Venture Publishing Inc.

Schalenghe, R. (1991). The joint commission's "agenda for change" as related to the provision of therapeutic recreation services. In B. Riley (Ed.). *Quality management: Applications for therapeutic recreation*, (29–42). State College, PA: Venture Publishing Inc.

Schnelle, J., Ouslander, J., Osterweil, D., & Blumenthal, S. (1993). Total quality management: Administrative and clinical applications in nursing homes. *Journal of the American Geriatric Society*, 41, 1259–1266.

Shank, J., & Kinney, W.B. (1991). Monitoring and measuring outcomes in therapeutic recreation. In B. Riely (Ed.). *Quality management: Applications for therapeutic recreation*, (69–82). State College, PA: Venture Publishing Co.

Touchstone, W. (1984). Fiscal accountability through effective risk management. *Therapeutic Recreation Journal*, 4th Quarter, 20–25.

Wagner, L. (1995). Survey to stress quality assurance. *Provider*, July, 37–38.

West, R. (1987). The role of quality assurance in the professionalization of therapeutic recreation. In B. Riley (Ed.). *Evaluation of therapeutic recreation through quality assurance*, (1–5). State College, PA: Venture Publishing Inc.

Wilhite, B., Terry, B., Yoshioka, C., & McLean, D. (1983). Exploring quality circles in the provision of therapeutic recreation services. *Therapeutic Recreation Journal*, 3rd Quarter, 6–13.

Wright, S. (1987). Quality assessment: Practical approaches in therapeutic recreation. In B. Riley (Ed.). *Evaluation of therapeutic recreation through quality assurance*, (55–66). State College, PA: Venture Publishing Inc.

C H A P T E R   1 5
Typical Problems and Solutions

OBJECTIVES..

After completing this chapter, you should:

- understand and prepare for common administrative problems that impact your job
- learn about typical programming issues and the solutions for them
- tackle miscellaneous concerns that have the potential to decrease the effectiveness of your program if left unchecked

INTRODUCTION

Managing your department in an effective manner means that you will frequently face problems that seem insurmountable. Issues that you will encounter usually fall into either an administrative or program planning category. Administrative problems concern your ability to manage your program through the organizational structure, whereas programming issues deal with the specifics of your activity department. Additionally, some typical problems fall into a third or miscellaneous category that are just as important to resolve as the other issues.

Learning how to deal with problems, especially those that recur regularly, will help you grow as an activity professional and as a person. You are not expected to know how to handle every situation perfectly, but you should learn from each experience to help you weather the next crisis. Becoming comfortable with your role and your facility will certainly assist you in dealing with challenging interactions, unpleasant issues, and difficult people.

Problem-Solving ....

The job of solving problems, a daily task for all managerial staff, can be handled alone or with help from peers or your administrator. Often, problems have to be solved alone when quick decisions are required. When time permits, assistance from peers or other staff members should be utilized. Curtis and Fine (1984) mention that peers can be a source of problem-solving assistance that is often overlooked. They further define the term "collaborative consultation" to mean a method of solving problems, especially interpersonal ones, in which all parties involved bring contributions to the solution. In this problem-solving model, one person acts as the consultant, who imparts the expert information, and the other party receives the information and considers it before rendering a decision. The advantage of this method is the increase in interpersonal peer relationships that help to improve a caregiver's job effectiveness.

Steps in the collaborative problem-solving model were documented by Gutkin and Curtis (1982). They list seven steps of problem-solving, using collaborative methods: problem clarification, review of the factors which influence the problem, brainstorming, looking at alternatives, assigning roles and responsibilities, implementation and, evaluation.

In a brief review of each step, Gutkin and Curtis state that the problem should be defined in ". . . clear, concrete behavioral terms. . ." and be "observable" and able to be "quantified." The outside factors that impact the problem, such as the environment or interpersonal issues, should also be considered. **Brainstorming**, another step in the problem-solving process, requires the parties to suggest numerous ideas as solutions to the problem. All suggestions, no matter how far-fetched, are all recorded for review. Once a problem-solving path has been chosen, assignments are made to all parties handling the solution. The process for solving the problem is then implemented, and the evaluation stage begins.

All problems, large or small, can be handled using this method. Obviously, long-standing, complex problems will take longer to move through the process, but the basic framework will provide guidance to help you manage your issues.

Administrative Problems ....

Many of the most perplexing problems fall into the category of administrative issues. Because you are faced with delivering a program to meet specific needs in an always changing facility environment, you are bound to be faced with frustration from time to time. Let's take a look at some of your more challenging issues.

Limited Resources

In most facilities, even where funding appears to be stable, there are always limited and sometimes even diminishing resources for programs. Your job is to do your best with what you have, but you need to be smart about your allocation of resources. First, accept the fact that you will be working in an environment where there are clear limitations on spending. Much of the financial changes that occur in health care frequently have a direct bearing on operational issues, such as staffing and programming supplies. There are many departments in need of equipment and supplies to function and your department is one of six or more service areas that requires a budget.

Remember that you can make a dynamic program without an ideal amount of funding. Your biggest resources are you and your staff. With a little ingenuity and constant but gentle pressure on administration for more funds, you will succeed in making your program fly.

Lack of Space and Time

Space constraints are a troublesome issue for many activity professionals. A fresh look at your facility could help you locate new spots for programs or to share areas that may have previously been designated for a single departmental service. With the advent of OBRA regulations that ask you to maximize the quality of life and individualize care in a facility, programs should not be held to the formal boundaries of a particular room or space. Wide hallways or other unused spaces may provide corner areas for reading, socializing or setting up music stations. Your use of space to meet needs is limited only by your imagination and the cooperation you generate from other departments.

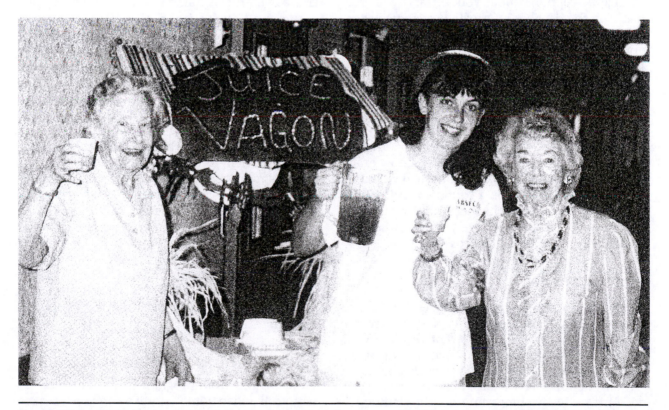

Figure 15–1   Designing a special drink cart solves an interdepartmental problem by providing for hydration, dietary, and social needs.

Organization is the key to solving time problems. If you are not organized, days and weeks will slip away from you, and many of your primary goals will not be accomplished. Planning is a job requirement for much of the work you do. Schedules are needed for programs, visits, documentation, and so forth. Without organization, none of these things will occur regularly. Write your plan for each day on paper (a few "to do" items) the night before. Your list will greet you in the morning before the day takes you away from the chance to think quietly. Be sure to include the unexpected things that might occur. If your day is jammed, you will be behind starting with the first item that took longer than anticipated. Help yourself by ridding yourself of the time-wasters on the job. Do your visiting at lunchtime, and use less busy, off-hours to do your creative thinking. With a little time management, you will be surprised at the positive results you reap.

Lack of Support from Administration

You may be fortunate to work with an understanding administrator, or you may be struggling along and feel misunderstood. If you fall into the latter category, you have some work ahead of you to change perceptions about yourself and your program. All the previous information presented about acting in a professional manner and conducting yourself as a respected department head will certainly help you in this area. Show your ideas to your administrator in an organized and meaningful way. It will have more clout than a sloppy, thrown-together presentation. If you feel that your department is considered an afterthought by your administrator, you may have to win your administrator over by the results you achieve. Show examples of your forward progress continually, and, of course, do not give up on a confident and positive image. Over time, even the most indifferent person will be hard pressed to dispute your overwhelming results in meeting resident needs!

Staffing Problems

Most activity managers would agree they are always in need of more staff, but often this cannot be accomplished with the current regulatory climate. You must have qualified staff to implement your programs. With luck, your administrator, owners, or both, have realized that in order to provide truly effective programming, the staffing levels need to be studied and adjusted. The facility layout or design may force the need for additional staff because of simple issues of transporting to multiple floors and being available to residents who are not often mobile. Other specialty programs will require more involved staffing patterns to meet increased program demands.

If your staffing patterns are not what you would like them to be, you do have a few options. First, be sure that the people you have working for you are really qualified so that your residents receive a full performance from each of them. Next, evaluate your program realistically to estimate where and how you could utilize others. If you are planning to speak to your administrator (a good next step), be specific in your request and the reasoning for your request. You will appear unprepared if you go in and say, "I need more staff" or "I can't provide adequate programs." Your request should detail your needs based on areas where improvements are required. For example, you may have studied the number of new admissions over the last six months and determined that you now have a fifty percent increase in the total resident population with cognitive impairments than you had last year. Point out the steps you have taken, from a programming standpoint, to address the increases of cognitive deficiencies (i.e., specialized dining situations, increased volunteers trained to run small group programs, and so forth). Your awareness of the changes in your population and the aggressive way you have addressed the problem, however, still leaves you with staffing problems on days between the hours of 4:30 p.m. to 6:00 p.m. Your request to the administrator should be specific, based on a thorough analysis of your problem area. You want the staffing hours allotted to the activity department to be increased by 1.5 hours per day. When you present this scenario to your administrator, along with your detailed research and attempted solutions, you increase your chances of receiving approval. Be prepared to accept alternate solutions to your staffing problem if your brainstorming session with your administrator shows that additional hours are not available. Do not be discouraged if your request is denied the first time around. Keep collecting your data and make another presentation as soon as you can.

Programming Problems ....

Problems with your program can, at times, be easier to solve than administrative concerns, because of your ability to control the area of programming. However, you still may be challenged by some of the issues that come your way in the form of problems with your program.

Inheriting a Weak Program

Many activity professionals face their first major hurdle on a new job by reviewing the existing program and realizing that the program in no way meets the needs of the resident population. Understanding that a big change has to occur to correct this situation, what do you do? The first step may be to speak to the administrator to find out the reasons why the program did not meet resident needs. (You now know why you were hired!) The reasons are not important to the solution, but will help you understand past facility issues. Discuss what you must do to implement a new program and schedule. Be honest in the areas of concern, but at the same time, maintain a professional attitude in any criticism of your predecessor.

Let your administrator know what you will be doing to identify and correct the problem. Meet and assess your new residents as quickly as possible. Using your assessment tools, make some broad recommendations as to how to redesign your program based on their needs. Time should be devoted to a chart audit to see if current documentation matches the actual resident picture that you find. Give your administrator a rough timetable for completing your research and implementing your changes. A discussion concerning the next expected visit from any regulatory agencies should also be a part of your conversation. With your administrator's approval, plans for evaluation and change should be shared with your fellow department heads, then the general staff for support and understanding. Contacts with a consultant (if you have one) or peers in your company or neighboring facilities could also be helpful as you tackle this major change.

Staff Burnout

Dealing daily with diverse problems and increasing demands takes its toll on even the strongest individual. Stress, a natural response to a challenge, is discussed by Kirsta (1986) as ". . . a feeling of not being in control of your life." A certain amount of stress is normal and a part of everyday life on the job. When the feelings of being out of control in your work life mount up, professional burnout occurs. **Burnout**, a term defined as ". . . exhaustion, lack of energy or loss of commitment" by Vessell (1980), reveals itself in a person's reduction of their performance or participation in the organi-

zation. In addition to decreasing morale, burnout leads to problems ranging from missed work time, lateness, and changes in the level of quality that an organization delivers to its clients. Solutions to burnout, suggested by Vessell, include making a detailed individual assessment and identification of the problem, setting up a system of support among professional colleagues, and providing an in-service or seminar schedule that provides necessary information about changes in the field of specialty. The experts agree that identifying the problem is the most crucial step in making a positive change. Having a mentor or other person to talk to about the issues of concern is also helpful.

Coping With Resident Discharges and Deaths

Changes in your resident population through discharges or deaths occur frequently, but that does not mean that these are easy situations with which to deal. Resident discharges, to home or a more independent situation, are positive separations, but still involve loss. A resident's death, especially one with whom a close relationship has formed, can be difficult to handle for staff as well as other residents. Adjusting to the transient nature of health care, even in long-term care, can be challenging for individuals, such as activity professionals, who pride themselves on compassion and understanding. We are happy to see a resident go to a more independent situation, but we are devastated to lose a resident to a lingering illness that results in death. Along with the discussion of dealing with death in Chapter 3, seek the solace of your peers in handling the death of residents in the facility. Often, just talking about the person in a positive way and sharing special things about that person helps you deal with the loss. Parry (1994) suggests that one way to handle the mourning experienced by staff as well as residents following a resident death is to hold a single session grief group. Some of the benefits identified in this group meeting of residents and staff held shortly after the resident's death are to provide an outlet for fear and anxiety, as well as a support system for the grieving process. Individual conferences with residents and staff allow for additional opportunities to voice feelings of grief.

Handling Unneeded Donations

The enthusiasm of a new job will leave you preoccupied and unprepared for the many unwanted or inappropriate "donations" you may receive in the course of your job. There are many gifts received that help your program, and you may be thinking, "what could be so terrible about people donating items?" First, the unsolicited items you receive may not fit your needs, such as old newspapers or chipped dishes. You may also find that the quantities of donations are more than your allotted storage space can handle (i.e., fifteen boxes of Reader's Digest books). Other donations, such as used medical equipment, are not permitted because of safety or sanitation reasons.

Some donated items, such as funeral flowers, pose an initial problem if they are received in quantity or if they are left in their original containers. The flowers could be offensive to many of your residents. The flowers should be taken apart and rearranged before being placed throughout the facility. Care must be used to ensure that flower displays are not placed in areas where some residents might consume them.

As part of your policy and procedure development, include a policy on the handling of donations and clearly indicate, with approval from your administrator, which items can be accepted for use in your facility. Review the policy with the other department heads, as well as your facility receptionist, who will probably receive the initial calls from donors.

Miscellaneous Problems ....

A few of the problems that are typical in your position cannot be defined by classification, but nonetheless require your attention. Some of the more common situations follow.

"No One Understands What I Do!"

You are correct! Many of the staff, residents, and families do not understand what you do in the course of a day to meet the residents' needs! Your best line of defense is to use every opportunity to educate others about your job and your profession. Schedule in-service time for staff, an educational session for your residents who may be interested, and a family night program for relative and friends. As your job responsibilities change with regulation shifts, update the staff, residents, and families with your new tasks. As more of your facility programs involve other departments, you will see a greater understanding of the things you do.

Rigid Thinking

If you have not already heard the two phrases, "We've always done it this way" and "We've never done it that way," you probably will. Staff and residents, unaccustomed to the creative process that allows for many chances to get an idea across or a program accomplished, may feel the need to challenge your attempts to try a new approach. As with many of the best ideas or program plans, it takes a great deal of trying (and failing) to launch a successful idea. The naysayers may be right. The idea did not work before, but take a new approach in different circumstances and try to make it happen. Most people are comforted by a steady routine, but taking a risk is one way to move a situation forward. Do not let your creativity die because some of your proposed plans are met with skepticism.

Infantilization

A key psychological issue in programming and the approach to residents is the issue of **infantilization**, defined as attributing child-like qualities to an elderly adult. Infantilization occurs among many categories of staff in the facility and usually happens because of the dependency state of an elderly resident during the process of institutionalization. Goldsmith (1994) reports that increased needs of the elderly for assistance with activities of daily living, such as dressing, eating, and toileting reminds staff of the needs of small children, and they react by slowly making a negative association between dependency needs and a child-like state. Infantilization is expressed by the way a resident is dressed or groomed, use of condescending language, or the way in which their environment is presented to them. Goldman gives examples: placing bows or pigtails in an elderly woman's hair, or dressing residents in brightly colored or inappropriate clothing for their age. Other examples include speaking to residents by their first name or using pet names such as "dearie" to refer to them. Professionals disagree on the "plush toy" controversy, that also relates to infantilization. Researchers such as Francis and Baly (1986) find that stuffed toys make a positive contribution in the psychosocial aspects of life whereas others, like Bowlby (1993), suggest that before using an item in a resident room, the professional should ask himself or herself the question, "Would you put this up in your home?" Dignity and resident rights issues may also be violated with such things as no privacy when providing minor care or presenting the environment in a child-like manner.

Bowlby (1993) discusses the term "**learned helplessness**" to describe a cycle of repeated experiences an individual has that shows he or she has no effect on the outcome of a situation. The individual then learns to become "helpless" in response to the new situation and experiences further loss of motivation or emotional difficulties each succeeding time it occurs.

With the advent of OBRA and its emphasis on the enhancement of quality of life for residents, a problem such as infantilization or learned helplessness must not be part of the activity programming that you offer or part of the facility climate. Goldsmith (1994) suggests the following ways to overcome and avoid infantilization in your facility. First, independence and adult-like behavior should be stressed in all facility programs. Staff must become sensitized to effects of infantilization through in-service programming, especially the teaching style that involves role-playing. Adapting the environment to increase residents' use of space and to act more independently in each area helps to curb infantile treatment. Finally, focusing on contributions of residents and their past successes in life definitely reduces the formation of helpless behaviors.

Dealing with Difficult People ....

You have organized your program to its desired level, and you are managing all the demands on your time. You are, however, confronted with the task of dealing with difficult people on the job. Difficult personalities may take any form from loud, impossible, and threatening to angry and unpredictable. A difficult person can include a colleague, a resident, a family member, or even your administrator! Sondak (1986) lists four guidelines to help deal with difficult personalities: accept that difficult people are a reality, give up trying to change them, accept that you are not the intended target of their negative behavior, and realize that you do not have to agree or like them to deal with them. Sondak goes on to state that by keeping others off balance, difficult people attempt to control situations, and are persistent in their behavior which also makes them difficult. A person responding to the behavior of a difficult individual must learn how to cope in order to continue with the business of the day. Depersonalizing the behavior is the first step, followed by a realization that becoming emotional yourself does not solve the situation. When difficult people learn that you will not react to their behavior, you keep your balance and set the stage for resolving issues. Do not run away from confronting or handling these types of encounters. They are part of your growth process as a manager and a fact of life in every facility.

Working with Corporate Consultants ....

Part of your experience as an activity professional may require you to work with an activity consultant from your own corporation or from the outside. If a consultant is assigned to your department, do not automatically assume that you will have problems with him or her. For many new activity professionals, having a consultant visit quarterly, monthly, or even more frequently is beneficial to problem-solving, not problem-creating. Consultants are usually brought in by management to assist someone new get through a difficult transition stage (new staff, new owners, and so forth), prepare for an upcoming survey, or improve the quality of programs. Conflicts, when they do arise, come from roles not clearly defined between activity director and consultant, "creative differences," or at times, a struggle for control within the department.

A consultant is a team member who observes, and based on experience, makes recommendations for improvement. Unless otherwise specified, a consultant does not participate in the actual operation of your department, but instead offers information for you to implement in your programs. The logical way to clear up confusion of roles is to review the consultant's contract and clarify any discrepancies with your administrator.

Other differences of opinion can arise when a consultant and activity director do not see eye to eye on creative approaches. This will be a tough problem to solve because recommendations coming from your consultant that do not blend with your style of leadership or program implementation may cause added confusion or frustration. Find a way to use suggestions and maintain your own presentation. Be open-minded to the fact that the consultant may be suggesting only that you try something new.

Some activity professionals feel threatened or experience a power struggle when faced with having to work with a consultant. You are still in charge of your department and responsible for the day-to-day operating decisions. A consultant should not be a threat to you, but viewed instead as another experienced person helping you and your program succeed. To counteract feelings of being excluded, try to develop a close rapport that will make you both feel more relaxed in carrying out your respective duties. Do not be afraid to ask for help or direction with your program. Also, ask your administrator if you can sit in on any conferences that your consultant has with him or her, or at the very least, request a copy of the consultant's report and review it in detail with your administrator.

SUMMARY

Having workable solutions to common problems that you face on the job allows you to focus on your primary task: helping the residents satisfy their needs. Gaining experience and confidence in the workplace further assists you to attain your program and personal goals.

R E V I E W Q U E S T I O N S

1. What are the seven steps of the collaborative problem-solving method?
2. What are three examples of infantilization?
3. How can stress and burnout be prevented?

4. Define learned helplessness.
5. What are some of the ways you can deal with a weak program?

O N Y O U R O W N

1. Design a strategy to deal with a difficult family member who visits you every day to complain about the lack of participation in programming by her family member.

2. How can you use your programs as a way to prevent learned helplessness?
3. What other ways can you help residents and staff cope with death in the facility?

R E F E R E N C E S

Bowlby, C. (1993). *Therapeutic activities with persons disabled by Alzheimer's disease and related disorders.* Gaithersburg, MD: Aspen Publishers, Inc.

Curtis, M., & Fine, A. (1984). A collaborative approach to problem-solving in therapeutic recreation. *Therapeutic Recreation Journal*, 1st Quarter, 18–26.

Francis, G., & Baly, A. (1986). Plush animals: Do they make a difference? *Geriatric Nursing*, Vol. 7, 140–142.

Goldsmith, S. B. (1994). *Essentials of long-term care administration.* Gaithersburg, MD: Aspen Publishers.

Gutkin, T., & Curtis, M. (1982). School based consultation: Theory and techniques. In C. Reynolds and T. Gutkin (Eds.). *Handbook of school psychology.* New York: John Wiley & Sons.

Kirsta, A. (1986). *The book of stress survival.* New York, NY: Fireside Books.

Parry, J. (1994). Another special group: The single session grief group. In I. Burnside & M.G. Schmidt (Eds.). *Working with older adults: Group process and techniques.* 3rd edition, (p. 346–351). Boston, MA: Jones and Bartlett Publishers.

Sondak, A. (1992). *Dealing with difficult people.* [training materials]. Edison, NJ: Personnel Management Services.

Vessell, R. (1991). The devastating costs of professional burnout. *Therapeutic Recreation Journal*, 3rd Quarter, 11–14.

F U R T H E R R E A D I N G

Kraus-Whitbourne, S., & Wills, K. (1994). Psychological issues of institutional care of the ages. In S. B. Goldsmith (Ed.) *Essentials of long-term care administration*, (p. 11–24). Gaithersburg, MD: Aspen Publishers, Inc.

LeSage, J., Slimmer, L., Lopez, M., & Ellor, J. (1989). Learned helplessness. *Journal of Gerontological Nursing*, Vol. 15, No. 5, 9–15.

Pearlman, R., & Uhlmann, R. (1991). Quality of life In elderly chronically ill outpatients. *Journal of Gerontology*, Vol. 46, No. 2, M31-M38.

C H A P T E R   1 6
Volunteers

OBJECTIVES ....

After completing this chapter, you should:

- understand how recognition of the needs of your department and the needs of volunteers are the first steps in volunteer management
- gain an awareness of the stages of management for volunteers including recruitment, interviewing, training, supervision and recognition
- increase your knowledge about use of resident volunteers and handling of unusual volunteer situations

INTRODUCTION

Faced with the challenges of providing a superior activity program on a modest budget with limited staff, many activity professionals have turned to volunteers as a source for enhancing their programs. Although the management of volunteers can be a time-consuming process, volunteers yield benefits to the entire facility. With the proper forethought and continuing vigilance, the volunteer program in your facility can be a wonderful way to multiply the benefits of your whole program.

The Role of the Volunteer ....

At one time or another, almost everyone has either been a **volunteer** or come in contact with volunteers. Volunteers are so much a part of life, particularly in health care settings, that we tend to take them for granted because often, we spend little time thinking about them. What is a volunteer, and what is the special role that a volunteer plays in the area of long-term care?

A volunteer in a long-term care setting is an individual willing to devote unpaid time and services to a facility and its residents. With proper training and supervision, volunteers can work in any department, but many individuals who feel the desire to volunteer in the long-term care setting often gravitate toward the activity department. The activity department, as we can verify, offers diverse challenges for volunteers, from personal resident visits to making party decorations, as well as many chances to interact with the residents at different times of the day and in numerous ways.

A volunteer performs at least three main functions in a long-term care facility. First, volunteers allow you to expand and enhance your program in the facility. With limited budgets and resources, having additional help to manage certain programs will give you the time to start other projects or increase the benefits of existing programs. Your volunteers may also have skills that match your program needs and can be assets by helping you get a new program off the ground. As you will discover, there are many ways that volunteers assist in extending your program.

Another reason to use volunteers in your programs is to bring additional nonstaff reinforcement to residents' goals and program plans. With structure and guidance from you, volunteers can engage residents in increased participation based on their identified needs, and support specialized and individual programs that you initiate. Having a different perspective, volunteers may, at times, motivate residents to participate more fully in an activity. Residents get used to seeing staff members, and often look forward to a visit from a volunteer which increases their socialization.

The most vital role that volunteers play in the facility is the obvious reminder to residents and staff that the residents are still bonded to their community. Cunninghis (1986) states: "Their help, day in and day out, visibly demonstrates to the residents that people outside are still concerned about them." As we see the trends toward aging in place continuing in the future, the concept of community members, such as volunteers, bridging the gap between the resident and the "outside world" becomes even more critical.

The Needs of Your Department

Having learned the general services volunteers can provide, your next task is to evaluate your program to determine logical places for volunteers to augment your schedule. Placing volunteers effectively should be based on the needs of your program and your residents, not on the whims of your volunteers. A volunteer may approach you with an idea for candlemaking classes, but if you have no resident interest for that kind of activity, re-evaluate this volunteer and try to channel his or her services into a more useful area.

As you review your calendar and project lists, sort your volunteers according to these broad categories: resident-centered programs, activity administrative projects, and special assignments. Resident-centered programs are group or individual programs that focus on interactions with residents in a variety of settings. Examples include transport-

ing residents to special events, assisting with small groups, or conducting individual activity programs at bedside. Volunteers performing any resident-centered programs require specialized training in acceptable resident interactions.

Activity administrative projects are those that do not demand resident interactions, are more behind-the-scenes, and may involve clerical or artistic abilities. Activity administrative projects include making decorations, setting up a room visit cart, typing letters, making telephone calls, or buying gifts for residents. Volunteers in activity administrative projects require training, but not as extensively as those interacting directly with residents.

The category of special projects is usually reserved for a seasoned volunteer in whom you have observed an ability to handle a unique project or someone with a specialized skill that you need for the project. Special volunteer project assignments include coordinating voter registration in the facility or working with the resident council on their color choices for the new activity room wallpaper. Provide the volunteer with whatever task-oriented training is required for each project.

Thinking of the volunteer task categories helps to identify potential uses for volunteers in your program. Using a **volunteer needs sheet** (see Figure 16–1) base your requirement for volunteers

PROGRAM	VOLUNTEER NEEDS TYPE		
	RESIDENT CENTERED	**ACTIVITY ADMINISTRATIVE**	**SPECIAL PROJECT**
Current Program			
Future Programs			

Completed by: _____   Date: _____

Figure 16–1 Determining your volunteer needs is the first step in planning a volunteer program.

in specific programs on a realistic view of your current schedule. For example, if you have evaluated your nature walk program and recently found that two new admissions would benefit from this event, seek a volunteer to help you increase your resident participation and avoid pulling staff off another project. You may realize that you need a volunteer who speaks and writes Portuguese, someone with moderate art skills to make new room identifiers, or a singer to help you motivate your morning music break. Both Cunninghis (1986) and the Indiana State Department of Health (1991) recommend that volunteer tasks should be specifically identified to avoid problems. As your volunteer needs change over time, update your volunteer need sheet at least monthly or quarterly. With this sheet in hand, you are ready to look at your potential volunteers.

The Needs of Your Volunteers

Volunteers of varying ages and backgrounds may come to your facility to give their time for a variety of reasons. Understanding the motivation of volunteers assists you in managing and nurturing them during their stay. In discussing one of the Gallop Organization polls, Wilson (1990) cites that one of the key reasons people choose to volunteer is to ". . . do something useful." The Gallop source on which Wilson reports concludes that enjoyment of the work and having a sense that a relative could profit from their efforts are also motivating factors for volunteers. Knoth (1989) mentions that reasons for volunteering include socialization, an opportunity for recognition and acceptance, a chance to obtain new abilities, to fulfill course requirements, or to relieve loneliness or boredom.

The ages and motivations of your potential volunteers will greatly effect the outcome of their success in your facility. Wilson (1990) suggests that sixty-six percent of the total volunteers in any setting already have paid employment and men and women are almost equally represented in that percentage. Trends in particular groups are interesting to note: teenage volunteers are declining whereas senior citizens (who Wilson refers to as the "chronologically gifted") are volunteering in increasing numbers. Special population segments, such as the "baby boomers" born between 1946–1964, volunteer in large numbers, but have increased demands on their time because of work and family commitments. These needs must be understood when they approach any organization to volunteer. The "sandwich generation" who struggle with multiple responsibilities, are finding that time is a shrinking commodity and, therefore, their numbers as volunteers are decreasing.

The needs of volunteers and the overall trends in volunteering should be analyzed along with your facility policies and your specific departmental needs to determine the number and type of volunteers that best suit your program.

Management and Use of Volunteers

The management and utilization of volunteers is similar to your efforts to oversee your employees. Although there are some cross-overs, the administration of volunteers has unique challenges because of their unpaid status and transient nature. Following the basics of management and organization, establish clear guidelines for your staff and the facility in obtaining, supervising, recognizing, and, if needed, removing volunteers from your facility. Your firm and structured approach to managing volunteers will bring efficiency and enhancement to your department.

Recruitment

Your efforts to determine the number and specific category of volunteers you need for your programs will pay off as you begin your recruitment drive. It is virtually impossible to successfully look for volunteers if you do not know who it is you need. Using your volunteer needs sheet, see if there are any areas where a number of similar requirements are needed. Many of the authors who have briefly written on the subject of volunteering agree that the following are some of the more common and practical ways to recruit volunteers:

1. Ask current volunteers to solicit friends. "Word of mouth" is considered the best way to recruit, according to Peckham & Peckham (1982).
2. Contact civic or community organizations. Because Wilson (1990) reported that over sixty percent of volunteers have paid employment, reaching them in the work or community setting may be best.
3. Media coverage by means of newspapers, cable television, and radio can also be effective. Some forms of coverage may be free because it is considered community publicity or a public service.

4. Organized slide shows or video presentations showing the special aspects of your facility may also help in recruiting. Both Knoth (1989) and Sander (1993) suggest slide shows as an excellent recruitment tactic.
5. Use mailings, flyers, or bulletins. You may find that sending targeted letters to specific organizations is effective or that an inexpensive advertisement placed in a church or synagogue bulletin reaches your core audience.
6. Design your own program to fit your needs. If, for example, you have determined that your programs would best be served by college-age students, make your recruitment efforts directly through a college placement office. Or, if you find that you need more volunteers similar to the ones you already have, consider doing a motivational recruitment effort in your own volunteer pool.

With any recruitment plan, think through what you want to have happen when your potential volunteers hear or see your message. Are you asking them to call? Be sure the contact name is clear in your message and the person screening the calls for you is aware of the recruitment effort. If you are contacting organizations in person, follow your visit with a thank you note and call again in a few weeks if you have not had a response.

Interviewing and the Application Process

If your efforts have reached their target audience and you have a response, you now face the prospect of determining whether or not your potential volunteer is the person you actually need. The simplest way to gather information about a prospective volunteer is through the use of a volunteer application (see Figure 16–2). The application form covers many aspects similar to an employee application, but expands on areas concerning time availability and interests. Volunteer applicants who call to schedule an appointment, or those who just drop in, should complete an application for your review. Once reviewed for thoroughness and compared against your current needs on your volunteer needs sheet, you can quickly determine if there is a match.

Opinions differ as to whether all prospective volunteers should be interviewed, especially if they have not called for an appointment. It appears that since volunteers are unpaid and have made the effort to stop in and complete an application, a courtesy interview should be conducted to see if there could be some program benefits.

The preferable situation is for a candidate to have responded by telephone and scheduled an appointment in advance. Allow at least fifteen to twenty minutes for an interview and time before or after your session to take the potential volunteer on a quick tour of the facility. The tour accomplishes two things: the volunteer gets a look at the facility operation, and you, as the activity professional, get a chance to gauge volunteer responses to resident encounters. This same technique works well with employee interviews. If you see an uncomfortable reaction or hesitation when meeting residents, consider that this candidate would be better off in activity administrative duties or possibly not in this type of setting at all.

The interview itself should be conducted in an office or other private area whenever possible. The application should have been completed before the interview and adequate time set aside to review it prior to the interview. The volunteer candidate should be made to feel comfortable during your discussion. Questions should focus on his or her experience in meeting the needs of your department, but general queries should include:

- why have you selected this facility as a place to volunteer?
- why do you like working with long-term care clients?
- what do you feel you have to offer the facility and the residents?

Be aware of body language and any other clues about potential problems. Anderson and Lauderdale (1986) mention three important qualities that all volunteers should possess: warmth, empathy, and genuineness. Finding volunteers who can relate to others in a nonjudgemental fashion and show concern for a resident's feelings in a down-to-earth way are certainly ideal. As we discussed earlier, people want to volunteer for many reasons, but some of the reasons are not suitable for your residents. For example, an individual who feels that volunteering can solve his or her problem of loneliness, but causes the residents to suffer because the volunteer is burdening them with his or her own problems. Match physical reactions you note against the information found in the application.

After discussing all the information contained on the application, make a quick determination as to whether the volunteer is suitable in general, and has skills or background to fill one of your positions. One of the biggest disservices done to volunteers is when they are not correctly placed during the initial process. If you have an opening

Name: _____   Date Application Completed: _____

Address: _____   Telephone Number: (   ) _____

_____

Type of volunteer projects you are most interested in:

_____ 1. Resident-centered (helping residents during programs, friendly visiting)

_____ 2. Activity administrative (making decorations, typing, errands)

_____ 3. Special projects (activity planning, committee, voter registration)

Time you can commit to the facility: (circle)

Day	Time Frame	Amount of Time
Sunday	Morning	$1/2$ Hour
Monday		1 Hour
Tuesday	Afternoon	1 to $1/2$ Hours
Wednesday		2 Hours
Thursday		Other: _____
Friday	Evening	
Saturday		

Please list any previous job or volunteer experience:

Do you have any special skills, talents, hobbies, or other experiences that may be of interest to our residents?

What are your reasons for wanting to volunteer?

How were you referred to the facility?

Do you have any medical restrictions or other issues that we should be aware of when considering your placement in the facility?

Personal or other references:

I understand that if I become a member of the volunteer team at the facility, I will be trained and assigned to a job based on my experience and the needs of the facility. I agree to abide by the policies of the facility for the health and safety of the residents.

Volunteer Applicant Signature _____ Date _____

FOR OFFICE USE ONLY

Interviewed by: _____   Comments: _____

_____

Placement Approved: Yes _____   No _____   If no, why? _____

Training Date: _____   First Assignment: _____

Figure 16–2   A sample volunteer application form.

for a particular volunteer, discuss the available spot in detail, and see if the volunteer is interested and can meet the time commitment you require. A brief job description should be prepared for a specific post and reviewed with the volunteer. If you and the candidate come to agreement about their duties, including amount of time per week, schedule a training and orientation session. Training prepares a person for a specific type of job, whereas orientation is a process of learning to adapt skills and training to a particular facility.

Plan training on how to be a good volunteer, as well as coverage of orientation items such as fire safety, door alarms, parking procedures, and so forth. Reilly (1985) adds that if available, a new volunteer should receive a handbook on policies and procedures of the home or operation that applies directly to them.

Training, Orientation, and Placement

Adequate training for volunteers is not only necessary for ensuring success with residents, but also has a bearing on a volunteer's feeling of satisfaction with his position. In a study of training experiences of volunteers, Ozminkowski, Supiano, and Campbell (1991) found that volunteers who were involved in the training offered by a facility were found to have higher levels of satisfaction than those who had not had training. Additionally, they also determined that satisfaction with the volunteer experience continues to increase as the amount of training increases.

Your training sessions (to acclimate volunteers to the unique qualities of volunteering) may be held once in a while or at the beginning of your total orientation session. Topics should include how to interact politely with residents, what goes on in a long-term care facility, the aging process, and tips on how to make visiting most effective. Glemby (1993) suggests that part of the training for new volunteers should include information explaining quality of life issues and Cunninghis (1986) adds that the sessions should cover expected behaviors of residents. An example of some of the training and orientation topics that should be covered with volunteers are shown in Figure 16–3.

There are a number of other factors to consider during an orientation phase. Merrill (1979) mentions using a probationary period as a means of determining a volunteer's effectiveness before an assignment is thought of as permanent. Establishing volunteer accountability for specific duties is suggested by Knoth (1989), and Eliasen and Feick (1989) talk about observing volunteers first before assigning them tasks. Clearing up any concerns about insurance coverage for volunteers, especially on trips outside the facility, as well as managing money or other valuable items, are raised by Murphy (1994) as issues to handle during the initial stages of orientation. If you detect potential problems, monitor the new volunteer and if necessary, provide additional training or remove the volunteer from the assignment.

Supervision

Spend time assisting and guiding new volunteers toward a good performance to ensure that the integrity of your program is maintained. Placing volunteers in their first assignment requires a time commitment from you or a member of the facility to be certain that they understand their responsibilities and are treating the residents properly. Supervision is one of the more time-consuming aspects of using volunteers, and may cause you to ask, "Why am I spending so much time with someone who is supposed to help me find more time?" The answer is that volunteers require much of your time before, during, and after programs to be effective, but the time allotted is worth the effort.

After you have developed a level of confidence with a particular volunteer and feel they can handle a situation alone, take the time to greet them and casually monitor their facility encounters.

Name of Volunteer: _____   Date of Training: _____

Name of Trainer: _____

    A. Training Issues

        1. Policies and procedures of the volunteer department: dress code, sign-in/sign-out policy, reporting absences, problems.

        2. Residents' rights

        3. "Dos" and "don'ts" of volunteering

        4. Brief overview of the aging process

        5. How to approach residents

        6. How to handle hostile or upset residents

        7. Medications and restraints

    B. Orientation Issues

        1. Fire/safety procedures/door alarms

        2. Introductions to staff and residents

        3. Handwashing/universal precautions

        4. Resident restrictions and precautions

        5. Parking and entering/exiting the facility

        6. Reporting unusual problems, incident reports

        7. Facility tour

I have received training and orientation on the above topics and I understand the responsibilities of my volunteer assignment.

Volunteer Signature _____   Date _____

Figure 16–3   The volunteer orientation and training form.

Your residents and other staff can also provide feedback on the progress of volunteers. Should a volunteer not meet your expectations, meet privately with the individual and outline a plan for changing the situation.

Time Maintenance

Measuring the time that individual volunteers and groups spend in the facility is important for two reasons. First, it helps you manage your programs better when you can monitor the amount of staff time and volunteer time in particular areas of your program. Second, logging volunteer time also serves as the basis for a system of recognition and rewards.

Facilities vary in the manner that volunteer time is managed, but most programs use a **volunteer log sheet**, either at a central point of entry to the building, such as a reception desk, or in the activity office (see Figure 16–4). Having a sheet for volunteers to date and sign when entering and leaving the facility makes your volunteer accountable and demonstrates to him or her that you feel they are important. By placing the log sheet in the activity office or main activity room, you are setting up a means for greeting by the activity staff. Some facilities have a requirement that a volunteer entering the building must be met by a staff member. Other facilities go a step further and require that the volunteer be escorted to their work area. These policies may seem strict, but they have been put in place to make the volunteer feel welcome and ensure that the volunteer and the residents are having a satisfactory experience.

Depending on how your statistics on volunteer time are to be used, you may have forms in place to calculate your annual totals for each individual volunteer. The data may be part of a quarterly or end of the year report to your administrator or you may use the calculated time as a basis for awards and recognition.

Recognition and Nurturing

Because volunteers are unpaid members of your team, much has been said about how to properly reward and motivate them. **Recognition** usually takes two forms: informal and formal. Informal recognition is spontaneous and can be simply thanking them for a job well done, highlighting them in the facility newsletter, remembering to ask about their grandchildren, or praising them in front of the residents or other staff. Formal recognition is planned and usually takes the form of a yearly function to honor volunteers, an article in the newspaper, or gifts or other awards presented publicly or privately. Some facilities have annual volunteer recognition traditions that are part of the special events of the community whereas others change the recognition approach from year to year. Any situation that is organized and allows the volunteers to be noticed and feel honored for their accomplishments will be appreciated. Be sure to ask your volunteers for their feedback after a function to ensure that your intentions were well received.

Honoring and rewarding volunteers helps to keep them in your facility. Volunteers may leave for many nonfacility related reasons, but be sure that you are doing everything possible to moti-

Date: _____

Volunteer Signature	Area Assigned	Time In	Time Out	# Hours /Comments

Figure 16–4 Record keeping for volunteers can be accomplished with the volunteer log sheet.

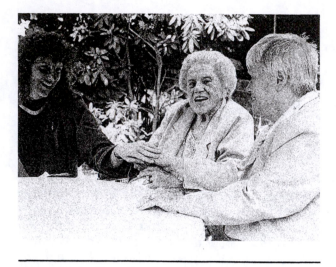

Figure 16–5 Spending time observing a new volunteer with a resident will assist in the orientation process.

vate them to stay. Cunninghis (1986) talks about what volunteers want from their volunteer placement, such as tasks that are purposeful, guidelines on where their job ends and another begins, participating in situations where their skills are used, and sensing that they are being listened to.

Resident Volunteers

A special group of volunteers may exist right in your midst and go unnoticed without prompting from you. Some of your residents are part of that senior citizen volunteer segment mentioned earlier and have a great desire to volunteer. Drew (1985) mentions reasons why nursing home residents feel a call to volunteer service. Residents may feel that having a needed role, fulfilled by volunteering, increases feelings of self-esteem and usefulness. Additionally, through volunteering, residents have an opportunity to channel the vast experiences of aging. In discussing innovative resident volunteer programs, Goodwin (1985) feels that structured resident volunteer situations ". . . allow the residents the opportunity of giving back something to others who have given to them."

Consider your resident volunteers as you do your community volunteers by matching their desires with your program needs and rewarding them for their efforts with praise and recognition. A common problem of resident volunteers is the feeling that payment should result from their efforts, according to Reginek (1993). This situation can be avoided if the resident volunteer program is formalized and discussed at a resident council meeting. Some of the resident volunteer activities that can be successful were cited by Seville (1985)

as community-oriented, such as reassurance telephone calls to other seniors in the area; resident-focused, such as mail delivery or letter-writing; and facility and/or program assistance, such as typing or making decorations. Goodwin (1985) also mentions including residents in fund-raising activities, such as babysitting or tutoring. It is important to note that, although there are many opportunities in your program planning to capitalize on the hidden talents of your residents, you should remember that the decision to participate belongs to the resident. The resident's physician should also be consulted to ensure that volunteering fits into the medical plan of care for the resident. When appropriate, residents should be encouraged to volunteer and all volunteer efforts should be taken into consideration when activity care planning takes place.

Growing Your Program ....

You may have the luxury of working in a facility that has a flourishing volunteer program and feel that growth of your program is unnecessary. Or, maybe you face starting from scratch. No matter what size program you have, look for new recruiting sources to keep your program thriving. Just when you think your program is stable, three of your best volunteers may move or experience family problems and drop out for a while. With a plan in place to keep your recruiting efforts active, you will not be caught short by sudden changes. If you keep a regular, year-round incentive program going for volunteers and staff to help you find new recruits, you will always have new faces and opportunities to enhance your program.

Working with groups of volunteers, instead of individual volunteers, is an easy way to increase your programs. The benefits of working with clubs that visit or volunteer performer groups is that they engage your residents by their sheer numbers. They are also of assistance to you because they help with transporting and clean-up. The downside of working with groups is the inflexibility of scheduling with so many members involved. Also, some residents love the chaos and flurry of activity; others do not.

Having an **auxiliary** group can also present challenges. An auxiliary group is a formal volunteer organization appointed by the ownership or board of directors to work on facility projects. The benefits are the same as working with large groups of volunteers, with an extra bonus of having this group dedicated to facility issues. The direction and guidance of the auxiliary is one area, however, where conflict may arise. If the majority of the auxiliary's time is spent with the activity department, but the activity department head does not have authority over the delegation of projects and assignments to the auxiliary, problems can surface. Your administrator should be consulted to resolve any questions about responsibilities and help you use the combined strengths of an auxiliary to build your program.

A word of caution about growing too big or too fast. You must observe and manage all the volunteers who support your program. If you have lost the ability to provide personal attention or knowledge about the activities of your volunteers, your program is no longer under your control, and your activities may become ineffective. Step back and analyze how your program should be tailored to fit your needs.

Unique Problems of Volunteers .....

The benefits of having volunteers certainly outweighs the negatives, but there are still a few other thorny problems that you may encounter with volunteers. As we saw earlier in the example of the volunteer who upset residents with news of his or her own problems, sometimes the reason a

volunteer comes to a facility initially impacts that person's success. There are other unfortunate situations created, at times, by volunteers who are demanding or unreliable. Cunninghis (1986) adds that problems such as not allowing residents to be independent or doting on a particular resident are common but usually preventable when volunteers are screened properly. Every case involving volunteer adjustment problems must be handled individually, and you will need to speak with the person privately and make a plan that best serves the resident and the facility.

SUMMARY

Volunteers add another dimension to the long-term care setting by allowing opportunities for the activity professional to expand and augment programs. By understanding the reasons why people volunteer and studying activity programming needs, a successful match may be made between volunteer and activity department task to benefit the residents. Proper screening, management, and recognition all serve to make the volunteer a full member of the team and add to the services that residents expect and enjoy.

REVIEW QUESTIONS

1. How can volunteers benefit the residents and the activity program?
2. What are some of the key reasons that individuals volunteer?
3. Name three kinds of informal volunteer recognition techniques.
4. What are the three categories of volunteer functions that you have available in your department?
5. What kind of training and orientation does a volunteer require?

ON YOUR OWN

1. Some of your residents and volunteers have complained about the conduct of one of your volunteers. You have seen no evidence of any problem; in fact, you feel this individual is an exceptional volunteer. How can you tactfully handle the situation?
2. You have a new specialty unit opening in your

facility in six months. What can you do now to begin planning for volunteer assistance, and how do you handle the situation with your current volunteers?
3. Plan a start-up campaign for using resident volunteers in a facility where none have existed to date.

REFERENCES

Anderson, S., & Lauderdale, M. (1986). *Developing and managing volunteer programs: A guide for social service agencies*. Springfield, IL: Charles C. Thomas Publisher.
Cunninghis, R. N. (1986). *The activity programming

handbook*. Holmes Beach, FL: Geriatric Educational Consultants.
Drew, L. S. (1985). Veteranship for nursing home residents: Integrating residents into volunteer services.

In J. D. Cook (Ed.), *Innovations in activities for the elderly: Proceedings of the 1994 national association of activity professionals convention*, (p. 79–85). Binghamton, NY: The Haworth Press.

Eliasen, K., & Feick, C. (1989). *The activity director as educator.* Nanaimo, British Columbia, Canada: E. & F. Education Services.

Glemby, J. (1993). The special magic of volunteers. In R. N. Cunninghis (Ed.). *Improving the quality of life in long-term care: A guide and sourcebook for the activity professional*, (p. 244–246). Holmes Beach, FL: Geriatric Educational Consultants.

Goodwin, D. (1985). Innovative "resident volunteer" programming. In J. D. Cook (Ed.), *Innovations in activities for the elderly: Proceedings of the 1984 national association of activity professionals convention*, (p. 69–71). Binghamton, NY: The Haworth Press.

Indiana State Department of Health (1991). *Nursing home activity directors course.* Indianapolis, IN: Division of Health Education, Indiana State Department of Health.

Knoth, M. (1989). *The professional activity director.* Lafayette, IN: Valley Press.

Merrill, T. (1979). *Activities for the aged and infirm.* Springfield, IL: Charles C. Thomas Publisher.

Ozminkowski, R., Supiano, K., & Campbell, R. (1991). Volunteers in nursing home enrichment: A survey to evaluate training and satisfaction. *Activities, Adaptation & Aging*, Vol. 15 (3), 13–43.

Peckham, C. W., & Peckham, A. B. (1982). *Activities keep me going.* Lebanon, OH: Otterbein Home.

Reginek, J. (1993). Resident volunteer program. In R. N. Cunninghis (Ed.), *Improving the quality of life in long-term care: A guide and sourcebook for the activity professional*, (p. 82). Holmes Beach, Fl: Geriatric Educational Consultants.

Reilly, B. A. (1985). Volunteers: The value to the total program of good volunteers. In E. S. Deichman & M. V. Kirchhofer (Ed.), *Working with the elderly: A training manual and teaching guide*, (p. 172–178). Buffalo, NY: Potentials Development Inc.

Sander, P. (1993). *Activity and volunteer service policies and procedures.* La Grange, TX: M & H Publishing Co.

Seville, J. (1985). The good samaritan program: Patients as volunteers. In J. D. Cook (Ed.). *Innovations in activities for the elderly: Proceedings of the 1984 national association of activity professionals convention*, (p.73–78). Binghamton, NY: The Haworth Press.

Wilson, M. (1990). *You can make a difference!: Helping others and yourself through volunteering.* Boulder, CO: Volunteer Management Associates.

F U R T H E R   R E A D I N G

Elliott, J., & Sorg-Elliott, J. (1991). *Recreation programming and activities for older adults.* State College, PA: Venture Publishing Inc.

Goodwin, D. (1982). *The activity director's "bag of tricks".* Snellville, GA: The "Activity Factory".

Hastings, L. (1981). *Complete handbook of activities and recreational programs for nursing homes.* Englewood, NJ: Prentice-Hall Inc.

Murphy, A. (1994). *Working with elderly people.* London, England: Souvenir Press.

Teaff, J. (1985). *Leisure services with the elderly.* St. Louis, MO: Times Mirror/Mosby.

CHAPTER 17
•••••••••••••••••••••••••••••
Establishing Community Ties

KEY TERMS...

community   intergenerational

OBJECTIVES..

After completing this chapter, you should:

■ recognize the benefits of establishing an internal community for your residents
■ understand the steps involved in formulating programs with the external community
■ perceive and utilize the advantages of intergenerational programs

INTRODUCTION

Providing a solid community for your residents, both internally and externally, is one of the tasks of progressive programming. The benefits of offering community bonds for residents are numerous. Special programs thought to be community-oriented, such as intergenerational programming, will lend joy and excitement to your already well-structured program schedule.

Building and Maintaining a Facility Community

Before we discuss how to utilize the internal and external community elements, an understanding must be established of what a community is, and why it is important in the long-term care setting. A **community** is defined as a group of individuals who share some common purpose in a particular location. A community has certain points in common that you should be aware of to help you begin the process of building an internal community for your residents. Adelman, Frey, and Budz (1994) suggest that a true community must possess a "collective identity," formed through meaningful interpersonal relationships. Residents who leave a home environment and come into the long-term facility have experienced many losses and adjustments discussed in previous chapters. Feeling comforted by the internal community and remaining in touch with the external community are two crucial components of adjustment to the new long-term care environment. Therefore, the benefits that a community atmosphere brings to the long-term care setting through your depart-ment is an integral part of your programming objectives.

Some researchers have studied the effects of community links, particularly as they relate to other care settings, such as rehabilitation or residential care, where the contact and bonding with the community remains strong. In looking at characteristics that define a high-quality community, McMillan and Chavis (1986) offer these factors as necessities: membership, influence, social integration, and emotional connection. Membership simply means a sense of belonging. Influence refers to members' opinions that may impact the behavior of other members. The benefits of living together is defined as social integration. Group interactions and shared tasks can provide an emotional connection.

If you think in terms of your town or a local organization as an example to understand the dynamics of establishing an internal community in the long-term care setting, a community should have four key elements to make it unique. The factors that define a community are shared experiences, availability of services, neighbors and friends, and familiar places and landmarks. Let's look at each factor individually to see how an activity department can foster the maintenance of an internal community.

First, a community has members that have some goals or objectives that are similar. For residents in long-term care, the common ground is the need for medical services and to be taken care of properly. The need for skilled care is the reason that residents have reached the institutional part of the long-term care continuum. The developers of a concept called longevity therapy, Graubarth-

Szyller and Padgett (1989), suggest that an internal community is built on the things that do not change during one's lifetime. Examples include the need to feel connected with others, to feel productive, and have a purpose. They propose that an internal community structure is built by creating a relationship between residents, staff, and administration that includes communication, learning, motivation, and support. The principles of longevity therapy are in line with support of community bonding, because a primary goal of the longevity therapy program is to view the aging process as a time of awakening, rather than a decline in functioning. As an activity professional, you may foster common bonds by offering programs with universal appeal, such as entertainment events.

Another factor in establishing an internal community for your residents is to consider providing all the available services that would normally be received if they were members of an external community group. Medical care is a given in the long-term care facility, but what about the professional services that most of us take for granted in our external community settings? Some of the life tasks that residents might expect include getting a haircut or set, going to the cleaners or shopping, stopping at the post office, attending religious services, buying and reading the newspaper, participating in leisure and recreational activities, walking the dog, and talking to neighbors. Designing an environment that responds to some of these familiar patterns of community involvement can add comfort and reassurance. An example of an activity that promotes a community spirit is establishing a store for residents, suggested by McClannahan and Risley (1973). Although the concept may not be appropriate for all facilities or residents, having a store or meeting place where residents can make personal decisions and purchases, can add to self-esteem and maintenance of other skills that might be lost in the institutional environment. Participation in the travelling clothing stores that bring shopping experiences in to the residents can be rewarding. Other services, such as a central area designated for mail pick-up and delivery, hairdressing/barber services, a spot for having coffee and reading the newspaper, purchasing minor items, and being able to get outside easily and safely for a morning or evening stroll, can be vitally important in delivering a community atmosphere.

The neighbors and friends of your internal community are staff, family members, visitors, and volunteers. Being interested in the physical changes, emotional, and social aspects of a resident's adjustment is the responsibility of all members of a caring community. The warm bonding of interpersonal relationships and repeated exposures to one another over time can build strong bonds that replace those left behind in the external community. As in the outside community, there will be "shut-ins" who may want periodic visits from a caring person. Residents may need gentle coaxing by their "neighbors" to come to programs. Acknowledging the unique aspects of all residents and understanding their potential common problems is the role of the compassionate internal community members.

Creating familiar places and comfortable landmarks to define the hometown community is suggested by Wilden (1994). She states "The secret of creating a sense of community within your facility is to become more than a home and become a hometown." Delivering the expected services that were part of the external community must be integrated into your facility environment through creative approaches. A community-oriented intervention for residents includes starting a "downtown" area in the facility, if space permits. There, familiar icons such as a mailbox or barber pole, reminds residents of the area's purpose and provides needed services. Wayfinding cues such as street signs for "main street," could be used to designate your central service area for residents or directional guidance to help residents feel at home. Large or obvious landmarks, such as a big clock or park bench setting, can also be used to give a community "feel" and present a memorable community spot.

Bringing the External Community Into the Facility ....

Maintaining strong ties with your external community is an important task of your department to ease the adjustment of your residents to the institutional environment. Mendell and Kincaid (1981) suggest that "the long-term care facility must not operate in isolation, but instead must view itself as part of the larger surrounding community." They offer that the objectives of an activity department of a long-term care facility in planning for a community program should be to provide services to the community in the form of recreation programs, as well as establish a vital link between facility members and the community for support. One of the most important links is the contact between the resident of the long-term care facility and established friends and other community members. Mendell and Kincaid comment that it is an often overlooked fact that a resident of a facility may still have many friends and contacts in the community that can offer a connection.

Assessing Resident Needs

During the normal assessment process, you will determine past and current interests of residents, hobbies, lifestyles, and other pertinent information to assist you in proper activity planning. One of the considerations you will make during assessment is the manner in which the resident participated in community life. Did the resident grow up in one town, marry, and raise a family there during his or her lifetime? Is the resident an immigrant, and considers the community the one he or she left sixty years ago in the home country? Was the resident part of a subcommunity, such as the military or of a religious group? Did the resident live in a thriving metropolis and never interact much with community offerings? These and many other questions should help you form a picture of the needs of some of your residents in terms of community involvement. Although needs are assessed for each resident on an individual basis, a broad look at how your residents could benefit from community contact is necessary. Based on your research, ask yourself "In what form will the resident population benefit from community intervention?"

Determining Community Needs

As you contemplate the needs of your residents, consider what issues your community may have and where your facility, residents, and department can make a difference. Trocchio (1994) suggests you evaluate the role your department or facility can play for your community by considering a few factors. She mentions that consideration should be given to whether or not community programs you might participate in with your residents are addressing known community needs. Additionally, the community participation should be in line with your facility's mission statement and objectives.

External community programs take different forms. You may work with community leaders to bring regular community services into your facility, such as voter registration. Or, you may ask entertainment groups to perform in the facility, reminiscent of times residents attended group programs where their children might have performed. More creative use of external community programming involves a partnership between the activity department and one or more community groups to solve an issue or fill a need. Determining the need is the first step. Examples of external community partnering efforts include planning a community health fair and allowing the long-term care facility to host the event, offering use of facility space for routine club meetings, helping to raise money for community projects and charities, and involving residents in outward volunteer efforts from which the community may benefit, such as reassurance telephone calls. There are endless numbers of community functions and projects of which you and your residents can be part. Joining the local Chamber of Commerce or calling other civic organizations will certainly put you in contact with the community members who may need help and may be able to help you.

Mendell and Kincaid (1981) offer guidelines for the activity department that wishes a rapport with community groups who will use facility space. Some of their suggestions include a registration procedure with a clear explanation of the program to be offered and orientation to existing facility policies and procedures. Following the event, good program management dictates an evaluation of the effectiveness of the event. Mendell and Kincaid propose that the evaluation of the community program use points such as whether or not the event met the set objectives and if the communication flow was effective.

Another community intervention is the use of trips to reaffirm a connection. Residents will enjoy going back to many familiar places if they are from the area. Sightseeing trips, outings for lunch, personal shopping, or attending a movie can be simple and effective ways of maintaining all-important community links.

Intergenerational Programming

As a natural offshoot of external community programs, **intergenerational** partnerings are very special programming events for all involved. Intergenerational means "between different generations" and an intergenerational program is one that is established for mutual benefits by more than one generation. Clark (1991) focuses on the community elements of intergenerational programming by stating "It is entirely possible, through intergenerational programming, that the nursing home may become the center of community involvement. For the children it becomes a living learning center, and for the elderly it becomes the new neighborhood."

A principal step in learning about intergenerational programming is to look at the benefits of participation by both the elderly and the children who each receive different and positive experiences. In general terms, Clark (1991) summarizes that the two key reasons why intergenerational programs are so successful is that the program ". . . helps to diffuse negative stereotypes of aging but also presents a more positive picture of long-term health care." Haber and Short-DeGraff (1990) offer that intergenerational programs "challenge typical stereotypes" about the aging process. The elderly gain the advantage of being able to continue and maintain activities during the span of aging. Benefits for the elderly are also seen in spontaneous affection, excitement, and periods of increased socialization. Haber and Short-DeGraff also report that researchers have determined that improvements in self-esteem, health, and satisfaction with life also are noted in elderly involvements with intergenerational programming. Keller and McArdle (1985) mention that as an elderly person establishes a new role as a resource to a younger individual, he or she may be compensating for loss of other societal roles. Additionally, Rapelje and Ventresca (1982) suggest that when elderly clients have the opportunity to assume responsible community roles, such as that of a teacher or resource person, self-worth increases. In looking at intergenerational successes in day care settings, Stremmel, Travis, Kelly-Harrison, and Hensley (1994) listed a number of beneficial factors found in most encounters. The positive factors were respect and "learn from each other," unconditional love and attention, opportunity to experience grandparent figures, and generational differences in interests and activity levels. McMahon (1987) proposes that a full study of the needs of the elderly would not be complete without a view of the emotional issues concerned with intergeneration contact. She looks at an intergenerational program as a positive structure to "counteract segregation by age" by stating, "There is a special need for the healthcare professional to focus on the relationships and expectations of different generations as they proceed along life's continuum." Prior to exposure to intergenerational programming, McMahon suggests that each generation viewed each other as more conservative than they really were, but attitude changes occurred during programming.

For children participating in intergenerational programs, they benefit by receiving attention, time, social and emotional growth, and love, according to Haber and Short-DeGraff (1990). Clark (1991) offers that for young people ". . . contact with persons in long-term care facilities is vitally important to the continued strength and revitalization of the family unit." She adds that the contact is important to the youth as a break from their normal pressure-filled schedule and a buffer against potential loneliness or bonding they feel. The elderly individual offers the child a positive role model of survival, the years of life experience a resource, and act as a sounding board to listen to issues. Smith and Newman (1993) suggest that benefits of this programming to children are found in three areas: physical, cognitive, and emotional. Physical contact, such as snuggling and nurturing touches, are common. The children increase their cognitive sense by directly experiencing the older life cycle. Emotionally, children see and feel caring, older adults who offer warmth and unconditional caring. Bowlby (1993) feels that appropriate goals of any intergenerational program that involves the cognitively impaired should promote a "normalized" atmosphere, encourage socialization, and offer a positive setting for caring physical contact.

Acknowledging the expected growth of the elderly population, McMahon (1987) feels that increased dependence between generations will grow and intergenerational programming will be an obvious by-product. There are three presentation methods that intergenerational programs can utilize to deliver an experience. The first method suggests that elderly persons act as a resource for younger persons. Examples of this are elderly volunteers in pre-school settings or foster grandparents programs. The second intergenerational model is for the child or adolescent to serve as a resource for the elderly person. Examples include regular visits or telephone calls, minor tasks (letter-writing), or shopping. The last model that demonstrates the most benefits is the exchange of resources and talent that comes when both old and young share skills equally during an event. Some examples include joint programming, such as newsletter productions, drama workshops, and participation in events specially tailored for a high-level experience.

Experiences from a good intergenerational program must be planned. In addition to meeting the needs of both age groups, Bowlby (1993) mentions that intergenerational encounters should preserve the dignity of all participants. West and Hutchinson (1992) feel that programming should build relationships, but are influenced both positively and negatively by such factors as the ". . . the personal characteristics of the elder and the child, the nature of the activity they are doing together and the interventions offered by the staff." Keller and McArdle (1985) outline an eight-step process to establish an intergenerational exchange. The first step is to establish mutual goals and objectives. In steps two and three, roles and responsibilities are outlined, and the participants are determined. In step four, volunteers and participants are interviewed, and in step five, training and orientation of all participants is completed. Steps six and seven involve management of the actual activity and offering recognition to all participants and volunteers. In the last step, an evaluation of the program is conducted. Langford (1993) proposes that a checklist of questions be offered to all colleagues and potential clients before an intergenerational project is started. The basic programming questions are who, what, how many, where, when, and how much? Haber and Short-DeGraff (1990) propose that programming elements to consider include respecting all participants, using activities that limit frustration, and providing appropriate training for all staff and participants. They suggest that consistent communication is vital and the understanding that all participants interact at different levels is important. Principles that apply to successful intergenerational programs, such as specific program goals for children, the elderly, and staff, are mentioned by McDuffie and Whiteman (1989). They feel that training, constant feedback, and communication are vital. Leitner and Leitner (1985) add that the regularity of programs fosters greater interrelationships between participants.

McDuffie and Whiteman (1989) elaborate on successful strategies for selecting appropriate participants and leaders. First, they advise that chil-

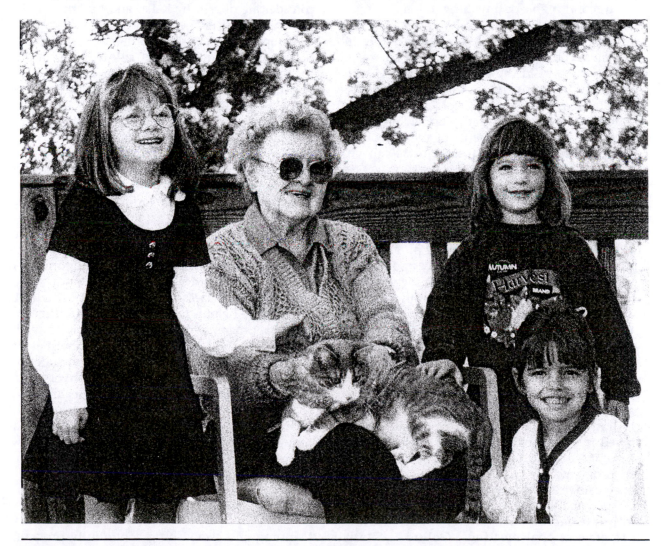

Figure 17–1   Cultivating intergenerational relationships that include pets help to maintain a community atmosphere for residents.

dren should be looked at individually, rather than as part of a class group. Considerations, such as the stage of development a child is experiencing, their health, and energy levels are all factors to weigh. Proper and empathetic preparation for children should occur through the use of stimulations, role-play, and discussions to determine their attitudes about elderly people and to educate them on the situations they will encounter. Even with individual assessment of participants, McDuffie and Whiteman recommend that whenever possible, an entire class should visit to allow a positive experience of meeting elderly residents. When reviewing residents, they feel that elements such as lifestyle and interests, confusion levels, and physical or mental status should have a bearing. Bowlby (1993) also mentions that cognitively impaired residents should be chosen with care and respect must be given to those who appear uncomfortable or unwilling to join.

According to McDuffie and Whiteman (1989), activity professionals selected for team leadership roles must complete some tasks to prepare for the interaction between the two generations. First, he or she should actively communicate with the schoolteacher, and share biographies of all planned participants. The activity professional should also attempt to involve the parents of the school children for feedback and information. Each visit should be planned in detail to avoid unpleasant surprises. Evaluation should conclude each session.

There are many programs that have been accomplished successfully with intergenerational groups. Obviously, age of the children has a bearing on level of activities, but many programs that interest your residents now may be modified for use with children. Allthorpe (1993) suggests using theatrical experiences based on reminiscences as a basis for intergenerational programs and Mason-Luckey (1985) and Sandel (1985) found success with the use of rhythmic games and folk songs. Nurturing and positive experiences were documented by Epstein and Greenberger (1990) and Hook (1988) in their horticultural therapy efforts with children and the elderly. Haber and Short-DeGraff (1990) propose that events can be designed in which elderly residents assist children as volunteers and in foster or adopt-a-grandparent programs. Newman and Ward (1993) found that positive behaviors in residents with dementia, such as increased extending of hands and appropriate tactile encounters, occurred during intergenerational meetings. Gollub & Shulkin (1978), McDuffie and Whiteman (1989), and many other researchers have developed engaging

program materials to assist in beginning effective intergenerational projects.

Because of the divergent needs of the two groups, however, problems may be encountered during programming. Suld (1973), in an early intergenerational effort, encountered problems with the sizes of groups and the variations among participants over the weeks of programming. When adjustments were made to control group size and specific participants, improvements were noted. Building relationships between groups took longer than anticipated, as reported by West and Hutchinson (1992). Additionally, some of the children in their study had trouble communicating with elderly residents and others had difficulty working with the elderly on projects. Cashmore (1994) feels that program problems are decreased when proper education is provided on the aging process and other expected characteristics. Other areas to consider are offered by Keller and McArdle (1985) and include remembering to properly assess resident capabilities, consider permissions, transportation, and insurance issues. Clark (1990) proposes the continual need for education in preproject start-ups and ongoing programs in the school systems to educate and prepare students for encounters with elderly people.

Evaluation, a necessary final step in any programming effort, should be completed following each intergenerational experience with every group. A summary of the encounter from the prospective of the children will yield one set of results whereas those of the elderly may show another. The activity professional and the teachers involved should formalize the event and document the reactions, as well as use the information to guide future programs. McDuffie and Whiteman (1989) devised a list of evaluation criteria that may be helpful as you evaluate your intergenerational programs. They suggest looking for "willing participation" and anticipation by both elders and children. Other positive factors include improved moods, smiling, increased conversation, emotional closeness, and comfortable feelings.

Intergenerational programming is an excellent way to build and bridge a community for your residents and offers programming value by allowing the children to become the "familiar faces" of the community.

SUMMARY

Planning and establishing community programs is a crucial part of your full program design. Looking at methods to build an internal community and integrate the external community into your facility will assist in providing vital links for residents. Intergenerational programming, an accessible and interesting form of external community involvement, will add a dimension to your active schedule.

R E V I E W   Q U E S T I O N S

1. What are some of the factors important in establishing an internal community for residents?
2. What are the kinds of external community formats?

3. What are the three different categories of intergenerational programming?

O N   Y O U R   O W N

1. What are some environmental adaptations you can use to help residents feel a community spirit?
2. How would you structure a three-week preproject educational program of 30-minute sessions for the preschool level in working with your moderate cognitively impaired residents?
3. Name five community groups you could contact, explain how they might enhance regular programming, and discuss how you both can benefit from special partnerships in programming.

R E F E R E N C E S

Adelman, M., Frey, L., & Budz, T. (1994). Keeping the community spirit alive. *The Journal of Long-Term Care Administration*, Vol. 22, 4–7.

Allthorpe, D. (1993). Theatre of memories. *Nursing Times*, Vol. 89(44), 70–71.

Bowlby, C. (1993). *Therapeutic activities with persons disabled by Alzheimer's disease and related disorders.* Gaithersburg, MD: Aspen Publishers Inc.

Cashmore, M. (1994). A lifetime of memories: A community development pilot project. *Perspectives*, Vol. 18(2), 2–5.

Clark, P. (1991). *Intergenerational arts in the nursing home.* New York, NY: Greenwood Press.

Epstein, S., & Greenberger, D. (1990). Nurturing plants, children, and older individuals: Intergenerational horticultural therapy. *Journal of Therapeutic Horticulture*, Vol. 5, 16–19.

Gollub, W., & Shulkin, S. (1978). *Family rituals: Short activities for family communication.* Philadelphia, PA: School District of Philadelphia.

Graubarth-Szyller, B., & Padgett, J. (1989). *Longevity therapy: An innovative approach to nursing home care of the elderly.* Philadelphia, PA: The Charles Press.

Haber, E., & Short-DeGraff, M. (1990). Intergenerational programming for an increasing age-segregated society. *Activities, Adaptation & Aging*, Vol. 14(3), 35–49.

Hook, P. (1988). Plant folklore: An intergenerational approach to developing activities. In R. H. Mattson (Ed.) *Proceedings of health through horticulture, horticulture therapy short course*, (49–52). Manhattan, KS: Kansas State University.

Keller, M. J., & M. McArdle (1985). Establishing intergenerational exchange opportunities. *Activities,*

Adaptation & Aging, Vol. 7(2), 31–43.

Langford, S. (1993). A shared vision. *Nursing Times*, Vol. 89(44), 67–69.

Leitner, M. J., and Leitner, S. I. (1985). *Leisure in later life: A sourcebook for the provision of recreational services for elders.* Binghamton, NY: Haworth Press.

Mason-Luckey, B. (1985). Intergeneration movement therapy: A leadership challenge. *Activities, Adaptation & Aging*, Vol. 9(3), 141–150.

McClannahan, L., & Risley, T. (1973). A store for nursing home residents. *Nursing Home* 22(6), 10–11.

McDuffie, W., & Whiteman, J. (1989). *Intergenerational activities program handbook,* 3rd edition. Binghamton, NY: Broome County Child Development Council, Inc.

McMahon, M. (1987). The value of intergenerational relationships. *Journal of Gerontological Nursing*, Vol. 13(4), 25–29.

McMillan, D., & Chavis, D. (1986). Sense of community: A definition and theory. *Journal of Community Psychology*,14, 6–23.

Mendell, R., & Kincaid, J. (1981). Cooperation needed between the long-term health care facility and the surrounding community. *Activities, Adaptation & Aging*, Vol. 1(3), 31–35.

Newman, S., & Ward, C. (1993). An observational study of intergenerational activities and behavior change in dementing elders at adult day care centers. *International Journal of Aging & Human Development*, Vol. 36(4), 321–333.

Rapelje, D., & Ventresca, D. (1982). Intergenerational programs: Untapped ideas. *Dimensions in Health Service*, 591, 28–29.

Sandel, S. (1985). Creating and playing: Bridges for intergenerational communication. *Activities, Adapta-*

tion & Aging, Vol. 9, (3), 133–139.

Smith, T., & Newman, S. (1993). Older adults in early childhood programs: Why and how. *Young Children*, March, 32–35

Stremmel, A., Travis, S., Kelly-Harrison, P., & Hensley, A.D. (1994). The perceived benefits and problems associated with intergenerational exchanges in day care settings. *The Gerontologist*, Vol. 34, 4, 513–519.

Suld, V. (1973). When the children come so does laughter. *Modern Nursing Home*, April, 45–47.

Trocchio, J. (1994). Oldest and newest promise is responding to community needs. *The Journal of Long-Term Care Administration*, 22(3), 22–24

West, M., & Hutchinson, S. (1992). Intergenerational geriatric remotivation. *Clinical Nursing Research*, Vol. 1(3), 221–235.

Wilden, V. (1994). Go beyond "home", Create a hometown. *Journal of Long-Term Care Administration*, 22(2), 9.

FURTHER READING

Campanelli. L., & Leviton, D. (1989). Intergenerational health promotion and rehabilitation: The adult health and development program model. *Topics in Geriatric Rehabilitation*, 4(3), 61–69.

Dunkle, R., & Mikelthun, B. (1982). Intergenerational programming: An adopt-a-grandparent program in a retirement community. *Activities, Adaptation & Aging*, Vol. 3, No. 2, 93–105.

Glass, B. (1982). Building activities into a network of community based supports. *Activities, Adaptation & Aging*, Vol. 3, No. 2, 55–60.

Glaser, M. (1994). "Grandma, please!" *The Journal of Long-Term Care Administration*, Vol. 22, 4–6.

Hargrave, T., & Anderson, W. (1992). *Finishing well: Aging and reparation in the intergenerational family.* New York, NY: Brunner/Mazel Publishers.

Hill, D. (1987). Promoting intergenerational programs: Triads with youth, elderly, and students: A case example. *Journal of Gerontological Social Work*, Vol. 10(3/4), 155–165.

Kennedy, G. (1992). Shared activities of grandparents and grandchildren. *Psychological Reports*, Vol. 70, 211–227.

Knoth, M. (1989). *The professional activity director.* Lafayette, Indiana: Valley Press.

Lee, G., & Ellithorpe, E. (1992). Intergenerational exchange and subjective well-being among the elderly. *Journal of Marriage and The Family*, Vol. 44, 217–224.

Lee, G. (1979). Children and the elderly: Interaction and morale. *Research On Aging*, Vol. 1(3), 335–360.

Oliphant, R. (1985). The american nursing home: A novelist's view. *Nursing Homes*, July/August, 19–23.

Poole, G., & Gooding, B. A. (1993). Developing and implementing a community intergenerational program. *Journal of Community Health Nursing*, 10(2), 77–85.

Rath, S., & Trocchia, J. (1981). Nursing home residents as surrogate grandparents for preschool children. *Activities, Adaptation & Aging*, Vol.1(4), 55–58.

Shulkin, S., & Gollub, W. (1979). *Grandparents and grandchildren: A whimsical, joyful sharing book.* Philadelphia, PA: Programs and Publications.

Tobiason, S. J., Knudsen, F., Stengel, J., & Giss, M. (1979). Positive attitudes toward aging: The aged teach the young. *Journal of Gerontological Nursing*, Vol. 5, No. 3, 18–23.

CHAPTER 18
In-service Programs and Other Education

KEY TERMS ....

in-service   sandwich generation
respite care   lesson plan

OBJECTIVES ....

After completing this chapter, you should:

- plan and execute in-service programs for activity staff, general staff, and family members
- understand suitable topics for each in-service group and to have the skills necessary to present community teaching events
- develop abilities as an instructor to make effective presentations

INTRODUCTION

Education, whether through in-service programs or community events, is an important promotional tool for the activity professional. This chapter covers preparation for reaching activity professional staff, general staff, and family members through in-service education. Educational community functions will also be discussed and appropriate suggested topics given for specific learning groups. Information on teaching style and preparation for instructing conclude the chapter.

An **in-service** program is defined as the continual on-the-job staff training required for any position in a facility. The ongoing training needs of one position, such as administrator, may be greater than another, but staff at all levels should continue to learn to improve job performance.

Although some staff education programs are mandated on a yearly basis by the state or federal regulations that govern your particular facility or position, benefits for attending in-service education programs are numerous. Participation in programs yields obvious advantages for employees such as increased knowledge in specific areas, but the subtle positives of in-service programs give staff members an opportunity to view other departments in a different way, increase understanding and communication between departments, and refocus staff to their main employment purpose; to serve the needs of the residents.

For activity professionals, you will plan in-service education programs to reach two distinct groups. The first group will be your own activity staff. Depending on the topic, you may wish to include your volunteers on occasion. The second group you want to reach is the general staff members from all departments. In addition to traditional in-service training for these two groups, you should organize education programs for family members, and, if required, the outside community.

Activity Department In-Services .....

Planned on a monthly or bi-monthly basis, ongoing education for the activity staff can be held as part of your regular monthly staff meeting or as a separate program. You may ask your staff to suggest ideas for sessions, as well as using your own knowledge of the field and departmental observations to develop topic areas.

Goals for Activity Department Programs

The goals of your programs will be vastly different from the sessions you prepare and present to the general staff. Goals for the programs for your activity professionals include:

1. Developing new skills by a review of innovative techniques.
2. Learning to cope with problems such as disruptive residents or stress.
3. Enhancing existing skills in areas such as professionalism or management.
4. Improving the overall effectiveness in meeting resident needs.

Carter and James (1979) felt that a recreation professional needs learning in both "personal and professional concerns" in order to keep up with industry changes.

Sample Topics

In a study of knowledge and basic skills for activity directors, Hunter (1984) found that activity directors rated the "problems of aging" as their most critical educational need. Hunter also discovered that knowledge in the areas of tailoring recreation programs to particular residents, understanding physical and psychological health needs and learning about general recreation and management issues were other areas of education in which activity directors expressed interest in learning. Concerned that health care workers may have varied or lower levels of knowledge about aging, Palmore (1977) designed a "Facts on Aging Quiz" that can be used as an initial training device for health care staff. Results of the "Facts on Aging Quiz" in trials with social workers as reported by Barresi and Brubaker (1979) have shown that despite educational efforts, respondents show a negative bias toward the elderly and their aging process. Further work on knowledge about aging should be conducted with activity personnel because Hunter's work (1984) indicates there is a need. The "Facts on Aging Quiz" can be used as a training device for activity, general staff, and modified for use with family groups. Patterson (1980) outlined the procedure for using "game-like activities," called simulation, to provide a reality-based learning experience.

In her work, Henderson (1981) found that recreation professionals who work with older adults needed more information on programming for special groups, activity analysis, innovative programming, and leadership techniques. When Maypole (1985) conducted a study with activity directors to determine their training needs, he concluded that information on working with residents with challenging medical conditions, such as dementia or mental health problems, ranked as ". . . the higher priority training needs. . . ." The study also identified less significant training requirements on educational topics such as working with families on issues concerning death and dealing with residents with mental health or other problems. The program needs of each activity department will be different, but the following list will help you to choose some sample areas for activity in-service programs based on general categories:

- *administration:* management, volunteers, interdepartmental relationships, regulations, policies and procedures, budgeting
- *programming:* new methods, determining needs, documentation, reaching a special population, trips, therapy interventions, resources

- *evaluation:* quality assurance, surveys, reports, studies
- *miscellaneous:* brainstorming, sensory training, role-play

In their book on in-service education, Eliasen and Feick (1991) suggest additional topics for activity professionals such as ethical responsibilities, adaptation of activities, and time management.

Another segment of learning with which you can provide your staff are any of the crucial, but often overlooked subjects involving other departments. You may request that another department head be a guest speaker at a future meeting to cover the topic if you lack the expertise to handle it on your own. It is vital that your activity professionals receive initial and ongoing training in the following key areas because often, they are exposed to these issues on a regular basis:

- *administration:* OSHA requirements, such as hazard communications, bloodborne pathogens; handwashing
- *dietary:* sanitation, food handling practices, therapeutic diets
- *nursing:* feeding residents, transporting and transferring residents, toileting techniques, range of motion and acceptable exercises, restraint usage and release protocol, identification of residents with potentially dangerous conditions (diabetics, combative behavior)
- *social services:* sexuality training, advance directives/living wills, coping with difficult residents

General Staff In-Services ....

Having the activity staff conduct specialized in-service training programs for all staff provides an opportunity for increasing awareness and improving job performance for the general staff. In his three-year study of in-service training required for gerontology workers, Hickey (1974) mentioned that some of the benefits of in-service training are ". . . Staff-patient and staff-staff communications expanded; staff role differences tended to recede in the context of discussing patients or patient care . . . staff meetings became more oriented toward function than structure . . . the learning process itself was reported and observed to continue in a variety of situations outside the classroom."

The programs planned for general staff members from other departments should occur on a quarterly or bi-annual basis, depending on facility needs. Include some specific repeat programs on certain topics that require reinforcing, such as the function of the activity department in the facility.

Goals for General Staff Programs

A program of in-service sessions for general staff members should address the following goals:

- increase visibility and understanding of the role of the activity department
- provide new ideas on how resident needs are met through activity programming
- offer suggestions for joint participation among departments to assist with resident goals and problems

The focus of your programs for general staff depend on your relationship with other departments as well as the general reception that the activity department receives in your facility. If you are experiencing difficulties with overall cooperation and understanding of the activity department, it may be necessary to provide repeated sessions that attempt to build up good will. On the other hand, if your relations with other departments are cordial, you may be able to tackle growth areas such as sensory training or role playing.

Tips for Connecting With a General Staff Audience

When planning a program for all staff members, be prepared that your audience may not be excited or alert. You may want to illicit as much participation as you can from this group by dis-

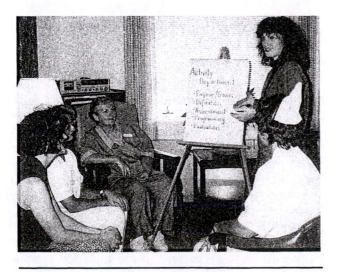

Figure 18–1 An in-service program for the general staff can be intimate to encourage participation.

carding the traditional presentation format and placing yourself as a "moving target" who speaks while walking throughout the group. You can also try group techniques of asking questions of specific group members whom you know to be comfortable with speaking or by breaking the larger group into smaller sections to work together on a project. In the work of Hickey (1974), he suggested that nontraditional teaching methods work best for reaching this audience because of the diverse backgrounds of the attendees. He also mentioned the use of active techniques such as ". . . role-play, video-tape exercises, psychodrama. . ." and passive method examples such as ". . . lecture, films, written exercises. . ." as helpful.

Using examples of specific residents or situations brings the issues into focus for many participants. When incorporating examples, be sure to avoid unintentionally embarrassing any specific individual and, of course, be careful not to divulge confidential information. Be upbeat, and whenever possible, use "show" rather than "tell" techniques. Keep things simple and avoid all medical jargon and abbreviations. If your audience appears sleepy or bored, they probably are! Switch gears and try another approach before you lose them altogether. In the week following your in-service presentation, talk to some of the attendees to see if you connected positively.

Sample Topics

Focusing on one of the benefits of in-service, Schwartz (1974) theorized that in order to boost morale, staff education programs should concentrate on factors that deal with the care of the elderly in areas such as adjusting to losses, providing necessary amounts of stimulation for all resident needs, and providing ". . . meaningfulness of residents' lives." Informational in-services on topics such as disease processes or physical conditions are helpful to staff because often, there is limited time during orientation to cover how a particular physical condition impacts the elderly. For example, in-service education on the subject of blindness was researched by Wineburg (1982). His work shows that not only are long-term care workers lacking basic skills to cope with a resident's blindness, but also collaborate efforts are not being sought between blind service agencies and facilities to provide adequate staff training. Although the availability of blind service referrals has increased in the last decade, the study illustrates that activity and general staff require better in-service training to properly work with long-term care clients.

The following list suggests some key areas that activity staff members can present to other staff to meet their educational needs:

1. Define an activity, and explaining what the activity department does to identify and meet resident needs through appropriate programming. Anderson (1990) discussed some ideas on presenting general information about activity planning and offered suggestions on hosting in-service training on group building, approaches, and problem solving to illustrate this point.
2. Develop better communication skills. James and Deichman (1981) suggested that all health care providers can benefit from therapeutic communication skills training that incorporates active listening, empathy, and appreciation.
3. Understand the aging process and the limitations that occur physically, cognitively, spiritually, and emotionally. There are many active methods for involving the staff in learning aspects of aging. Williams (1985) reviews a simulation game called "Into Aging." It is an example of a participatory type of learning that can be used with all staff to illustrate expected parts of the aging process.
4. Confront issues on death and dying. The work of Kubler-Ross (1969) presents an effective overview of death and dying. In-service planning on the subject of death, dying, and loss has been explored by Hughes (1993) with guidelines for both residents and staff.
5. Empathize with resident losses and adjust staff behavior accordingly. Both Anderson (1990) and Hughes (1993) suggest holding an in-service on understanding resident losses that may be a result of the process of institutionalization.
6. Learn and practice group problem-solving techniques. Berger (1982) designed an in-service training program technique for problem-solving that follows six steps: "general orientation, defining the situation, identifying positive and negative thoughts, brainstorming, decision-making, and carrying out the solution." This procedure can be used for any type of problem on which staff may need to work.
7. Deal with stress and staff burnout.

Family Programs ....

Although educational programs for family enrichment are not traditionally part of your formal in-service program, consider and plan for these programs in the same way you have for your own department and the general staff. The family members, friends, religious contacts and other visitors that make up your residents' outside support group have special needs that can be filled in part by your programs. In her research on families coping with institutionalization, Soloman (1983) observed that "Middle-aged children are experiencing their own life crises at the same time they experience the crises of their parents' lives." Soloman also found that there are four distinct and difficult episodes that families must adjust to concerning the institutionalized resident: decision made to enter a facility, actual admission to the facility, change to a higher level of care, and finally, death. These and other family support issues you could address in programs should include dealing with separation from loved ones, coping with chronic illness, handling guilt over facility placement, and adjusting to the long-term care environment.

Goals for Family Programs

Presenting a talk or seminar to families can be planned as a free-standing program, as part of larger facility educational effort, or as a result of requests from family members during family council meetings. Any family educational event should have the following goals:

■ inform and educate to gain greater understanding of resident care issues
■ decrease anxiety about the resident's placement
■ increase bonding between residents, staff, and family members to allow for the highest levels of care to be delivered

Challenges and Sample Topics for Family Programs

Reaching family members in an educational setting can be a challenge for activity professionals. Initially, there might be some reluctance of family members to see the activity professional as an educator because their exposure to activity staff is usually as the facilitator of programs for residents. You may present the program for a specific educational session or you may have arranged for a speaker. If you are the presenter, fine-tune your teaching abilities.

Family programs require a firm structure to avoid conflicts. With a clearly defined agenda and department heads present in the audience, specific questions on resident care that have no bearing on the subject matter can be taken up with specific staff members at the conclusion of the program. This avoids ruining a program by an individual who may be in attendance for noneducational reasons, such as the airing of complaints. A study by Burks, Lund, and Hill (1991) illustrates that the factors that most influence a caregiver's attendance at a support meeting are ". . . greater perceived helpfulness from the meetings, long time providing care, and lower life satisfaction. . . ."

There may also be some program planning overlaps with other departments in the material you wish to present to families. Be sure that social services did not present a similar issue under a different heading a few weeks back. Additionally, be cautious on interpreting facility policies for other departments if questions should arise.

Many of the same topic areas listed for use by the general staff can be tailored to fit the needs of family members. Some other areas you might consider include understanding a specific disease process, determining realistic expectations for long-term care, explaining the benefits of an activity program, assisting the resident as an outside caregiver, and dealing with feelings of grief, anger, and frustration.

Community Programs ....

Reaching out to the community through education can be a wonderful way to improve the facility's image and provide needed information about activity programming and long-term care. By inviting the public into the facility, you normalize the institutional environment for both residents and community members. Educational programs that include the community are most likely to be an offshoot of your whole plan for community involvement in your activity programming. By analyzing the needs of your community members (who may later require the services of the facility) and providing them with the educational information they lack, you offer a unique service. Indirectly, you also give people in the surrounding area a positive perception of how a long-term care facility looks and operates.

Goals For A Community Program

To be successful, a community speaking event should foster the following objectives:

- promote a positive experience in a long-term care facility
- receive information to decrease anxiety and stress

- allow the community the opportunity to be a larger part of the residents' every day life

Preparation and Sample Topics

Preparation for your presentation should be carefully done for a community-wide event. Your target audience may be less definable than a family group or your own general staff members. With a community group, you will most likely have a diverse representation of educational levels and backgrounds, and you will have to proceed accordingly. You stand the most chance of success if you keep your presentation simple and repetitive, at least on the key points. This audience may prefer hand-out materials that they can review at home with other relatives. Therefore, you may wish to distribute photocopied materials at the end of your presentation. Another factor you may have to deal with at a community program is the presence of the media. Become familiar with the need for press coverage. When you are the featured speaker, be careful of overstating or misstating any facility policies or answering any "tricky" questions during your presentation. If you anticipate any problem areas, review your materials in advance with your administrator.

As stated in the family programming section, many of the topics useful in staff programs have applications for community programs. Some additional areas are: activity planning ideas for home care givers, defining and discussing **respite care** from an activity perspective, presenting the challenges of the **sandwich generation** (those middle-aged adults responsible for the care of their own children and their elderly parents), senior health education, and activity planning for hospice care.

Informal caregivers at home have a variety of needs that can be addressed in community programs. Respite care is an important, short-term program that some facilities offer in which family members are spelled for a week or two from their normal home care duties. The resident is admitted to the long-term care facility for a brief time to allow the caregiver a rest or vacation. Families need reassurance and understanding of the respite process, especially the steps that the staff takes to follow the guidance of the caregiver concerning daily activities and routines. Many of the caregivers in need of respite care may also be members of the sandwich generation. In their article on this group, Dobson and Dobson (1985) describe the sandwich generation's experience of raising a family along with caring for a parent, and note, "these middle-aged adults are becoming aware of their own mortality, which heightens the sense of running out of time." They are experiencing what Dobson and Dobson term "middlescence," a transition period in which responsibilities for caregiving increase. Extra time with children, friends, or other activities diminish, causing resentment and frustration. Schmidt (1980) commented on another phenomenon, similar to the sandwich generation, of ". . . parent-child pairs in which the children themselves are at or near retirement, and the parents, in their mid-80s or beyond." Observations are made by Schmidt concerning the crisis the "young old" (the child) faces because of limited finances and depleted strength; however, caregiving responsibilities still exist for the "old old" (the parent) with high probability of increasing future care needs.

According to the CARE-NET (West Central Georgia Caregivers Network) study, a research effort of caregivers described by Carter and Golant (1994) in their book about caregiving, stated that informal caregivers (family member or other unpaid help) were citing "specialized training" and "information" as some of their most important needs.

Another community group that activity professionals can impact in programming are youth groups. DeBolt (1991) reminds activity professionals that offering young people positive experiences with the elderly and teaching them about the aging process is a responsibility. As the baby boomers age, new generations will be entering the health care professions to care for the over sixty-five population, and their influences will be positively felt if they are exposed to early teaching experiences.

As another way to meet community needs, Butler (1981) proposes the establishment of a teaching nursing home that could aid in geriatric research and use the nursing home for outward services into the surrounding area.

By offering alternatives and education to your community, you are assisting your community members with their current medical challenges.

Conducting an Effective In-Service or Educational Program ....

Similar to your successful planning of an activity program for your residents, your preparation for any in-service or group educational seminar will be the key to a smooth and well-received program.

Materials

After defining your target audience as discussed above, select your topic, outline your presenta-tion, and gather all the appropriate resources. Research the topic area and tailor the materials to your target group. Attention must be paid to the type of presentation method appropriate to the objectives of your particular session. In their work on the activity director as an educator, Eliasen and Feick (1991) define three specific areas that an activity professional wishes an in-service attendee to accomplish during a session: ". . . acquire information, apply knowledge . . . or acquire a skill and/or develop an attitude." Eliasen and Feick further describe the instructional techniques that an activity educator can use to attain a particular learning objective. In order to "acquire information," they suggest that teaching techniques such as lectures, visual demonstrations, or question and answer periods may work best. To learn to "apply knowledge," the authors propose that methods such as group discussion or case study situations are suitable to understand the learning objectives. Eliasen and Feick offer learning approaches such as process demonstration, practice opportunities, role-play, and experiential activities as a plan for achieving "acquiring a skill and developing or modifying an attitude" objectives.

With any teaching plan, take adequate time to gather your class materials. Prepare overhead transparencies and hand-out information that is easy to read and understand. Be sure to document any sources you use and request permissions ahead of time for use of copyrighted materials. Anticipate questions and problem spots and plan for them in advance. Vary your presentation methods by including lecture with a visual portion (a film or video), then close with ample time for audience participation through questions and answers. Give appropriate credit, both verbally and in writing, for any assistance you may have received in preparing your presentation.

Room Preparation

Ensure that your room can handle seating, lighting, and equipment ahead of time. On the day of your presentation, double check the area well in advance of your program and be sure everything is in order. Whenever possible, set up the traffic pattern in the room to minimize distractions for the speaker (late arrivals should not walk in front of the speaker). Refreshments could be provided before or after your program to assist with the mingling process of your attendees.

Your Teaching Style

Your background may have included educational training, but if it did not, you need some tips on developing a teaching style. First, and most important, be prepared, organized, and start on time! Consider the issues that may be working against you and prepare for them. In her book, Leary (1994) mentions four barriers to learning that can impact a teacher's success: instructor attitude, emotional and social cultural attitudes, competition, and good conditions for learning. Each of these may cause the learning experience to be more or less successful, and you should be prepared for each contingency.

Eliasen and Feick (1991) describe an instructor as ". . . able to create an atmosphere conducive to learning," and that a teacher should strive to display information in a unique way. They also remind instructors to consider the qualities of the "adult learner." They note that each adult comes to a learning session as a person with a "lifetime of different experiences" that created "different attitudes, values. . . and educational backgrounds which affect their ability and desire to learn."

Use a **lesson plan**, notes, or other reminders to stay on track. Break your presentation into parts to keep the audience interested. Circulate a sign-in sheet or have attendees sign in at the entrance. Summarize the key points in simple hand-outs, but remember to distribute materials at the end of your talk to avoid losing the attention of your audience. Work with a time frame that is reasonable for the topic at hand. Be aware of bored attendees and adjust accordingly. Close your talk by reiterating your key thoughts. Allow enough time for a question and answer period. When appropriate, ask for a written evaluation of the program from the attendees' perspective, and ask your colleagues and departmental staff for their important feedback.

Figure 18–2 illustrates a sample in-service/educational schedule for a long-term care facility.

SUMMARY

As a key staff member, the activity professional has responsibilities as an educator to the activity staff under his or her direction. In-service programs presented by the activity staff to the general staff and family members are important to promote the objectives of the activity department and to provide further educational opportunities to these groups. Reaching the community through educational events is also vital to forging relationships and problem-solving issues. Acquiring the necessary skills to become an educator is another step in the professional growth process.

Program	January	February	March	April	May	June	July	August	September	October	November	December
In-service												
Activity Department Staff	Sensitivity Retraining	Special Events Planning	Horticultural Therapy	Volunteer Recruitment	MDS and Care Planning	Presentation by Interns	Using Community Resources	Quality Assurance Report/ Follow-up	Physical Aspects of Aging	Assessment Skills	Management Through Objectives	Alzheimer's Disease Update
General Staff	Handling Residents with dementia			The Role of the Activity Department			Dealing with Anxious Residents				Aging Simulation Exercise	
Education												
Family Program			Dealing with Grief and Loss			Join the Care-Giving Process			Humor Therapy			Stress Reduction
Community Program				Activities Planning for the Home Caregiver					Psychological Aspects of Aging			

Figure 18–2   An in-service and educational schedule for a calendar year.

• •
R E V I E W   Q U E S T I O N S

1. Based on the research, what are some of the identified educational needs of activity professionals that in-service programs should address?
2. What are some of the benefits of in-service training for the general staff discussed by Hickey?
3. What is respite care, and what are some of the educational needs of informal caregivers?
4. What are the stages that families experience during the institutionalization process?
5. Why are simulation programs effective for many educational programs?

O N   Y O U R   O W N

1. What other topics could be planned that would help community members deal with the problems of the sandwich generation?

2. Plan an in-service for the activity staff concerning myths about aging, then modify your presentation to be suitable for general staff and family members.

3. You are the new activity director in a large facility with four staff members relatively new to the field. They have received basic activity training, but they lack confidence and adequate management skills to cope on the job. How would you plan your annual in-service calendar to increase learning and improve their job performance?

R E F E R E N C E S

Anderson, D. R. (1990). *A professional guide for activity inservices*. Sarona, WI: Rosewood Publishing.

Barresi, C. M., & Brubaker, T. H. (1979). Clinical social workers' knowledge about aging: Responses to the "facts on aging" quiz. *Journal of Gerontological Social Work*, Vol. 2(2), 137–146.

Berger, R. M. (1982). A problem solving model for in-service training. *Journal of Gerontological Social Work*, Vol. 4(3/4), 21–33.

Burks, V. K., Lund, D. A., & Hill, R. D. (1991). Factors associated with attendance at caregiver support group meetings. *Activities, Adaptation and Aging*, Vol. 15(3), 93–108.

Butler, R. N. (1981). The teaching nursing home. *The Journal of the American Medical Association*, Vol. 245, No. 14, 1435–1437.

Carter, R., & Golant, S. K. (1994). *Helping yourself help others: A book for caregivers*. New York, NY: Time Books, Random House.

Carter, M., & James, A. (1979). Continuing professional development program for therapeutic recreators. *Therapeutic Recreation Journal*, 3rd Quarter, 12–15.

DeBolt, N. (1991). Teach and reach the future. *Activities, Adaptation and Aging*, Vol. 15(3), 67–71.

Dobson, J. E., & Dobson, R. L. (1985). The sandwich generation: Dealing with aging parents. *Journal of Counseling and Development*, Vol 63, 572–574.

Eliasen, K., & Feick, C. (1991). *The activity director as educator: Guidelines for planning inservice sessions*. Nanaimo, British Columbia, Canada: E. & F. Education Services.

Henderson, K. (1981). Continuing education needs of therapeutic recreation professionals. *Therapeutic Recreation Journal*, 1st Quarter, 36–43.

Hickey, T. (1974). In-service training in gerontology: Toward the design of an effective educational process. *The Gerontologist*, 14, 57–64.

Hughes, M. (1993). *Dying, death, and loss in long-term care*. La Grange, Texas: M & H Publishing Company Inc.

Hunter, H. C. (1984). The activity director in a nursing care facility: How does she fit in? *Activities, Adaptation and Aging*, Vol. 4(4), 13–44.

James, F., & Deichman, E. S. (1981). To listen and to hear: Guidelines for the development of a communications skills course for nursing home personnel. *Activities, Adaptation and Aging*, Vol. 2(1), 69–80.

Kubler-Ross, E. (1969). *On death and dying*. New York, NY: Collier Books, Macmillan Publishing Co.

Leary, S. (1994). *Activities for personal growth*. Sydney, Australia: MacLennan & Petty Pty Ltd.

Maypole, D. E. (1985). Activity therapist continuing education needs assessment. *Activities, Adaptation and Aging*, Vol. 7(2), 15–23.

Palmore, E. (1977). Facts on aging: A short quiz. *The Gerontologist*, 17, 315–320.

Patterson, P. (1980). Simulations in therapeutic recreation training programs. *Therapeutic Recreation Journal*, 3rd Quarter, 15–20.

Schmidt, M. G. (1980). Failing parents, aging children. *Journal of Gerontological Social Work*, Vol. 2(3), 259–268.

Schwartz, A. N. (1974). Staff development and morale building in nursing homes. *The Gerontologist*, 14, 50–53.

Soloman, R. (1983). Serving families of the institutionalized aged: The four crises. *Journal of Gerontological Social Work*, Vol. 5(1/2), 83–96.

Williams, J. (1985). Into aging: A simulation game. *Activities, Adaptation and Aging*, Vol. 6(3), 13–16.

Wineburg, R. J. (1982). The elderly blind in nursing homes: The need for a coordinated in-service training policy. *Journal of Gerontological Social Work*, Vol. 4(3/4), 67–77.

F U R T H E R   R E A D I N G

Bullock, C., & Carter, M. (1981). Status report: Continuing professional development program for therapeutic recreators. *Therapeutic Recreation Journal*, 2nd Quarter, 46–49.

Coffey, F. (1986). Continuing professional development. *Therapeutic Recreation Journal*, 3rd Quarter, 11–20.

Deck, M. (1995). *Instant teaching tools for healthcare educators*. St. Louis, MO: Mosby.

Hughes, M. (1987). *In-service on loss: Family, aging & staff stress.* La Grange, TX: M&H Publishing Co.

Killian, K. (1984). Respite care and the therapeutic recreator. *Therapeutic Recreation Journal,* 1st Quarter, 27–30.

Lian, M., Bowen, M., & Egger, K. (1985). In-service training in therapeutic recreation for persons with severe handicaps. *Therapeutic Recreation Journal,* 1st Quarter, 27–35.

O'Morrow, G., & Reynolds, R. (1989). *Therapeutic recreation: A helping profession.* Englewood Cliffs, NJ: Prentice Hall.

Munson, W., Zoerink, D., & Stadulis, R. (1986). Training potential therapeutic recreators for self-efficacy and competency in interpersonal skills. *Therapeutic Recreation Journal,* 1st Quarter, 53–61.

Pike, R. W. (1989). *Creative training techniques handbook: Tips, tactics and how-to's for delivering effective training.* Minneapolis, MN: Lakewood Books.

Stumbo, N. (1986). A definition of entry-level knowledge for therapeutic recreation practice. *Therapeutic Recreation Journal,* 1st Quarter, 15–30.

Unterreiner, C. (1979). A study of continuing education needs of personnel delivering therapeutic recreation services in the state of Missouri. *Therapeutic Recreation Journal,* 1st Quarter, 44–49.

C H A P T E R   1 9
Advancing Your Career

OBJECTIVES.......................................

After completing this chapter, you should:

- gain insight as to how to assess your career goals and advance in your facility
- increase your professional image

INTRODUCTION

Career planning and professional advancement are areas of development that managers consider at different stages of employment. Assessment of career objectives and professional image enhancement allow successful growth in other career areas such as multifacility activity director, consultant, or administrator. Degrees or credentialing through professional organizations is another path to advancement.

Your success on the job may cause you to consider advancement to either a higher level in your present career track or further growth into a related management position. Congratulations on having the foresight to realize that you can continue to grow and develop your skills! To make a suitable career change, you should devote time time to explore the exact manner in which you wish to advance.

Assessing Your Goals

Switching gears into a different area or position requires planning. If you are an activity assistant, you will not wake up one day and find yourself hired as a activity director if you have not been working toward that goal beforehand. The first step in any career change is to research and explore options for yourself. You may have reached this "option consideration" stage after feeling restlessness in your position, or you may have your employment goals all mapped out. Knowing that you want to look into other areas, ask yourself the following questions:

- what aspects of my current job do I like and why? Which ones do I dislike and why?
- do I enjoy working with people or do I favor tasks that I can work on alone?
- do I like managing projects and people? Am I comfortable being a leader?
- is a change in routine a favorite part of my day or do I like to have things the same?
- what are my job strengths and what are my weaknesses?
- where do I see myself in five years?

Your answers may surprise you. Looking at your likes and dislikes, a clearer picture should emerge concerning the direction you may wish to take. There are three distinct paths you can consider when making a career change from your current activity position:

1. Moving up to a different position in your existing facility or organization.

2. Increasing your education or credentials for a variety of job change options.
3. Advancing into administration as either a regional activity professional, an assistant administrator, or an administrator.

Moving Up in Your Facility or Organization

If you have decided that your facility or parent company has opportunities that meet your goals, you should pursue a career change without changing your employer. Some long-term care operations are large enough to offer many career choices in a large activity department, in a related department, such as social services, or in a combined departmental setting, such as resident services. Other facilities may be part of a bigger chain of homes and may have corporate opportunities for you or a new position in a larger or smaller setting, whichever is your preference. In any case, take a look at your on-the-job image before you consider a career change.

Standards of Practice. For retooling your professional behavior, especially in the area of activities, join one of a few prominent organizations in the field of activities and recreation. The **National Association of Activity Professionals (NAAP)** is a Washington, D.C.-based organization that promotes a high degree of ethics and standards for their membership of activity professionals who work in a variety of settings. Included in its code of ethics for members, the NAAP (1989) lists the following expected standards of practice: "The Activity Professional shall demonstrate professionalism by the programs they design or the services they offer; . . . Ensure that credit is given to others for the use of their ideas, materials and programs. Participate in continuing education opportunities to strive for professional competence . . ."

Another organization is the **National Certification Council for Activity Professionals (NCCAP)** that determines certification credentials for activity professionals. The NCCAP (1990) mandates a code of ethics that addresses exemplary performance expectations, including:". . . To seek competency rather than fulfill minimum requirements. . . . To be a high quality provider of activities that enhances the lives of the residents . . . To function at the highest practical level of one's ability and skills to the benefit of the residents . . . ."

In the area of recreational therapy, The **American Therapeutic Recreation Association (ATRA)** is another national organization that sets strict standards of excellence for recreation therapists working in long-term care facilities and other settings. Among the goals for recreation therapy professionals, the ATRA (1991) states the following: ". . . to develop and promote professional standards for therapeutic recreation, to advocate for the advancement of recreational therapy services through education, habilitation, rehabilitation, and medical treatment of individuals in need of services, . . . to serve as a resource for practicing recreational therapy professionals." The **National Council for Therapeutic Recreation Certification (NCTRC)** provides the necessary certification process for verifying that therapeutic recreation standards have been met.

In the related area of leisure, the **National Therapeutic Recreation Society (NTRS)** (1993) is a branch of the National Recreation and Parks Association founded in 1967. Its vision statement suggests that ". . . leisure and recreation should be available to all people, especially those with disabilities or limiting conditions. . . ." The National Recreation and Parks Association National Certification Board monitors a certification process for leisure professionals within this organization.

Professionalizing Your Image. There are a number of things you can do to upgrade your image on the job that will help prepare you for an internal job change. The list of suggestions that follows is a common sense approach to improve your status at your facility:

1. Look the part! Dress neatly and professionally when not engaged in programs that require special attire.
2. Remind yourself that as an activity professional, you are an equal member of the health care team and that you have much to contribute. Do not perpetuate the image that an activity program or activity staff member is any less a part of the facility.
3. Master effective speaking skills. Opportunities abound for you to speak in front of residents, fellow department heads, staff, families, and other invited guests. It is natural to be fearful the first few times, but the fear diminishes with each opportunity to hone your skills.
4. Come prepared to meetings and other official functions. Amazingly, numerous people attend prescheduled meetings without writing materials, prepared questions, or opinions.
5. Accept and welcome more responsibility. Your sincere efforts to increase your departmental or facility duties will provide positive exposure for you to welcome new challenges and a

chance to show your administrator just how versatile you can be. Remember, adding responsibilities should be in areas where your abilities will be stretched, but you can still envision succeeding. Requesting additional duties is not necessarily related to salary upgrades or other monetary rewards. Enjoy the opportunity to try something new with little regard for any future acknowledgement.

6. Learn as much as you can about anything and everything in your facility. Your observations and knowledge will be invaluable in understanding the larger scope of facility operations and in recommending any positive changes you may envision to your administrator.

7. Develop strong personal and job-related ethics for your conduct, and serve as an example to your staff and co-workers. A high degree of personal integrity is essential for continued respect and trust from your peers.

8. Focus on building good interpersonal skills with other department heads, residents and their families, activity co-workers, and general staff. Use tact and diplomacy in your every-day dealings with others. From time to time it may be difficult, but the rewards will be worth the effort.

9. Share information and successes with others. Too often, we hear of individuals not sharing the specifics of a program because someone may copy it. When you are confident in yourself and your abilities, an opportunity to have another facility adopt aspects of one of your programs will be satisfying.

10. Assert yourself when necessary to have your ideas and opinions known. You never want to hear, "I had no idea you felt that way" after a decision has been made that may affect your programs. There are many ways to express your thoughts that are effective but nonthreatening.

11. Try for goals you truly believe in. Do not let the comments of others force you to give up on something you feel strongly about.

12. Seek new challenges or create your own. A self-motivated person finds ways to keep the job stimulating for the residents and himself or herself.

13. Accept defeat gracefully. You will have many chances to practice this, and your professional image will be shaped by your ability to move ahead after defeats or even failures.

Along with testing the image enhancement techniques above, your quest to advance should include an ongoing dialogue with key employment decision-makers such as your administrator or corporate consultant. Developing a **mentor** relationship with your administrator or other key staff member will certainly be helpful. A mentor is someone established in your field who takes an interest in you and guides or advises you. During your employee evaluation or in other meetings, alert your contact to your decision to seek advancement in the company or organization. Discuss the obstacles that may prevent you from moving up immediately, such as lack of proper experience, education, or funding. Work with your supervisor to set a plan to achieve your goals, including a specific time frame.

Increasing Your Education and Credentials

Adding to your knowledge base as an activity professional is necessary for personal growth, as well as for preparing for potential job changes. There are three areas that you can work on to improve your marketability: degreed programs, certification programs, and continuing education courses.

Degreed Programs. There are a host of two-year community colleges, four-year colleges and universities, as well as graduate schools that offer a wide range of academic courses in the field of recreation and activities. Depending on your career interests, you can choose from courses in one

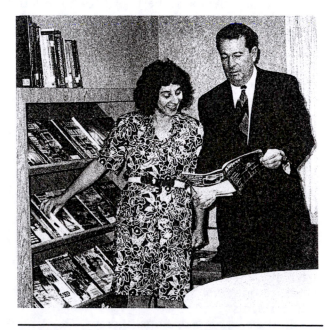

Figure 19–1 Developing a mentor relationship with your supervisor will be helpful as you advance your career.

particular area (i.e. working with the cognitively impaired) as a nonmatriculating student, or you may want to pursue a program that will lead you to a college degree in therapeutic recreation. There are also some correspondence schools that offer courses in activities and recreation by mail. Be sure to investigate thoroughly any program before enrolling to ensure that it meets your needs.

Certification Programs. Another road to recognition as an activity professional is through certification from either the NCCAP or the NCTRC.

In their certification information, NCCAP (1994) offers a procedure for activity certification based on academic achievements and experience in three professional categories: **Activity Assistant Certified (AAC)**, **Activity Director Certified (ADC)**, and **Activity Consultant Certified (ACC)**. An AAC is defined by NCCAP as ". . . one who meets NCCAP standards to assist in carrying out, with supervision, an activity program." An ADC is categorized by NCCAP as an individual " . . . who meets NCCAP standards to direct/coordinate/supervise an activity program, staff and department primarily in a geriatric setting." Within the different education and experience categories for the ADC, there exists a special classification called **Activity Director Provisional Certified** for individuals who are in the process of completing their ADC requirements. The final classification for the ACC is for a person who equaled the NCCAP requirements " . . . to be a consultant, trainer and instructor for an activity program, staff, department or coursework." Official documents verifying strict qualifications and experience are submitted by interested individuals to the Certification Review Committee along with an application fee. No formal testing is involved. The information is analyzed by the Review Committee based on the level of certification sought and a decision is rendered within a few months. If certification is granted, renewal is conducted every two years based on completion of the required continuing educational credits. This mode of qualification has started to gain acceptance with many Department of Health officials on the state level. The certification offers a recognized alternative to those individuals who may have entered the activity profession through nontraditional or nonacademic channels.

The National Council for Therapeutic Recreation Certification (1994) conducts the qualifica-tion and review process necessary to receive a **Certified Therapeutic Recreation Specialist (CTRS)** Professional certificate. A CTRS is defined as an individual who " . . . selects activity modalities. . . to treat or maintain the physical, mental and emotional well being of patients." There are two primary requirement categories in order to obtain this special certificate: educational and testing. The educational standards are detailed and require a minimum level of coursework directly in therapeutic recreation courses and other related classes. There is an examination given after the educational requirements have been met. Successful completion of both segments, along with proper fees paid, is necessary to receive the certificate of CTRS.

Those individuals trying to determine which type of certification is the most appropriate should consider that the CTRS is an academically focused credential because a major requirement is a degree in therapeutic recreation or the required therapeutic recreational coursework. Additionally, an internship or length of paid experience is required. The CTRS credential has applications in many recreational settings, including long-term care. Many CTRS workers come into the recreation profession first, then may discover long-term care as a career option later, as opposed to the AAC or ADC worker who often enjoys the long-term care setting first and may require further experience or additional training for credentialing. The AAC and the ADC certification is based on education and experience, but allows for a broader base of academic majors as long as key coursework requirements are met. No examination is required for these certification categories. Although experience may come from different areas, one of the reasons for developing the AAC, ADC, and ACC classifications was for activity and recreation professionals trained on the job or from other disciplines, to have a method to judge and recognize their professional merit in the activity profession. Those seeking the AAC or ADC certification are often from long-term care, residential, or rehabilitation settings.

Another avenue for certification is the **National Therapeutic Recreation Society (NTRS)**. It offers three levels of certification through the National Recreation and Parks Association National Certification Board. These certification categories, also applicable to professionals working in the activity field in long-term care, are **Certified Leisure Professional (CLP)**, Provisional Professional, and **Certified Leisure Associate (CLA)**.

Continuing Education Courses. A further method of enhancing credentials is through participation in continuing education courses. Colleges, professional development groups, and seminar leaders all offer classes that may be accredited as continuing education by monitoring organizations such as the NTCRC or NCCAP. Some professional organizations or individual seminar leaders may partner with two- or four-year colleges to offer certificate programs in areas such as therapeutic recreation or other specific activity fields. NCCAP, which recognizes a ninety-hour activity course as a minimum training requirement for new activity professionals, sees this course being offered around the country in many different ways. At times, the ninety-hour course is held by a seminar leader with continuing education credits available, or it may be part of a community college course where college credits can be obtained. Participating in continuing education programs offer a quick way to increase knowledge or determine a new area to further explore.

Advancing into Administration

One of the pathways of professional growth from a position as an activity professional would be into formal long-term care administration. Positions in administration include regional activity director, assistant administrator, and administrator. Consider a move in this direction carefully. These are demanding professions and will require all your interests and job skills, as well as an investment of time.

Your background as an activity professional allows you to face the challenges of nursing home administration or a regional activity director's position in a unique way. Coming up through the ranks and observing an administrator or assistant administrator in action is the best way to see the joys and pitfalls of the business. In activity programming, you have been interacting with your administrative team and have absorbed more about the daily operation of the facility than you realize. As a department head and member of the interdisciplinary care team, you have sharpened your management skills such as empathy, listening, sharing, and directing. You also have the advantage of knowing the residents; you have shared their joyful moments as well as their sadnesses.

Finding a mentor or sympathetic administrator to advise you would also be of great benefit. If you cannot count on your current administrator for guidance on this type of career matter, network with colleagues to find someone who can help. Visiting as many other facilities as you can during this time will serve you well; seeing how other facilities handle problems will add to your knowledge base.

The actual choice to upgrade your skills is more important than the job or career path you take. Continue to learn, and set a good example for your staff at the same time.

SUMMARY

Advancing in your career or on the job requires analysis, preparation, and planning. Objectively considering your goals and taking steps to increase your knowledge by enrolling in degreed programs or continuing educations classes can be accomplished through desire and discipline. Joining some of the key activity organizations also assists you in your quest to advance. Moves into administration or consulting are also a consideration. You are limited only by your own goals and dreams.

R E V I E W   Q U E S T I O N S

1. Name three professional organizations that may be helpful in the activity field.
2. What are three ways to improve your professional image as your prepare for a job change?

3. What do the letters ADC and CTRS stand for? What are the differences between the two?

O N   Y O U R   O W N

1. What areas have you identified in the recreation or activity field that you would like to pursue?

2. How can you achieve your long-term goals?
3. What are your reasons for wanting to advance into an administrative position?

R E F E R E N C E S

American Therapeutic Recreation Association (1991). *ATRA standards of practice task force.* [Brochure] . Hattiesburg, MD: author.

National Association of Activity Professionals (1989). *NAAP code of ethics.* [Brochure]. Washington, DC: author.

National Certification Council for Activity Professionals (1990). *NCCAP code of ethics.* [Brochure]. Park Ridge, IL: author.

National Certification Council for Activity Professionals (1994). *NCCAP certification application.* [Brochure]. Park Ridge, IL: author.

National Council for Therapeutic Recreation Certification (1994). *NCTRC certification information.* [Brochure]. Thiells, NY: author.

National Therapeutic Recreation Society (1993). *NTRS vision statement.* [Brochure]. Alexandria, VA: author.

F U R T H E R   R E A D I N G

American Therapeutic Recreation Association (1995). *ATRA college and university therapeutic recreation programs directory.* Hattiesburg, MS: author.

Compton, D. M. (1989). *Issues in therapeutic recreation: A profession in transition.* Champaign, IL: Sagamore.

National Association of Activity Professionals, Professional Development Committee (1994). *Correspondence courses: A guide to self-study programs available to the activity staff person.* Washington, DC: author.

CHAPTER 20

Self-Assessment Exam

To test your ability in the fundamentals of your position, use this self-assessment exam as a guide. The answers can be found in Appendix E. Good luck!

TRUE OR FALSE

1. The "wear and tear theory" of physical aging assumes that the human body wears out over time because of stress due to use. T F

2. Using visual cues and landmarks is an example of wayfinding. T F

3. Reminiscence is a process of recalling past memories that may involve family participation. T F

4. A standard OBRA survey is usually conducted in each facility every twelve to fifteen months. T F

5. The desire for spiritual fulfillment is one of the most prevalent needs among the elderly. T F

6. Members of the community benefit from in-service programming. T F

7. Speaking to your administrator is a good step in solving staffing problems. T F

8. Qualities of the ideal volunteer are warmth, empathy, and genuineness. T F

9. Resident information on therapeutic diets and restraint use is not necessary for activity planning. T F

10. Petty cash and check requests are two systems used to help manage the activity supply budget. T F

11. A quality improvement program does not have to involve the entire facility. T F

12. Group dynamics is a process in which a group of individuals takes on a unique identity in working through issues. T F

13. An acute disease may last over six months before recovery. T F

14. The work of Florence Nightingale is important because she set up the first nursing home. T F

15. Validation therapy should be administered by a highly trained therapist. T F

16. UTI is a medical abbreviation for urinary tract infection. T F

17. Practitioner behavior or standards are set in each facility, instead of by a professional organization. T F

18. Tuberculosis is no longer a threat in health care facilities. T F

19. Building an internal community is as important as keeping residents in touch with the external community. T F

20. Holding a single session grief group is one way to help residents adjust to the death of others. T F

21. Affective needs are those that involve the stimulation of the mind. T F

22. A CCRC is defined as a Continuing Care Retirement Community. T F

23. Activity analysis is a process in which specific programs are reviewed and judged for effectiveness of specific needs. T F

24. An OSCAR report contains a list of the regulations on which a facility is surveyed. T F

25. An in-service/educational calendar for the activity department should be set up annually. T F

26. A community resource file is a list of all the volunteers in your local community. T F

27. One of the three parts of the recreation service delivery model is recreation evaluation. T F

28. Stress is a normal part of life. T F

29. The use of the Resident Assessment Protocols (RAPs) is the first step in the assessment process. T F

30. A longitudinal study provides the most valuable research information on the aging process. T F

31. One of the differences between quality assurance and total quality management is that prevention instead of inspection is part of TQM. T F

32. A mentor is a person who guides you and offers advice on your job or career.　　　　T　F
33. The cellular genetic theory of aging suggests that dangerous toxins have accumulated in the body over time.　　T　F
34. A revenue budget is made up of operating expenses and capital expenses.　　　　T　F
35. An orientation checklist is another name for your job description.　　T　F
36. Volunteers who participate in facility training are shown to have increased levels of satisfaction.　　T　F

37. If a resident qualified, Medicare Part B could be used to pay room and board at a long-term care facility.　　　　T　F
38. Consultants are usually on the facility payroll and conduct programs for you.　　T　F
39. Alzheimer's disease and multi-infarct dementia are examples of reversible dementia.　　T　F
40. Activity pursuit patterns are a key area of responsibility for activity professionals in documentation on the MDS.　　T　F

F I L L   I N   T H E   B L A N K

1. Doing right things right and making continuous improvements is one definition of _____.
2. The _____ system contains the hair, nails, and skin.
3. _____ _____ is a term used to describe middle-aged individuals balancing the responsibility of their lives and those of an aging parent.
4. A classification of activities, called _____ activities, are those which provide opportunities for self-expression and choice.
5. A process in which reminiscence and memory are used to reflect on aspects of one's life is called _____ _____.
6. Program planning should incorporate the ethnicity or _____ _____ of a resident.
7. A quality tool that weighs the benefits of something against its cost is called _____ _____.
8. An institution that operates to make a financial profit is called a _____ facility.
9. A person who studies the aging process is called a _____.
10. The number of staff members or departmental hours approved in each pay period by administration are called a _____ _____.
11. _____ is a stress-related term that refers to exhaustion, lack of energy, and lack of commitment.
12. The four areas of the OBRA survey process are: review of resident rights/quality of life, environmental quality assessment, dietary services system assessment, and _____ _____ _____ _____.
13. _____ _____ _____ is a method of monitoring volunteer time in the facility.

14. The act of an employee leaving a position involuntarily is called _____.
15. Special programs between generations that offer unique benefits are called _____ programs.
16. An interdisciplinary form that outlines key responsibilities for an event or meeting is called a _____ _____ _____.
17. Resident responses that are recorded for particular MDS items and require follow-up are called _____.
18. The _____ theory proposes that large amounts of social involvement in valued roles can produce increased self-satisfaction and esteem.
19. ACC written after a person's name stands for _____ _____ _____.
20. A budget that includes items which depreciate over time is referred to as a _____ _____.
21. An expected practice of all interdisciplinary team members, _____, is the discreet use of resident and other information to provide care but maintain privacy.
22. A 1987 act that created nursing home reform through a revised survey process is called the _____ _____ _____ _____ _____.
23. One of the most commonly seen medical conditions that has serious programming implications is called _____.
24. _____ _____ is the name for the first sheet of the medical record that contains vital resident data.
25. Agnosia and aphasia are conditions related to the _____ system.
26. _____ is the first step in the program planning and documentation process.

27. During the management act of _____, a supervisor gives tasks to an employee and follows up on their completion.
28. A form of therapy that uses expressive movement is called _____ _____.
29. Provided by product manufacturers, _____ _____ _____ _____, give product, safety, and emergency procedures information for worker safety.
30. Record retention requirements for the RAI state that information must be kept on the medical chart or accessible by computer for at least the last _____ months.
31. _____ is the written recording by interdisciplinary team members of assessments, evaluations, orders, or updates on the medical record.
32. Formal and informal _____ can be used to honor and thank volunteers for their contributions of time.
33. _____ is a term used to describe the stereotyping of older people.

34. A unified or _____ system of organizing the delivery of your activity programs uses a main area for most events.
35. A written marketing technique that packages the who-what-where-when-how is called a _____ _____.
36. Using the five senses as a means of activating emotions is called_____ _____.
37. A _____ _____ _____ manual provides written documentation for every function in your department, and is usually kept in the activity office for easy reference.
38. A state agency established to handle complaint and abuse reporting for the elderly is called the _____ office.
39. The inability to control bladder or bowel function is called _____.
40. Data collection is done through the use of a standardized form called the _____.

M U L T I P L E C H O I C E

Circle the correct letter

1. The Medical-Clinical Model of service delivery
   a) focuses on the whole person
   b) looks at the treatment of specific disease
   c) is geared for the mentally ill
   d) has categories of treatment, leisure education, and recreation participation
2. Which theory of social aging suggests that as age increases and social roles decline, individuals may withdraw from society to prepare for their own death?
   a) activity theory
   b) stress theory
   c) disengagement theory
   d) free radical theory
   e) continuity theory
3. The Americans With Disabilities Act has mandated compliance in the areas of
   a) the employment application process
   b) nondiscrimination toward the disabled
   c) environmental modifications
   d) all of the above
4. Program adaptations for working with cognitively impaired residents includes
   a) presenting increasingly more difficult tasks
   b) focusing on maintaining existing skills
   c) creating a busy environment
   d) centering on developing new skills

5. A CTRS receives certification from the
   a) NAAP
   b) ATRA
   c) NCCAP
   d) NCTRC
6. The following is not associated with good management skills
   a) accomplishing tasks through the work of others
   b) recruitment and supervising
   c) aggression and conflicts
   d) hiring and terminations
7. The budget process for the activity department involves these steps
   a) cost depreciation and accounting
   b) revenue calculations and projections
   c) planning, implementing, and documenting expenditures
   d) using provider agreements as a guide to spending
   e) none of the above
8. Effective recruiting of volunteers can be accomplished by
   a) incentive programs to current volunteers
   b) directing residents to help
   c) letters to civic organizations
   d) waiting for drop-ins
   e) a and c only
   f) all of the above

9. The following charting forms relate to the activity department
   a) photo release
   b) trip release
   c) medication orders
   d) physician orders
   e) all of the above
   f) none of the above

10. Quality that is active rather than re-active describes
    a) benchmarking
    b) critical pathways
    c) total quality management
    d) quality assurance

11. Behavior modification is
    a) a method for changing behavior
    b) a technique that uses positive and negative reinforcement
    c) a method that works on targeted behaviors
    d) all of the above

12. What is the difference between a regulation and a standard?
    a) standards have monetary penalties; regulations do not
    b) positive outcomes are looked at in regulations; negative outcomes in standards
    c) a standard is a guideline used by accreditation groups; regulations are used as a measure in state and federal agencies
    d) regulations have a plan of correction process; standards have remedies

13. The definition of activities of daily living (ADLs) is
    a) The sum total of all activity programs that a resident attends each day
    b) Skills required to perform bathing, dressing, toileting, and feeding
    c) The percentage of time that a resident is not at rest during the day
    d) The criteria used by physicians to test cognitive skills

14. Replacing an employee can be
    a) done through recruiting and interviewing
    b) a normal part of management
    c) a difficult task to face
    d) accomplished quickly to ensure program continuity
    e) all of the above

15. Establishing a climate of acceptance in a group by welcoming and thanking members is a part of
    a) remotivation
    b) reminiscence
    c) sensory stimulation
    d) reality orientation

16. Which of the following is not a way to deal with difficult people?
    a) accept that they are a reality
    b) try to change them
    c) realize that you are not the target
    d) acknowledge that you do not have to like them

17. Researchers have identified the requested training needs for activity professionals as
    a) residents with specific medical needs and the problems of aging
    b) what survey teams are looking for this year
    c) interrelations between facility departments
    d) infection control, handwashing, and advanced directives

18. Which statement is not a stereotype or myth about aging?
    a) chronological age determines the true age of an individual
    b) the majority of older people suffer from dementia
    c) hopelessness is a major part of aging
    d) nonproductiveness and inflexibility occur routinely with aging
    e) all of the above
    f) none of the above

19. The goals of a resident council may include all but one of the following
    a) provide a formal link to administration for residents
    b) give a forum to all resident issues
    c) provide an opportunity for learning about resident interests and using them in activities
    d) provide a chance for department heads to run a meeting for residents

20. Researchers have found that some of the benefits of intergenerational programs for the elderly include
    a) reducing stereotypes
    b) maintenance of skills and activities
    c) increasing scores on cognitive tests
    d) establishing a community link
    e) none of the above
    f) all of the above

21. Leisure may be defined as
    a) unobligated, free time
    b) time when no work or other necessary functions are being performed
    c) a period of time when recreation or activities may be planned
    d) all of the above

22. Environmental modifications can help residents in many ways. Which is an example of a successful environmental modification?
    a) high-tech designs
    b) minimize contrasts between floors and walls
    c) acoustic tiles to absorb sound
    d) long corridors

23. Denial, anger, bargaining, depression, and acceptance are stages of
    a) Maslow's hierarchy of needs
    b) Erikson's stages of development
    c) Kubler-Ross' model of grieving
    d) Gunn & Peterson's therapeutic recreation service model

24. Which of the following is not associated with activity service delivery?
    a) wellness model and therapeutic milieu model
    b) the manner in which activity services can be brought to residents
    c) experiential bonds and continuum model
    d) therapeutic recreation service model

25. When designing appropriate bedside programs, all the following factors should be considered except
    a) group dynamics
    b) resident comfort
    c) timing and supplies
    d) space or area for program

26. An advance directive can be interpreted as
    a) a health care proxy only
    b) living will or durable power of attorney
    c) power of attorney
    d) none of the above

27. Which of the following are benefits of horticultural therapy?
    a) a link to past skills
    b) caretaking of a living thing
    c) exposure to beauty
    d) observation of growth
    e) none of the above
    f) all of the above

28. Which of the following is not a goal of the hospice process?
    a) pain management
    b) maintenance of a resident's lifestyle
    c) comfort and listening
    d) isolation
    e) none of the above
    f) all of the above

29. Formalizing a resident volunteer program can make residents feel comfortable. Which of the following is not an example of a typical facility volunteer job?
    a) mail delivery
    b) leading a children's swim meet
    c) typing a newsletter
    d) making reassurance telephone calls
    e) all of the above

30. A chronic illness would not be represented by which of the following
    a) influenza
    b) diabetes
    c) asthma
    d) heart condition

31. Some of the quality tools to use in the TQM process include
    a) fishbone and brainstorming
    b) analysis and execution
    c) action plans and flowcharts
    d) performance objectives and monitoring
    e) b and d
    f) a and c
    g) none of the above

32. Section N of the MDS 2.0 Full Assessment Form contains all but which item
    a) space for signature, title, and date
    b) general activity preferences
    c) time awake
    d) average time involved in activities
    e) none of the above

33. A plan of correction may need to be prepared for a
    a) deficiency
    b) tag number
    c) regulation
    d) interpretive guideline

34. Institutional long-term care represents which services on the continuum of care, and at what level?
    a) rehab services and subacute at the high end of the continuum
    b) CCRC or personal care home at the midrange of the continuum
    c) in own home at the low end of the scale
    d) home-based services and senior housing at mid to high end of the scale

35. Which of the following are not identified as problem behaviors?
    a) wandering and pacing
    b) hostility and anger
    c) mobility and ambulation
    d) noise-making and rummaging

36. Two negative situations for residents that are a possible result of being in a non-nurturing institutional environment are
    a) mentoring and termination
    b) infantilization and learned helplessness
    c) burnout and tinnitus
    d) sundowning and suspicion

37. The following diseases, COPD, pneumonia, and emphysema, are reflective of which body system?
    a) musculoskeletal
    b) respiratory
    c) integumentary
    d) nervous
    e) none of the above

38. The digestive system is characterized by disease or conditions such as
    a) myocardial infarction
    b) diverticulosis
    c) multiple sclerosis
    d) dementia
    e) none of the above

39. Care planning
    a) follows the RAP process
    b) uses goals and approaches
    c) may involve improvement or prevention interventions
    d) uses time frames and measurable objectives
    e) all of the above
    f) none of the above

40. Hormone production in glands is the function of which body system
    a) reproductive
    b) nervous
    c) circulatory
    d) endocrine
    e) none of the above

41. Which of the following are useful methods of stretching your activity department budget?
    a) use of family members as volunteers
    b) fund raising
    c) bartering and garage sales
    d) contests and raffles
    e) all of the above

42. The musculoskeletal system is composed of
    a) bones, cartilage, and tendons
    b) nerves, ligaments, and bones
    c) joints, tendons, and skin
    d) tendons, glands, and muscle

43. Which of the following is not a characteristic of a psychotropic drug?
    a) may be over-the-counter
    b) used in psychiatric treatment
    c) could be considered a chemical restraint
    d) anti-anxiety and antidepressant drugs

44. Residents rights were written to
    a) inform staff and protect residents
    b) add length to regulations and the survey process
    c) uphold dignity, self-determination, and choice factors for residents

d) extend duties of ombudsman's office
e) a and c only
f) b and d only

45. Psychosocial aging changes may be characterized by
    a) decrease in response time
    b) personality and self-esteem issues
    c) cultural attitudes
    d) stress
    e) none of the above
    f) all of the above

46. Breaking a program down into component parts to determine the skills required to accomplish it is called
    a) activities of daily living
    b) force-field analysis
    c) activity theory
    d) activity analysis

47. Files of important information should be housed in the activity office. Which of the following should not be kept in the office?
    a) Material Safety Data Sheets
    b) completed Minimum Data Sets
    c) entertainer information
    d) inservice education records

48. Which of the following is not associated with total quality management?
    a) customer focus
    b) performance objectives
    c) continuous improvement
    d) support of management

49. Defense mechanisms used to handle stress are
    a) projection and denial
    b) mutation and withdrawal
    c) replacement and rationalizing
    d) selection and projection
    e) none of the above
    f) all of the above

50. The RAI involves all except
    a) episodic notes
    b) assessment and data collection
    c) RAPs and triggers
    d) Basic Assessment Tracking

A P P E N D I X   A
Activity Professional Staffing Requirements

NATIONAL

Alabama
Activities 420-5-10-.14

(3) Activities Coordinator

(a) There shall be a patient activities coordinator, who shall direct and supervise the recreation program in the facility. The program coordinator, if not qualified, must function under the supervision of a consultant who shall provide a minimum of five hours of consultation., if less than 75 beds, and eight hours of consultation; if 75 or more, each month until the coordinator is qualified.

Source: Rules of Alabama State Board of Health
Division of Licensure and Certification
Chapter 420-5-10
Effective Date: December 26, 1988

Alaska
7ACC 12.285 Activity Program

N039 The Activity program coordinator shall consult as necessary with an occupational or recreation therapist, unless the activity program coordinator meets the requirements of CFR 483.5 (1) (2) revised as of October 1, 1991

Source: State of Alaska
Department of Health and Social Services
Division of Medical Assistance
Health Facilities Licensing & Certification

Arizona
Health Care Institutions, Chapter 4

§ 36-447.11. Patient activities; requirements.

B. Each nursing care institution shall designate an activities coordinator to implement the program established pursuant to subsection A. The activities coordinator may serve in other employment capacities at the nursing care institution. Added by laws 1981, Ch. 320, § 3.

3. A registered recreational therapist, occupational therapist or other activity related therapist is on staff or on contract.

Source: Arizona Administrative Code Title 9, Ch. 10.
Department of Health Services—Health Care Institutions: Licensure

Arkansas
Defers to federal regulations.
Has 36 hour training course.
Source: Arkansas Health Care Association

California
72385 Activity Program-Staff

(a) Activity program personnel with appropriate training and experience shall be available to meet the needs and interests of patients.

(b) An activity program leader shall be designated by and be responsible to the administration. An activity program leader shall meet one of the following requirements:

(1) Have two years of experience in a social or recreational program within the past five years, one year of which was full-time in a patient activities program in a health care setting.

(2) Be an occupational therapist, art therapist, music therapist, dance therapist, recreation therapist, or occupational therapy assistant.

(3) Have satisfactorily completed at least 36 hours of training in a course designed specifically for this position and approved by the Department and shall receive regular consultation from an occupational therapist, occupational therapy assistant, or recreational therapist who has at least one year of experience in a health care setting.

Source: Sections 208(a) and 1275, Health and Safety Code. Reference: Section 1276, Health and Safety Code

Colorado
9.2 Staffing.

The facility shall employ activities staff sufficient in number to meet resident needs and qualified as either:

(1) an activity professional certified by the National Certification Council for Activity Professionals as an Activity Director Certified or Activity Consultant Certified;

(2) an occupational therapist or occupational therapy assistant meeting the requirements for certification by the American Occupational Therapy Association and having at least one year of experience in providing activity programming in a long term care facility;

(3) a therapeutic recreation specialist (registered by the National Therapeutic Recreation Society) having at least one year of experience in providing activity programming in a long term care facility;

(4) a person with a Master's or Bachelor's degree in the social or behavioral sciences who has at least one year of experience in providing activity programming in a long term care facility;

(5) a person who has completed, within a year of employment, a training course for activity professionals in an accredited state institution (if available) and who has at least two years of experience in social or recreational program work, at least one year of which was full-time in an activities program in a health care setting; or

(6) a person with monthly consultation from a person meeting the qualifications set forth in subsections (1) through (5). The consultation shall be sufficient in amount to assist the activity staff members to meet resident needs.

Source: Colorado Department of Health

Connecticut

(2) Each facility shall employ therapeutic recreation director(s).

(A) Persons employed as therapeutic recreation director(s) in a chronic and convalescent nursing home and rest home with nursing supervision on or before June 30, 1982 shall have a minimum of a high school diploma or high school equivalency, and shall have completed a minimum of 80 hours of training in therapeutic recreation. As of July 1, 1992, persons who met these criteria but who have not been employed as therapeutic recreation director(s) in a chronic and convalescent nursing home and/or rest home with nursing supervision for two continuous years immediately preceding reemployment in such capacity shall be required to meet the requirements of Section 19-13-D8t (r) (2) (c).

(B) Persons beginning employment as therapeutic recreation director(s) in a chronic and convalescent nursing home and/or rest home with nursing supervision between July 1, 1982 and June 30, 1992 shall have the following minimum qualifications:

(i) An Associates Degree with a major emphasis in therapeutic recreation; or

(ii) Enrollment in a Connecticut certificate program in therapeutic recreation; or

(iii) A Bachelors Degree in a related field and one year of full time employment in therapeutic recreation in a health care facility; or

(iv) A Bachelors Degree in a related field and six credit hours in therapeutic recreation; or

(v) An Associates Degree in a related field and two years of full time employment in therapeutic recreation in a health care facility; or

(vi) An Associates Degree in a related field and nine credit hours in therapeutic recreation.

(vii) As of July 1, 1992, persons who met these criteria but who have not been employed as a therapeutic recreation director in a health care facility for two continuous years immediately preceding reemployment in such capacity shall be required to meet the requirements of Section 19-13-D8t (r) (2) (C).

(C) Persons beginning employment as therapeutic recreation director(s) in a chronic and convalescent nursing home and/or rest home with nursing supervision on or after July 1, 1992 shall have the following minimum qualifications:

(i) An Associates Degree with a major emphasis in therapeutic recreation; or

(ii) A high school diploma or equivalency and enrollment within six months of employment in a Connecticut certificate program in therapeutic recreation. Each facility shall maintain records of the individual's successful completion of courses and continued participation in a minimum of one course per semester; or

(iii) A Bachelors Degree in a related field and one year of full time employment in therapeutic recreation in a health care facility; or

(iv) A Bachelors Degree in a related field and six credit hours in therapeutic recreation; or

(v) An Associates Degree in a related field and two years of full time employment in therapeutic recreation in a health care facility; or

(vi) An Associates Degree in a related field and nine credit hours in therapeutic recreation.

(D) "Related field" in subparagraphs (B) and (C) of this subdivision shall include but not be limited to the following: sociology, social work, psychology, recreation, art, music, dance or drama therapy, the health sciences, education, or other related field as approved by the commissioner or his/her designee.

(3) Therapeutic recreation directors(s) shall be employed in each facility sufficient to meet the following ratio of hours per week to the number of licensed beds in the facility:
1 to 15 beds, 10 hours during any three days;
16 to 30 beds, 20 hours during any five days;
Each additional 30 beds or fraction thereof, 20 additional hours.

Source: Section 19-13-D8t of the Regulations of Connecticut State Agencies

Delaware

Defers to federal regulations.

Source: Nursing Home Regulations for Skilled Care, Delaware State Board of Health

District of Columbia

Defers to federal regulations.

Source: District of Columbia Health Care Association

Florida

Defers to federal regulations.

Has superior rating system with incentives for activity credentials.

Georgia

290-5-8-.16 Recreation

(1) An individual shall be designated as being in charge of patient activities. This individual shall have experience and/or training in group activities, or shall have consultation made available from a qualified recreational therapist or group activity leader.

Source: Authority Ga. L. 1964, pp. 507, 612, as amended by Ga. L. 1969, p. 715 et seq; and Ga. L. 1972, p. 1015 et seq. Administrative History. Original Rule was filed on October 26, 1976; effective November 15, 1976

Hawaii

11-94-4 Activities program.

(c) A staff member, qualified by experience or training in directing group activities or recreation, shall be responsible primarily for the activities program.

(d) There shall be sufficient, appropriately qualified activities or recreation staff and necessary supporting staff to carry out the various activities in accordance with stated goals and objectives.

Source: (Auth: HRS §§321-9, 321-11) (Imp: HRS §§321-9, 321-11) (Eff. May 3, 1985)

Idaho

03.02151, Activities Program

03. Coordinator. The facility shall designate an Activities Program Coordinator who shall: (1-1-88)

a. Coordinate and supervise the program. (1-1-88)

Source: IDAPA 16.03.02150,02.d

Indiana

410 IAC 16.2-3-9 Activities program

(2) An activities director shall be designated and must be one of the following:

(A) A recreation therapist.

(B) An occupational therapist or a certified occupational assistant.

(C) An individual who has satisfactorily completed or will complete within six (6) months an activities director's course approved by the council.

Source: Authority: IC 16-10-4-5; IC 16-10-4-6
Affected: IC 16-10-4

Illinois

Subpart G: Resident Care Services

Section 300.1410 Activity Program

(c) Activity Director and Consultation

(1) There shall be a trained staff person responsible for planning and directing the activities program. This person shall be regularly scheduled to be on duty in the facility at least four days per week.

(2) If this person is not a Registered Occupational Therapist, a Therapeutic Recreation Specialist, or a Certified Social Worker with specialized coursework in social group work, the facility shall have a written agreement with a person from one of those disciplines to provide consultation to the Activity Director at least monthly, in order to make sure that the activity programming meets the needs of the residents in the facility.

(3) Any person designated as Activity Director who is responsible for planning and directing the activities program hired after December 24, 1987, shall have a high school diploma or equivalent.

(4) The activity director shall have a minimum of ten hours of continuing education per year pertaining to activities programming.

(5) Consultation will be required only every six months when the activity director meets or exceeds the criteria in Appendix E: Criteria for Activity Directors Who Need Only Minimal Consultation. (See Section 300.830 for consultant services when required.)

Source: Illinois Administrative Code, Title 77, Ch. 1, Sec. 300.140. Amended at 13 Ill. Reg. 4684, effective March 24, 1989

Section 300. Appendix E: Criteria For Activity Directors Who Need Only Minimal Consultation.

1. High school diploma or equivalent, 6 years total experience in Activities, 3 years experience as Activity Director. Basic training: completion of a basic orientation course of at least 36 hrs.

2. 2 year associate degree, 4 years total experience in Activities, 3 years experience as Activity Director. Basic training: completion of a basic orientation course of at least 36 hrs.

3. Therapeutic Recreation Assistant or Certified Occupational Therapy Assistant, 2 years total experience in Activities, 2 years experience as Activity Director. Basic training: completion of a basic orientation course of at least 36 hrs.

4. 4 year degree, 2 years total experience in Activities, 2 years experience as Activity Director. Basic training: completion of a basic orientation course of least 36 hrs.

The basic orientation course for activity shall include material related to life span changes; resident rights; etiology and symptomatology of aged, developmentally disabled, and mentally ill residents; therapeutic approaches; communication; philosophy and design of activity programs; activity program resources; standards and regulations; documentation; and management and administration.

Source: Illinois Administrative Code, Title 77, Ch. I, Sec. 300.TABLE B, Added at 12 Ill. Reg. 1052, effective December 24, 1987

Iowa

481-58.26(135C) Resident activities program.
58.26(2) Co-ordination of activities program.

(a) Each intermediate care facility shall employ a person to direct the activities program. (III)

(b) Staffing for the activity program shall be provided on the minimum basis of thirty-five minutes per licensed bed per week. (II, III).

(c) The activity co-ordinator shall have completed the activity co-ordinators' orientation course offered through the department within six months of employment or have comparable training and experience as approved by the department. (III)

(d) The activity co-ordinator shall attend workshops or educational programs which relate to activity programming. These shall total a minimum of ten contact hours per year. These programs shall be approved by the department. (III)

(e) There shall be a written plan for personnel coverage when the activity co-ordinator is absent during scheduled working hours.

Source: Iowa, Administrative Code 7/15/87

Kansas

28-39-144 Definitions.

(a) "Activities Director" means an individual who meets one of the following requirements:

(1) Has completed the requirements for certification as a therapeutic recreation specialist by the national therapeutic recreation society, as in effect May 1, 1991;

(2) has two years of experience in a social or recreational program within the last five years, one of which was full-time in a patient activities program in a health care setting;

(3) is registered in Kansas as an occupational therapist or occupational therapy assistant;

(4) has a bachelor's degree in a therapeutic activity field in art therapy, horticultural therapy, music therapy, special education or a related therapeutic activity field; or

(5) is a nurse aide who has completed a course approved by the Kansas department of health and environment in resident activities coordination and who receives consultation from a therapeutic recreation specialist, an occupational therapist or an occupational therapy assistant.

Source: Kansas Nursing Home Regulation 29-39-144

Kentucky

902 KAR 20:300. Operation and services; nursing facilities.
Section 6. Quality of Life.

(5) Activities.

(b) The activities program shall be directed by a qualified therapeutic recreation specialist who is:

(1) Eligible for certification as a therapeutic recreation specialist by a recognized accrediting body; or

(2) Has two (2) years of experience in a social or recreational program within the last five (5) years, one (1) of which was full time in a patient activities program in a health care setting; or

(3) Is a qualified occupational therapist or occupational therapy assistant; or

(4) Has completed a training course approved by the state.

Source: Kentucky Administrative Regulations, Title 902, Chapter 20, Health Services and Facilities, effective 5/3/91

Louisiana

J. Activities Coordinator

(1) The facility shall designate a staff member as Activities Coordinator, also known as Patient Activities Coordinator (PAC). The Activities Coordinator shall be responsible for providing a full, varied, independent, and group activities program in accordance with the physician's or-

ders and appropriate to the diversified needs and interests of each applicant/recipient.

(2) An Activities Coordinator may be one of the following individuals:

(a) A qualified therapeutic recreation specialist; or

(b) A person have the following experience:

(i) Two (2) years of experience in a social or recreational program within the last five (5) years; and

(ii) One (1) year of the experience shall have been gained as a full-time employee in a health care setting involving patient activity programs. or

(c) A qualified occupational therapist or occupational therapy assistant; or

(d) An individual who has completed the State approved Patient Activities Coordinator (PAC) Training Course; or

(e) A staff member otherwise trained or experienced in leading group activities.

(3) The time factor required in meeting the activity needs will vary according to the number participating. The following criteria shall be adhered to in meeting these needs:

(a) Facilities with eighty (80) beds or less shall have a part-time Activities Coordinator. Part-time is defined as a minimum of twenty (20) hours per week.

(b) Facilities with eighty-one (81) beds or more shall have a full-time Activities Coordinator. Full-time is defined as a minimum of forty (40) hours per week.

(c) The Activities Coordinator's hours shall not be limited only to the daytime hours. Many programs are better for participation if scheduled in the early evening hours.

Source: Louisiana Dept. of Health 10/1/85

Maine

15. A. 1. Activities Coordinator

The Activities Coordinator shall be qualified by training or experience as evidenced by:

a. Having completed, or is currently enrolled in, a training course approved by the Department of Education and Cultural Services; or having completed an approved course prior to the effective date of these regulations.

b. Is a registered occupational therapist or an occupational therapy assistant; or

c. Is a qualified therapeutic recreation specialist.

Source: Regulations governing the licensing and functioning of skilled nursing facilities and nursing facilities, Chapter 15

Maryland

.19 Patient Activities

B. Staffing. A staff member qualified by experience or training shall be appointed to be responsible for the activities program. If the designee is not a qualified patient activities coordinator as defined in Regulation .01Y, the Department may approve the designee based on the person's education, performance, and experience.

(31) "Patient activities coordinator" means a person who:

(a) Is a qualified therapeutic recreation specialist;

(b) Is a qualified occupational therapist;

(c) Is an occupational therapy assistant; or

(d) Has 2 years of experience in a social or recreational program in a licensed health care setting within the last 5 years, 1 year of which was full time in a patient activities program with guidance from a qualified consultant in a health care setting.

Source: Department of Health and Mental Hygiene Code of Maryland Regulations 10.07.02 Comprehensive Care Facilities and Extended Care Facilities, November 1994

Massachusetts

150.012 Activities and Recreation

(B) All facilities shall provide an activity director who is responsible for developing and implementing the activity program.

(1) The activity director shall possess a high school diploma or its equivalent; have the interest and ability to work with the ill, aged, and disabled; and have at least one year's experience or training in directing group activity.

(2) In total, all facilities shall provide at least 20 hours of activity per week, per unit.

(3) In a SNCFC activity programs shall be developed by the supervisor of therapeutic recreation services.

(4) The activity director of CSF shall in addition to possessing a high school diploma; have an ability to work with the elderly; have at least one year of experience or training in directing group activities; and possess documented experience and training in the planning and providing of special activities and programs for the elderly mentally ill which are geared toward enhancing resocialization and community integration of residents.

Source: 105 CMR: Department of Public Health 7/1/87

Michigan

R 325.20712 Diversional activities.

Rule 712.(2) There shall be a qualified staff member and such additional staff as necessary to plan, conduct and evaluate individual and group activities. Individual and group activities shall be available 7 days a week.

Source: State of Michigan Nursing Home Rules

Minnesota

4658.0900 Activity and Recreation Program.

Subpart 3. Activity and recreation program director. The activity and recreation program director must be a person who is trained or experienced to direct the activity and recreation staff and program at that nursing home.

Subpart 4. Staff assistance with activities. Sufficient staff must be assigned to assist with the implementation of the activity and recreation program, as determined by the needs of the residents and the nursing home.

Source: Minnesota Department of Health
Nursing; Boarding Homes: Operation
Effective date: June 1996

Mississippi

Section B—Patient Activities

702.1

Activity Coordinator. An individual shall be designated as being in charge of patient activities. This individual shall have experience and/or training in group activities, or shall have consultation made available from a qualified recreational therapist or group activity leader.

Source: Minimum Standards of Operations for Institutions for the Aged or Infirm, Mississippi State Dept. of Health, Division of Licensure and Certification

Missouri

Defer to federal regulations.
Source: Dept. of Social Services, Division 15, Page 198.

Montana

Defer to federal regulations.
Source: Montana Health Care Association

Nebraska

014 Resident Activities

014.02 Staffing and Qualifications

014.02A The nursing home administrator must designate a qualified resident activities director, a person who meets one of the following qualifications:

014.02A1 A qualified therapeutic recreation specialist with one year of experience in a long term care facility or geriatric setting; or

014.02A2 A licensed occupational therapist with one year of experience in a long term care facility or geriatric setting; or

014.02A3 A qualified therapeutic recreation assistant with one year of experience in a long term care facility or geriatric setting; or

014.02A4 A licensed occupational therapy assistant with one year of experience in a long term care facility or geriatric setting; or

014.02A5 An individual who has a Bachelor of Arts (B.A.) or Bachelor of Science (B.S.) degree in social or behavioral sciences with one year of experience in the provision of recreational services in a long term care facility or geriatric setting; or

014.02A6 An individual who has successfully completed a course of instruction in recreational services of at least 36 hours established by the Nebraska Health Health Care Association or the Nebraska Association of Homes for the Aged, or a substantially equivalent course established by any other health care association or entity; or

014.02A7 Has two years full-time experience in a resident activities program in a health care setting.

014.02B If the designated person is not fully qualified as an activities director as previously defined, the facility must have a written agreement with a qualified consultant for consultation and assistance on a regularly scheduled basis, reflecting the needs of the residents.

　　The qualified consultant must meet the eligibility requirements for activities director and have a minimum of one year experience in long term care facility or geriatric setting.

Source: Title 175 Chapter 12
Regulations and Standards for Skilled Nursing Facilities
Effective: June 27, 1987

Nevada

Defers to federal regulations.
Source: Chapter 449, Nevada Administrative Code (NAC), October 25, 1982

New Hampshire

He-P 803.03 Personnel and Staffing

(p) The recreational activities program shall be directed by a professional who shall be a therapeutic recreation specialist either:

(1) Licensed or registered, if applicable, by the State of New Hampshire and eligible for certification as a therapeutic recreation specialist by a nationally recognized accrediting body on August 1, 1989; or

(2) Has 2 years of experience in a social or recreational program within the last 5 years, 1 of which was full-time in a patient activities program in a health care setting; or

(3) Is an occupational therapist or occupational therapy assistant; or

(4) Has completed a training course approved by a state agency.

Source: Rules for Nursing Homes, Effective July 13, 1993

New Jersey

Subchapter 7. Mandatory Resident Activities

8:39-7.2 Mandatory staff qualifications for resident activities

(a) The facility shall have a director of resident activities who holds at least one of the following *[three]* **four* qualifications:

1. A baccalaureate degree from an accredited college or university with a major area of concentration in recreation, creative arts therapy, therapeutic recreation, art, art education, psychology, sociology, or occupational therapy; or

2. A high school diploma and three years of experience in resident activities in a health care facility and satisfactorily completion of an activities education program approved by the New Jersey State Department of Health after a review of the specific curriculum, consisting of 90 hours of training, and incorporating the following elements:

i. Overview of the activity profession;

ii. Human development: the late adult years;

iii. Standards of practice: practitioner behavior;

iv. Activity care planning for quality of life; and

v. Methods of service delivery in the activity profession; or

3. Served as director of resident activities on June 20, 1988, and has continuously served as activities director since that time.

4. Holds current certification from the National Certification Council for Activity Professionals (National Certification Council for Activity Professionals, 520 Stewart, Park Ridge, Illinois, 60068) or the National Council for Therapeutic Recreation Certification (National Council for Therapeutic Recreation Certification, Inc., P.O. Box 479, Thiells, NY 10984-0479).

(b) Currently employed activities directors who have completed an activities education course which was previously approved by the Department will not be required to complete the course described at (a)2 above.

8:39-7.3 Mandatory staffing amounts and availability for activities

At least 45 minutes of resident activities staff time per resident per week shall be devoted to resident activities. (This is an average. It is equal to one full-time equivalent staff member for every 53 residents.)

Source: New Jersey Administrative Code, Subchapter 7

New Mexico

1600. Activities

1602. Staff

A. Definition

1. "Qualified activities coordinator" means, in a skilled nursing facility, a person who:

a. Has a bachelor's degree in recreation therapy and is eligible for registration as a therapeutic recreation specialist with the National Therapeutic Recreation Society; or

b. Is an occupational therapist or occupational therapy assistant who meets the requirements for certification by the American Occupational Therapy Association; or

c. Has two (2) years of experience in a social or recreational program within the last five years, one year of which was full-time in a patient activities program in a health care setting; or

d. Has completed a state approved program.

Source: New Mexico HED 89-2

New York

415.5 Quality of life.

(2) The activities program shall be directed by a qualified professional who:

(i) Is a qualified therapeutic recreation specialist who is eligible for certification as a therapeutic recreation specialist by a recognized accrediting body on or after August 1, 1989; or

(ii) Has 2 years of experience in an age-appropriate social or recreational program within the last 5 years, 1 of which was full-time in a patient or resident activities program in a health care setting; or

(iii) Is a qualified occupational therapist or occupational therapy assistant.

Source: New York Health Regulations,Volume 10, Subvolume C., Document 10C-415.5

North Carolina

.1204 Designated Person

The facility administrator shall designate an activities and recreation services director who shall be under the administrative supervision of the administrator, be responsible for the activities and recreation services for all patients and who shall have appropriate management authority. Any director hired on or after the effective amended date of this Rule shall be a qualified professional who:

(1) Is a therapeutic recreation specialist or therapeutic recreation assistant certified by the North Carolina State Board of Therapeutic Recreation Certification pursuant to G.S. 90C-9 or is eligible for certification as a therapeutic recreation specialist by a recognized accrediting body; or

(2) Has two years of experience in a social or recreation program within the last five years, one of which was full-time in a resident activities program in a health care setting; or

(3) Is a qualified occupational therapist or occupational therapy assistant licensed as such by the North Carolina Board of Occupational Therapy pursuant to G.S. 90-270.70; or

(4) Is certified by the National Certification Council for Activity Professionals; or

(5) Has completed an activities training course approved by the state.

Source: North Carolina Authority G.S. 131E-104; 143B-165(10); 42 U.S.C. 1396 C.F.R. 483.15(f); Eff. March 1, 1983
Amended Eff. May 1, 1993; March 1, 1990

North Dakota

33-07-03.2-2120. Activity services.

The facility shall provide an ongoing program of activity services to meet the needs and interests of each resident which promotes or maintains each resident's physical, mental, and psychosocial well-being.

1. The facility shall employ a qualified activity coordinator who is responsible for the direction and supervision of the resident activity services. A qualified activity coordinator is:

a) An individual certified as a therapeutic recreation specialist by a recognized accrediting body;

b) An individual who is eligible for certification as a therapeutic recreation specialist by a recognized accrediting body for the first year the individual is eligible;

c) An individual who is activity director certified by a recognized accrediting body;

d) An individual who is activity consultant certified by a recognized accrediting body;

e) A qualified occupational therapist as defined in North Dakota Century Code chapter 43-40;

f) A certified occupational therapy assistant;

g) An individual who has the equivalent of two years of full-time experience in a social or recreational program within the last five years, one of which was in a resident activity program in a health care setting; or

h) An individual who has completed an activity training program approved by the department as meeting the requirements in section 33-07-03.2-22, and

(1) Has one year of full-time experience in the past five years in an activity program in a health care setting; or

(2) Receives monthly on site consultation for a minimum of one year after the completion of the program from an individual meeting the qualifications described in subdivision a, d, e, f, or g.

2. The facility shall have sufficient activity staff to provide an ongoing program of meaningful, stimulating, therapeutic, and leisure time activities to meet the needs and suited to the interests of each resident.

Source: North Dakota Administrative Code, General Authority: NDCC 23-01-03, 28-32-02, Law Implemented: NDCC 23-16-01, 28-32-02
Effective date: July 1, 1996

Ohio

Defers to federal regulations.
Source: Ohio Health Care Association

Oklahoma

310:675-9-10.1. Activity Services

(b) Activities director. There shall be a designated staff member, qualified by experience or training, responsible for the direction and supervision of the activities service. The activities director shall develop appropriate activities for each resident with identified needs. Activities staff hours shall be sufficient to meet the resident's needs.

Source: Oklahoma State Department of Health
Special Health Services — 0501, Chapter 675
Revised: February 17, 1994
Effective: June 25, 1994

Oregon

411-86-230 Activity Services

(2) Activity Director. The facility shall employ an Activity Director. He/she shall have a written job description which identifies the duties

and responsibilities of the position, including the requirements set forth by this rule.

(a) Qualifications. The director shall meet one of the following:

(A) Have two years experience in a social or recreational program within the past five years, one of which was full-time in a patient activities program in a health care setting; or

(B) Be eligible for certification as a therapeutic recreation specialist by a recognized accrediting body; or

(C) Be a qualified occupational therapist or occupational therapy assistant; or

(D) Have completed a 36-hour activities workshop. The workshop must be conducted by an individual with a master's or bachelor's degree in recreation therapy or a closely related field, or by a registered occupational therapist. Such individual must have at least one year of experience in long term care services. The course must cover the subject matters identified in Exhibit 86-1, which is attached to and made a part of these rules.

Source: Oregon N.F. Licensing DIV 86 PAGE 21

Pennsylvania

211.17 Patient activities.

b) A full-time member of the facility's staff shall be designated as responsible for the patient activities program. If he is not a patient activities coordinator he shall function with frequent regularly scheduled consultation from a person so qualified.

Source: Pennsylvania Licensing Regulations, June 1987

Rhode Island

Defers to Federal regulations
Source: Rhode Island Association of Facilities for the Aging

South Carolina

Statutory Authority: 1976 Code Section 44-7-250
N. (1). Resident Activities.

(b) A staff member shall be designated as a director of the resident activities program. This staff member shall have sufficient time to provide and coordinate the activities program so that it fully meets the needs of the residents. The individual shall have expertise or training and/or experience in individual or group activities.

Source: South Carolina Department of Health and Environmental Control
Regulation Number 61-17, February 28, 1992
Standards for Licensing Nursing Homes

South Dakota

44:04:12:02. Activities program.
An activities coordinator must be in charge of the activities programs.
Source: SL 1975, ch 16 § 1; 6 SDR 93, effective July 1, 1980; 14 SDR 81, effective December 10, 1987

Tennessee

Defers to federal regulations.
Source: Tennessee Health Care Association

Texas

19.702 Activities.

(b) The activities program must be directed by a qualified professional who:

(1) Is a qualified therapeutic recreation specialist or an activities professional who is:

(A) Licensed or registered, if applicable, by the state in which practicing; and

(B) Eligible for certification as a therapeutic recreation specialist, therapeutic recreation assistant, or an activities professional by a recognized accrediting body, such as the National Council of Therapeutic Recreation Certification, on October 1, 1990; or

(2) Has two years of experience in a social or recreational program within the last five years, one of which was full-time in a patient activities program in a health care setting; or

(3) Is a qualified occupational therapist or occupational therapy assistant; or

(4) Has completed an activity director training course approved by any state. The Texas Department of Human Services (DHS) does not review or approve any courses. DHS accepts only training courses approved by the National Certification Council for Activity Professionals or the National Therapeutic Recreation Society.

Source: Texas Dept. of Human Services, NFR/LMC 95-0

Utah

R432-150-14. Activities.
(1) The activities program shall be directed by a qualified recreational therapist licensed in accordance with Title 58, Chapter 40, Recreational Therapy Practice Act.
Source: Utah Department of Health

Vermont

Defers to federal regulations.
Source: Vermont Health Care Association

Virginia

Section 21.0 Patient Activities
21.2 There shall be a designated staff member re-

sponsible for patient activities. This individual shall have experience and/or training in directing group activity. Fullest possible use should be made of community, social and recreational opportunities.

Source: Rules and Regulations for the Licensure of Nursing Homes in Virginia

The Commonwealth of Virginia, Department of Health, Bureau of Medical and Nursing Facilities Services, Richmond, VA. October 15, 1980

Washington

(7) Activities

(c) The activities program must be directed by a qualified professional who:

(i) Is a qualified therapeutic recreation specialist or an activities professional who:

(A) Is licensed or registered. If applicable, by Washington state: and

(B) Is eligible for certification as a therapeutic recreation specialist or as an activities professional by a recognized accrediting body on or after October 1, 1990: or

(ii) Has two years of experience in a social or recreational program within the last five years, one of which was full-time in a patient activities program in a health care setting: or

(iii) Has completed a training course approved by the state.

Source: Washington Administrative Code Chapter 97: Nursing Homes, WAC 388-97-080

West Virginia

Defers to federal regulations; Activity director must complete a state-approved basic course.

Source: West Virginia Health Care Association

Wisconsin

HSS 132.69 Activities

(2) Staff. (a) Definition. "Qualified activities coordinator" means:

1. In a skilled nursing facility, a person who:

a. Has a bachelor's degree in recreation therapy and is eligible for registration as a therapeutic recreation specialist with the national therapeutic recreation society;

b. Has 2 years of experience in a social or recreational program within the last 5 years, one year of which was full-time in a patient activities program in a health care setting; or

c. Is an occupational therapist or occupational therapy assistant who meets the requirements for certification by the American Occupational Therapy Association; and

2. In an intermediate care facility, a staff member who is qualified by experience or training in directing group activity.

Source: 426-30 HSS 132 Wisconsin Administrative code

Wyoming

Section 20. Patient activities.

A. Responsibility for patient activities. A member of the facility's staff shall be designated as responsible for the patients or residents activities program.

1. The designated staff members responsible for patient activities shall be a qualified therapeutic recreational specialist, a qualified occupational therapy assistant or have had two years experience in a social or recreational program within the past five years, one of which was full-time in a patient activities program in a health care setting.

2. Frequent, regular consultation from a qualified patient activities coordinator shall be provided to the designated staff member if she is not qualified.

Source: Wyoming Statutes, Title 33, Professions and Occupations and Title 35, Public Health and Safety

INTERNATIONAL

Bermuda

(1) There should be a staff member responsible for managing activities, and supervising volunteers. The staff who provide recreation activities shall be qualified by education and/experience for the responsibilities of the position.

Qualifications of the staff member responsible for managing recreation should include:

- courses in recreation, gerontology
- demonstrated leadership skills
- excellent communication skills
- 3–5 years experience in longterm care
- knowledge of programs and techniques in recreation

Source: Guidelines for the Operation of Activities Programs in Bermuda Nursing Homes

Department of Health—Bermuda

Canada—Alberta

The Nursing Homes Act does not mention any specific provisions concerning the employment of recreation or activity staff members.

Source: Province of Alberta, Nursing Homes Act, Assented to June 5, 1985, Chapter N-14.1

Canada—British Columbia

In British Columbia an activity director is a designated person. There are no criteria choosing their professional service staff. Each facility writes their own policies and procedures and are governed by few guidelines.

Source: Description of Long Term Care Services in Provinces & Territories of Canada

Canada—New Brunswick

x. Recreation

9. When there is a formally organized Recreation Service, the manager of the service is qualified by education and experience commensurate with the demands of the position.

9.1 The qualifications of the manager include: degree or diploma in recreation, experience in recreation program delivery, management education and/or experience.

10. When there is no organized Recreation Services, a staff member and/or committee is designated responsible for the management of recreation activities.

10.1 The authority and responsibilities of the individual/committee are clearly delineated.

Source: New Brunswick National Standards for Survey and Accreditation, Vol. 1

Canada—Nova Scotia

Schedule "A" Regulations made Pursuant to Section 22(1)

Chapter 12 of the Statutes of Nova Scotia, 1976

19. (e) Administrators Responsibilities: Planning and implementing programs and activities in the home and community which provide social, educational, vocational, religious and recreational opportunities for the residents.

20. In addition to the requirements set out in sections 18 and 19, every home for special care shall have adequate and competent food service staff, domestic and maintenance staff, program and activity staff, administrative support staff, and such other staff as the Minister may prescribe.

Source: Homes for Special Care Act, Chapter 203 of The Revised Statutes, 1989

Her Majesty the Queen in right of the Province of Nova Scotia

Canada—Ontario

Ministry of Community and Social Services

Standard 1: Service Provision, E. Recreation and Leisure Services.

Recreation Services Staff E1.11 The staff who provide recreation and leisure programs shall be qualified by education and/or experience for the responsibilities of their position.

Qualifications of the staff member responsible for managing recreation and leisure services should include:

- a diploma in recreation/leisure studies from a recognized community college or university
- courses in gerontology
- demonstrated leadership and organizational skills
- knowledge of programs and techniques in recreation
- excellent communication skills
- 3 to 5 years experience in long-term care
- knowledge of community resources
- knowledge of program development

Source: Nursing Homes and Charitable and Municipal Homes for the Aged are governed by either the Nursing Home Act, the Charitable Institutions Act, or the Homes for the Aged and Rest Homes Act, as amended by Bill 101, The Long Term Care Statutes Law Amendment Act, 1993

Canada—Saskatchewan

4.6 Recreational Services

Staffing

The staff person designated by the board as responsible for recreational services should allocate his/her time entirely to such services. Where indicated, staff should seek input from others e.g. therapists, physicians and family members into individual resident programming. Certain activities may be prescribed for individuals as part of their treatment regimen.

Source: Saskatchewan Continuing Care, Special-Care Homes Division

Programming Section. Index Ref. 4.6. Date of issue May 1986

A P P E N D I X B
List of Vendors

Equipment, Supplies, and Educational Materials

adaptAbility
P.O. Box 515
Colchester, CT 016415-0515
800-243-9232

Benton-Kirby
14650 28th Avenue North
Plymouth, MN 55447
800-558-9917

Briggs Health Care Products
7887 University Boulevard
P.O. Box 1698
Des Moines, IA 50306-1698
800-247-2343

Care Source
500 Seattle Tower
1218 Third Avenue
Seattle, WA 98101-3021
800-448-5213

Castings By Creative Artworks
1601 Third Avenue
Suite 21AW
New York, NY 10128
212-410-9600

Clotilde, Inc.
2 Sew Smart Way B8031
Stevens Point, WI 54481-8031
800-772-2891

Craft King Inc.
P.O. Box 90637
Lakeland, FL 33804
800-769-9494

Creative Crafts International
16 Plains Road
Essex, CT 06426
800-666-0767

Cromers
1235 Assembly Street
P.O. Box 163
Columbia, SC 29202
800-322-PNUT

Department of Education Resources
Education Division
National Gallery of Art

4th and Constitution Avenue NW
Washington, DC 20565
202-737-4215

ElderSong Inc.
P.O. Box 74
Mt. Airy, MD 21771
800-397-0533

Gary Grimm & Associates
82 S. Madison Street
P. O. Box 378
Carthage, IL 62321-03478
800-442-1614

Geriatric Resources, Inc.
931 South Semoran Boulevard #200
Winter Park, FL 32792
800-359-0390

The Geri-Tones
430 East Illinois Road
Lake Forest, IL 60045
708-234-7108

Great Western Supply
2828 Forest Lane, Suite 2000
Dallas, TX 75234
800-527-2782

Golden Horizons, Inc.
P.O. Box 193
Sullivan, IL 61951
800-218-8182

Grow Lab
National Gardening Association
180 Flynn Avenue
Burlington, VT 05401
802-863-1308

Hammatt Senior Products
1 Sportime Way
Atlanta, GA 30340-1402
800-428-5128

Happy Products, Inc.
103 Elise Avenue
Crest Hill, IL 60435
800-OK-HAPPY

Health Edco
P.O. Box 21207
Waco, TX 76702-1207
800-299-3366, Ext. 295

Imaginart Communication Products
307 Arizona Street
Bisbee, AZ 85603
520-432-5741

Incentives for Learning Inc.
111 Center Avenue, Suite 1
Pacheco, CA 94553
510-682-2428

Independent Printing Consultant
4020 State Road 3
Sunbury, OH 43074
614-965-9663

Kipp Brothers, Inc.
240-242 So. Meridian Street
P.O. Box 157
Indianapolis, IN 46206
800-832-5477

Le Trend Enterprises, Inc.
P.O. Box 64073
St. Paul, MN 55164
800-328-5540

M & H Publishing Company, Inc.
P.O. Box 268
La Grange, TX 78945-0268
800-521-9950

M & N International, Inc.
13860 W. Laurel Drive
Lake Forest, IL 60045
800-727-8966

Medical & Activities Sales
P. O. Box 12476
Omaha, NE 68112
800-541-9152

Melody House, Inc.
819 N.W. 92nd Street
Oklahoma City, OK 73114-2701
405-840-3383

Nasco
901 Janesville Avenue
Fort Atkinson, WI 53538-0901
800-558-9595

NCM Consumer Products Division
P.O. Box 6070
San Jose, CA 95150
800-235-7054

News Currents
P.O. Box 52
Madison, WI 53701
800-356-2303, Ext. 3033
608-831-1570 (Fax)

North Coast Medical
187 Stauffer Boulevard
San Jose, CA 95125-1042
800-821-9319

Oriental Trading Company, Inc.
P.O. Box 2308
Omaha, NE 68103-2308
800-228-2269

Paradise Products, Inc.
P.O. Box 568
El Cerrito, CA 94530-0568
800-227-1092

Potentials Development Inc.
40 Hazelwood Drive, Suite 101
Amherst, NY 14228
800-691-6602

Professional Printing & Publishing, Inc.
P.O. Box 5758
Bossier City, LA 71171-5758
800-551-8783

Pun American Newsletter
1165 Elmwood Place
Deerfield, IL 60015
708-945-1790

Radio Memories
P. O. Box 193
Yorktown Heights, NY 10598
914-245-6609

S & S Arts & Crafts
P.O. Box 513
Colchester, CT 06415-0513
800-243-9232

Schulmerich Handbells
Carillon Hill
P. O. Box 903
Sellersville, PA 18960-0903
800-423-7464

Sea Bay Game Co.
P.O. Box 162
Middletown, NJ 07748
800-568-0188

Senior's Needs, Inc.
68 Stiles Road
Salem, NH 03079
800-777-2006

Shillcraft
8899 Kelso Drive
Baltimore, MD 21221
410-682-3060

The Speech Bin
1965 Twenty-Fifth Avenue
Vero Beach, FL 32960
407-770-0007

Stumps
One Party Place
P.O. Box 305
South Whitley, IN 46787-0305
800-348-5084

Support Source
420 Rutgers Avenue
Swarthmore, PA 19081
610-544-3605

Tandy Leather Co.
P. O. Box 791
Fort Worth, TX 76101
817-551-9771

Trend Enterprises Inc.
P. O. Box 64073
St. Paul, MN 55164
800-328-5540

Vanguard Crafts
P. O. Box 340170
Brooklyn, NY 11234-0003
800-662-7238

Voice Of The Rockies
P.O. Box 1043
Boulder, CO 80306
303-444-8334

West Music
1208 Fifth Street
Coralville, IA 52241
800-397-9378

Worldtone Music, Inc.
230 Seventh Avenue
New York, NY 10011
212-691-1934

Games

Sportime International
1 Sportime Way
Atlanta, GA 30340-1402
800-283-5700

Talicor, Inc.
190 Arovista Circle
Brea, CA 92621
800-433-GAME

Worldwide Games
P. O. Box 517
Colchester,CT 06415-0517
800-243-9232

Miscellaneous

Access to Recreation, Inc.
2509 E. Thousand Oaks Boulevard, Suite 430
Thousand Oaks, CA 91362
800-634-4351

Activity Management Systems Inc.
1713 E. 14th Street
The Dalles, OR 97058
503-298-7770

Adamo Industries Inc.
1182 Pallwood Road
Memphis, TN 38122
800-682-7702

Brennan Associates
237 Springfield Street
Wilbraham, MA 01095
413-596-2525

CAT/UB Products
Center for Assistive Technology
515 Kimball Tower
University at Buffalo
Buffalo, NY 14214-3079
716-829-3141

Companion Radio
NetWorx Corporation
1794 Penfield Road
Penfield, NY 14526
800-445-2449

Find/SVP
The Information Catalog
625 Avenue of the Americas
New York, NY 10011
800-346-3787

Independent Printing Consultant
4020 St. Rt. 3N
Sunbury, OH 43074
614-965-9663

Mary E. Miller & Associates
P.O. Box 53182
Cincinnati, OH 45253-0182
513-385-5329

The National Council on the Aging, Inc.
409 Third Street SW
Washington, DC 20024
800-867-2755

National Gallery of Art
Education Division
4th & Constitution Avenue NW
Washington, DC 20565
202-737-4215

TFH (USA) Ltd.
4537 Gibsonia Road
Gibsonia, PA 15044
800-467-6222

Stimulation

Bifolkal Productions, Inc.
809 Williamson Street
Madison, WI 53703
800-568-5357

Cross Creek
Recreational Products Inc.
RR #1 Box 409A
Amenia, NY 12501
800-645-5816

Eldergames
11710 Hunters Lane
Rockville, MD 20852
800-637-2604

Flaghouse, Inc.
150 No. MacQuesten Parkway
Mt. Vernon, NY 10550
800-793-7900

Geriatric Resources, Inc.
931 South Semoran Boulevard #200
Winter Park, FL 32792
800-359-0390

Tapes—Video/Musical

Anchor Audio Inc.
913 W-223rd Road
Torrance, CA 90502
310-533-5984

Armchair Fitness Videos
8510 Cedar Street
Silver Spring, MD 20910

Bible Alliance, Inc.
P.O. Box 621
Bradenton, FL 34206
813-748-3031

Captioned Films/Videos
Modern Talking Picture Service, Inc.
5000 Park Street North
St. Petersburg, FL 33709
800-237-6213

Choice Magazine Listening
85 Channel Drive
Port Washington, NY 11050
516-883-8280

Heartwarmers
6N534 Glendale Road
Mendinah, IL 60157
708-893-5383

International Folk Rhythms
P. O. Box 1402
Northbrook, IL 60065-1402
708-564-2880

LMER Video Productions
4600 Valley Road
Lincoln, NE 68510
402-483-4581

Points of Light Foundation
P. O. Box 66534
Washington, DC 20035
202-223-5001

Positive Communication, Inc.
P.O. Box 15
Bellvue, CO 80512-0015
970-484-3511

Presta Sounds
877 Will Scarlet Way
Macon, GA 31210
912-471-7194

Recordings for Recovery
National Headquarters
222 1/2 E. Main Street
P.O. Box 270
Midland, MI 48640
517-832-0784

Sentimental Productions
P. O. Box 14716
Cincinnati, OH 45250
513-244-6542

Therapy Resources, Inc.
P.O. Box 452
Ambler, PA 19002-0452
215-628-2603

A P P E N D I X   C
Publishers of Activity Books, Newsletters, and Journals

Publishers

Alpha Affiliates, Inc.
103 Washington Street
Morristown, NJ 07960-6813
201-539-2770
201-644-0610 (Fax)

Alzheimer's Care Guide
Box 11885
Reno, NV 89510
800-354-3371

American Guidance Service
4201 Woodland Road
P.O. Box 99
Circle Pines, MN 55014-1796
800-328-2560

American Health Care Association Publications
Department C1
P.O. Box 96906
Washington, DC 20090-6906
800-321-0343

American Hospital Publishing, Inc.
P.O. Box 92683
Chicago, IL 60675-2683
800-AHA-2626

Aspen Publishers, Inc.
7201 McKinney Circle
P.O. Box 990
Frederick, MD 21701
800-638-8437

Brady
Paramount Publishing Education Group
113 Sylvan Avenue, Route 9W
Englewood Cliffs, NJ 07632
201-592-3271

Charles C. Thomas Publisher
2600 South First Street
Springfield, IL 62794-9265
217-789-8980

Consumer Information Catalog
Consumer Information Center—5C
P.O. Box 100
Pueblo, CO 81002
719-948-3334

Creative Forecasting, Inc.
P.O. Box 7789
Colorado Springs, CO 80933-7789
719-633-3174

Creative Resources
P.O. Box 328
Etowah, NC 28729
704-891-2919

Delmar Publishers Inc.
P.O. Box 15015
Albany, NY 12212-5015
800-998-7498

Dover Publications, Inc.
31 East 2nd Street
Mineola, NY 11501
516-294-7000

Echo Publishing
614 East Grant Street
Minneapolis, MN 55404-1413
800-264-ECHO

The Eden Alternative
RR #1, Box 31B4
Sherburne, NY 13460
607-674-5232

ElderSong Publications Inc.
P.O. Box 74
Mt. Airy, MD 21771
800-397-0533

Eymann Publications, Inc.
P.O. Box 3577
Reno, NV 89509
702-358-1554

F.A. Davis Company
1915 Arch Street
Philadelphia, PA 19103
800-523-4049

Gary Grimm & Associates
P.O. Box 378
Carthage, IL 62321-0378
800-442-1614

Geriatric Educational Consultants
P.O. Box 1178
Holmes Beach, FL 34218
813-778-7050

Geriatric Resources, Inc.
9831 South Semoran Boulevard #200
Winter Park, FL 32792
800-359-0390

Gold Timers
A Division of Incentives for Learning
111 Center Avenue, Suite 1
Pacheco, CA 94553
510-682-2428

Guideposts
Carmel, NY 10512
800-431-2344

The Haworth Press, Inc.
109 Alice Street
Binghamton, NY 13904-1580
800-342-9678

Health Care Facility Educational Services
404 S. Lincoln, L3
P. O. Box 1453
Aberdeen, SD 57402-1453
800-357-6735

Healthcare Marketing Concepts
P.O. Box 167
Hinckley, OH 44233
216-278-2516

Heaton Publications
627 East Main Street
Albertville, AL 35950
800-221-2469

Ideals
P. O. Box 148000
Nashville, TN 37214
615-333-0478

Idyll Arbor, Inc.
P.O. Box 720
25119 S.E. 262 Street
Ravensdale, WA 98051
206-432-3231

Jossey-Bass Publishers
350 Sansome Street
San Francisco, CA 94104
415-433-1767

Keepsake Publishers
P.O. Box 21
Plover, WI 54467

Lindner/Harpaz
P.O. Box 993
Woodside, NY 11377

M & H Publishing Company, Inc.
P.O. Box 268
La Grange, TX 78945-0268
800-521-9950

Medical & Activities Sales
P.O. Box 12476
Omaha, NE 68112
800-541-9152

Mosby-Year Book, Inc.
11830 West Line Industrial Drive
St. Louis, MO 63146
800-325-4177

National Association for Senior Living Industries
184 Duke of Gloucester Street
Annapolis, MD 21401
410-263-0991

National Institute of Mental Health
5600 Fishers Lane
Rockville, MD 20857
301-443-4513

National Recreation & Park Association
2775 South Quincy Street, Suite 300
Arlington, VA 22206-2204
703-820-4940

Onward Publishing Inc.
10 Lewis Road
Northport, NY 11768
516-757-3030

Potentials Development, Inc.
40 Hazelwood Drive, Suite 101
Amherst, NY 14228
800-691-6602

Publicare Press
c/o Professional Printing & Publishing, Inc.
P.O. Box 5758
Bossier City, LA 71171-5758
800-551-8783

Prometheus Books
59 John Glenn Drive
Amherst, NY 14228-2197
800-421-0351

Recreation Therapy Consultants
6115 Syracuse Lane
San Diego, CA 92122
619-546-9003

Reminisce
Box 572
Milwaukee, WI 53201
414-423-0100

Rutgers University Press
109 Church Street
New Brunswick, NJ 08901
800-446-9323

S.N.A.P. Publications
P.O. Box 574
San Anselmo, CA 94979
415-453-6029

Springer Publishing Co.
536 Broadway
New York, NY 10012
212-431-4370

Twin Peaks Press
P. O. Box 129
Vancouver, WA 98666-0129
360-694-2492

Valley Press
P. O. Box 5224
Lafayette, IN 47903
317-447-5592

Venture Publishing, Inc.
1999 Cato Avenue
State College, PA 16801
800-234-4561

Volunteer Guide
P.O. Box 3577
Reno, NV 89509
702-358-1554

Whale Publishing
139 Lincoln Avenue
Harrisburg, PA 17111
717-564-6371

Winslow
Telford Road
Bicester, Oxon OX6 0TS, United Kingdom
+44-1869-355644

Related Journals

AARP Bulletin
American Association of Retired Persons
3200 E. Carson Street
Lakewood, CA 90712
310-496-2277
Founded: 1959
Published: Monthly

Activities, Adaptation and Aging
(The Gerontological Journal of Activities)
The Haworth Press
6549 S. Lincoln Street
Littleton, CO 80121
303-794-7676
Founded: 1980
Published: Quarterly

Abstracts in Social Gerontology
Sage Periodical Press
2455 Teller Road
Thousand Oaks, CA 91320
805-499-0721
Founded: 1957
Published: Quarterly

AIDS Education & Prevention
Guilford Publications Inc.
School of Public Health
University of South Carolina
Columbia, SC 29208
803-777-6217
Founded: 1989
Published: Bimonthly

Aging
U.S. Government Printing Office
Superintendent of Documents
Washington, DC 20402-9322
202-783-3238
Founded: 1951
Published: Quarterly

Aging: Generations
Journal of The American Society on Aging
833 Market Street, Suite 511
San Francisco, CA 94103
415-974-9600
Founded: 1976
Published: Quarterly

Aging Today
American Society on Aging
833 Market Street, Suite 511
San Francisco, CA 94103
415-974-9600
Founded: 1979
Published: Bimonthly

Alzheimer's Disease & Associated Disorders
Raven Press
1185 Avenue of the Americas
Mail Stop 3B
New York, NY 10036
212-930-9500
Founded: 1987
Published: Quarterly

American Horticulturist
American Horticultural Society
7931 E. Boulevard Drive
Alexandria, VA 22308
703-768-5700
Founded: 1922
Published: Monthly

American Journal of Art Therapy
Vermont College of Norwich University
Montpelier, VT 05602
802-828-8540
Founded: 1961
Published: Quarterly

The American Journal of Hospice Care
Prime National Publishing Corp.
470 Boston Post Road
Weston, MA 02193
617-899-2702
Founded: 1984
Published: Bimonthly

American Journal of Nursing
American Journal of Nursing Co.
555 W. 57th St.
New York, NY 10019
212-582-8820
Founded:1900
Published: Monthly

The American Journal of Occupational Therapy
American Occupational Therapy Association
4720 Montgomery Lane
P.O. Box 31220
Bethesda, MD 20824-1220
301-652-2682
Founded: 1947
Published: Monthly

American Journal of Physical Medicine &
Rehabilitation
Williams & Wilkins
428 E. Preston Street
Baltimore, MD 21202
410-528-8553
Founded: 1921
Published: Bimonthly

American Journal of Psychology
University of Illnois Press
1325 S. Oak Street
Champaign, IL 61820
217-333-8935
Founded: 1887
Published: Quarterly

Canadian Journal on Aging
University of Guelph
Francois Belance
Faculté de Medecine, Université de Montreal
C.P. 6128, SUCC.A.
Montreal, PQ, Canada H3C 3J7
514-343-6185
Founded:1982
Published: Quarterly

The Canadian Journal of Geriatrics
STA Communication Inc.
955 St. Jean Boulevard, Suite 306
Pointe-Claire, PQ, Canada H9R 5K3
514-695-7623
Founded: 1985
Published: 8x/yr.

Canadian Nursing Home Journal
Health Media
14453 29A Avenue
White Rock, BC, Canada V4P1P7
604-535-7933
Founded: 1985
Published: Quarterly

Contemporary Long Term Care
Bill Communications Inc.
355 Park Avenue South
New York, NY 10010-1789
212-986-4800
Founded: 1975
Published: Monthly

Federal Register Index
Office of the Federal Register
Washington, DC 20408
202-523-5227
Founded: 1936
Published: Monthly

Federal Register
U.S. Government Printing Office
Code of Federal Regulations
U.S. Government Printing Office
Superintendent of Documents
Washington, DC 20402-9322
202-783-3238
Founded: 1936
Published: Daily

Geriatrics
Advanstar Communication Inc.
7500 Old Oak Boulevard
Cleveland, OH 44130
216-896-2839
Founded: 1946
Published: Monthly

Geriatric Medicine Quarterly
MPI Medical Publishing Inc.
14 Ronan Avenue
Toronto, ON, Canada M4N, 2X9
416-481-6384
Founded: 1985
Published: Quarterly

Geriatric Nursing
Mosby-Yearbook, Inc.
11830 West Line Industrial Drive
St. Louis, MO 63146
800-325-4177
Founded: 1980
Published: Bimonthly

The Gerontologist
The Gerontological Society of America
1275 K. Street NW, Suite 350
Washington, DC 20005-4006
202-842-1275
Founded: 1961
Published: Bimonthly

Gerontology & Geriatrics Education
The Haworth Press Inc.
10 Alice Street
Binghamton, NY 13904-1580
607-722-5857
Founded: 1980
Published: Quarterly

Health Care Management Review
Aspen Publishers Inc.
7201 McKinney Circle
Frederick, MD 21701
301-417-7500
Founded:1976
Published: Quarterly

The Health Care Supervisor
Aspen Publishers Inc.
7201 McKinney Circle
Frederick, MD 21701
301-417-7500
Founded: 1982
Published: Quarterly

Health Facilities Management
American Hospital Publishing Inc.
737 N. Michigan Avenue, Suite 700
Chicago, IL 60611
312-440-6800
Founded: 1988
Published: Quarterly

Health Management Quarterly
The Haworth Press
P.O. Box 8566

Berkeley, CA 94707
607-722-5857
Founded: 1983
Published: Quarterly

International Journal of Aging & Human
Development
Baywood Publishing
26 Austin Avenue
P.O. Box 337
Amityville, NY 11701
516-691-1270
Founded: 1973
Published: 8x/yr.

Journal of Aging & Health
Sage Periodicals Press
2455 Teller Road
Thousand Oakes, CA 91320
805-499-0721
Founded: 1989
Published: Quarterly

Journal of Aging & Social Policy
The Haworth Press, Inc.
10 Alice Street
Binghamton, NY 13904-1580
607-722-5857
Founded: 1989
Published: Quarterly

Journal of Aging Studies
J.A I. Press Inc.
55 Old Post Road, No. 2
Greenwich, CT 06836-1678
203-661-7602
Founded: 1987
Published: Quarterly

Journal of American Ethnic History
Transaction Periodicals Consortium
Rutgers—The State University of New Jersey
New Brunswick, NJ 08903
908-932-2280
Founded: 1981
Published: Quarterly

Journal of the American Geriatrics Society
Williams & Wilkens
428 E. Preston Street
Baltimore, MD 21202
410-528-8553
Founded: 1953
Published: Monthly

Journal of Gerontological Nursing
Slack Inc.
6900 Grove Road

Thorofare, NJ 08086-9447
609-848-1000
Founded: 1975
Published: Monthly

Journal of Gerontological Social Work
The Haworth Press
10 Alice Street
Binghamton, NY 13904-1580
607-722-5857
Founded: 1978
Published: Quarterly

Journal of Health & Social Behavior
American Sociological Association
1722 N Street NW
Washington, DC 20036
202-833-3410
Founded: 1959
Published: Quarterly

Journal of Head Trauma Rehabilitation
Aspen Publishers Inc.
200 Orchard Ridge Drive, Suite 200
Gaithersburg, MD 20878
301-417-7500
Founded: 1986
Published: Quarterly

Journal of Long-Term Care Administration
American College of Health Care Administrators
325 S. Patrick Street
Alexandria, VA 22314-3571
703-549-5822
Founded: 1962
Published: Quarterly

Journal of Nursing Administration
J.B. Lippincott Co.
277 E. Washington Square
Philadelphia, PA 19106
215-238-4492
Founded: 1971
Published: 11x/yr.

Journal of Pastoral Care Publications
Journal of PC Publications Inc.
1068 Harbor Drive SW
Colabash, NC 28467
404-320-0195
Founded: 1947
Published: Quarterly

Journal of Poetry Therapy
Human Services Press
233 Spring Street
New York, NY 10013
212-620-8000
Founded: 1986
Published: Quarterly

Journal of Management Education
Sage Periodicals Press
2455 Teller Road
Thousand Oakes, CA 91320
805-499-0721
Founded: 1977
Published: Quarterly

Journal of Religion & Health
Human Sciences Press
233 Spring Street
New York, NY 10013
212-620-8000
Founded: 1961
Published: Quarterly

Journal of Social Behavior & Personality
Select Press
P.O. Box 37
Corte Madera, CA 94976
415-924-1612
Founded: 1986
Published: Quarterly

Journal of Women & Aging
The Haworth Press
10 Alice Street
Binghamton, NY 13904-1580
607-722-5857
Founded: 1989
Published: Quarterly

McKnights Long Term Care News
McKnights Medical Communications Co.
2 Northfield Plaza, Suite 300
Northfield, IL 60093-1217
708-441-3700
Founded: 1980
Published: Monthly

Provider
American Health Care Association
1201 L Street NW
Washington, DC 20005
202-842-4444
Founded: 1975
Published: Monthly

Psychology & Aging
American Psychology Association
750 First Street NE
Washington, DC 20002-4242
202-336-5500
Founded: 1979
Published: Quarterly

PT, Magazine of Physical Therapy
American Physical Therapy Association
1111 N. Fairfax Street
Alexandria, VA 22314

703-684-2782
Founded: 1993
Published: Monthly

Recreation Canada
Canadian Recreation & Parks Association
1600 James Naismith Drive
Gloucester, ON, Canada k2B 5NY
613-748-5651
Founded:1947
Published: 5x/yr.

Research on Aging
Sage Periodicals Press
2455 Teller Road
Thousand Oaks, CA 91320
805-499-0721
Founded: 1979
Published: Quarterly

Strategies
American Alliance for Health,
Physical Education & Dance
1900 Association Drive
Reston, VA 22091
703-476-3495
Founded: 1987
Published: 9x/yr.

Therapeutic Recreation Journal
National Recreation & Park Association
2775 S. Quincy Street, Suite 300
Arlington, VA 22206-2204
703-820-4940
Founded: 1967
Published: Quarterly

Topics in Geriatric Rehabilitation
Aspen Publishers Inc.
7201 McKinney Circle
Frederick, MD 21701
301-417-7500
Founded: 1985
Published: Quarterly

A P P E N D I X   D

List of Information Resources—Organizations and Groups

Aging Organizations

American Association of Retired Persons (AARP)
601 E Street NW
Washington, DC 20049
800-424-3410

Age Concern Scotland
54A Fountainbridge Edinburgh EH3 9PT
0131-228-5656

American Society on Aging
833 Market Street, Suite 511
San Francisco, CA 94103-1824
415-543-2617

Centre for Policy on Ageing
Patron: HM Queen Elizabeth the Queen Mother
25-31 Ironmonger Row
London EC1V 3QP
071-253-1787
071-490-4206 (Fax)

Children Of Aging Parents (CAPS)
Woodbourne Office Campus, Suite 302-A
1609 Woodbourne Road
Levittown, PA 19057
215-945-6900

Federal Council on the Aging
330 Independence Avenue SW, Room 4280
Washington, DC 20201
202-619-2451

Health Care Finance Administration (HCFA)
200 Independence Avenue SW
Washington, DC 20201
202-690-6726

International Federation on Aging
Headquarters-International Federation on Aging
380, rue St-Antoine Quest
Bureau 3200
Monteal, Quebec, Canada H2Y 3X7
514-287-9679
514-987-1567 (Fax)

National Aging Dissemination Center
1225 I Street NW, #725
Washington, DC 20005
202-898-2578
800-989-6537

National Council on the Aging (NCOA)
409 3rd St. SW
Washington, DC 20024
202-479-1200

National Institute on Aging
ADEAR Center
P.O. Box 8250
Silver Spring, MD 20907-8250
800-438-4380

National Institute on Aging Information Center
P.O. Box 8057
Gaithersburg, MD 20898-8057
800-222-2225

The National Council on Aging
Age Concern England
Astral House, 1268 London Road
London SW16 4ER
081-679-8000
081-679-6069 (Fax)

U.S. Department of Health and Human Services
330 Independence Avenue SW
Washington, DC 20201
202-619-0403

U.S. Department of Health and Human Services
Public Health Service
Agency for Health Care Policy and Research
Executive Office Center, Suite 501
2101 East Jefferson Street
Rockville, MD 20852
800-358-9295

Long-Term Care Organizations

American Hospital Association
325 Seventh Street NW
Washington, DC 20004
202-638-1100

Concerned Relatives of Nursing Home Patients
P.O. Box 18820
Cleveland, OH 44118-0820
206-321-0403

Elder Care Locator
Administration on Aging
U.S. Department of Health and Human Services
330 Independence Avenue SW
Washington, DC 20201
202-619-1006

National Association for Home Care
519 C Street NE
Washington, DC 20002-5809
202-547-7424
202-547-3540 (Fax)

National Association of Board Of Examiners for Nursing Home Administrators
808 17th Street NW
Washington, DC 20006
202-223-9750

National Association of Directors of Nursing Administration in Long Term Care
10999 Reed Hartman Highway, Suite 229
Cincinnati, OH 45242
513-791-3579

National Association of Professional Geriatric Care Managers
1604 N. Country Club Road
Tucson, AZ 85716
520-881-8008

National Institute on Community-Based Long-Term Care
C/O National Council on the Aging
409 3rd Street SW, 2nd Floor
Washington, DC 20024
202-479-6683

Special Constituency Section for Aging and Long Term Care Services
C/O American Hospital Association
840 N. Lake Shore Drive
Chicago, IL 60611
312-280-6372

Organizations for Specific Diseases and Conditions

AIDS

CDC National AIDS Clearinghouse
P.O. Box 6003
Rockville, MD 20849-6003
800-458-5231
301-738-6616 (Fax)

Visiting Nurses Association and Hospice of San Francisco
401 Duboce Avenue
San Francisco, CA 94117
415-861-8705

Alcohol and Substance Abuse

National Clearinghouse For Alcohol and Drug Information
P.O. Box 2345
Rockville, MD 20852
800-729-6686

National Council on Alcoholism & Drug Dependence
12 West 21st Street
New York, NY 10010
800-NCA-CALL

Alzheimer's Disease

Alzheimer's Disease and Related Disorders Association, Inc.
919 North Michigan Avenue, Suite 1000
Chicago, IL 60611-1676
800-272-3900

Alzheimer's Disease Education and Referral Center
P.O. Box 8250
Silver Spring, MD 20907-8250
800-438-4380
301-495-3334 (Fax)

National Foundation for Medical Research
1360 Beverly Road, Suite 305
McLean, VA 22101
703-356-8417

Amputation

American Amputee Foundation
P. O. Box 250218, Hillcrest Station
Little Rock, AR 72225
501-666-2523

National Amputation Foundation
73 Church Street
Malverne, NY 11565
516-887-3600

Asthma

Asthma and Allergy Foundation of America
1125 15th Street NW, Suite 502
Washington, DC 20005
202-466-7643

ALS

The Amyotropic Lateral Sclerosis Association
21021 Ventura Boulevard, Suite 321
Woodland Hills, CA 91364-2206
818-340-7500

Arthritis

Arthritis Foundation
P.O. Box 19000
Atlanta, GA 30326
800-283-7800

National Arthritis and Musculoskeletal and Skin Disease Information Clearinghouse
1 AMS Circle
Bethesda, MD 20892-3675
301-495-4484

Blindness

American Council of the Blind
1155 15th Street NW, Suite 720
Washington, DC 20005
202-467-5081
202-467-5085 (Fax)

American Foundation for the Blind
11 Penn Plaza, Suite 300
New York, NY 10001
212-470-7301

National Library Service for the Blind and
   Physically Handicapped
Library of Congress
Washington, DC 20542
202-707-5100

Cancer

American Cancer Society
1599 Clifton Road NE
Atlanta, GA 30329-4251
800-227-2345

Cancer Information Service
800-4-CANCER

National Cancer Institute
9000 Pockville Pike
Bethesda, MD 20892
800-422-6237

Coma

Coma Recovery Association
377 Jerusalem Avenue
Hepstead, NY 11550
516-486-2847
516-486-3815 (Fax)

Cystic Fibrosis

Cystic Fibrosis Foundation
6931 Arlington Road
Bethesda, MD 20814
800-FIGHT-CF

Developmental Disabilities

Administration on Developmental Disabilities
200 Independence Avenue SW
Suite 349D-HHH Building
Washington, DC 20201
202-690-6590

Diabetes

American Dietetic Association
216 West Jackson Boulevard
Chicago, IL 60606-6995
312-899-0040

National Diabetes Information Clearinghouse
1 Information Way
Bethesda, MD 20892-3560
301-654-3327

Digestion

Crohn's and Colitis Foundation of America
444 Park Avenue South, 11th Floor
New York, NY 10016-7343
800-932-2423

Epilepsy

Epilepsy Foundation of America
4351 Garden City Drive
Landover, MD 20785
301-459-3700

Head Injury

National Head Injury Foundation
1776 Massachusetts Avenue NW, Suite 100
Washington, DC 20036-1904
202-296-6443
202-296-8850 (Fax)

Hearing Impairments

Alexander Graham Bell Association for the
   Deaf, Inc.
3417 Volta Place NW
Washington, DC 20007
202-337-5220

National Association of the Deaf
814 Thayer Avenue
Silver Spring, MD 20910-4500
301-587-1788

National Information Center On Deafness
Gallaudet University
800 Florida Avenue NE
Washington, DC 20002-3695
202-651-5051

Heart

American Heart Association
National Center
7320 Greenville Avenue
Dallas, TX 75231-9990
214-373-6300

National Heart, Lung & Blood Institute
Information Center
7200 Wisconsin Avenue
P. O. Box 329
Bethesda, MD 20814
301-251-1222

Hypertension

National Hypertension Association, Inc.
324 East 30th Street
New York, NY 10016
212-889-3557
212-447-7032 (Fax)

Incontinence

National Association for Continence
P.O. Box 8310
Spartanburg, SC 29305-8310
800-BLADDER

Kidney

American Kidney Fund
6110 Executive Boulevard, #1010
Rockville, MD 20852
410-381-3052

National Kidney Foundation, Inc.
30 East 33rd Street
New York, NY 10016
800-622-9010

Lungs

American Lung Association
1740 Broadway
New York, NY 10019-4374
800-LUNG-USA

National Association for Ventilator Dependent
Individuals
3601 Poplar Street
P. O. Box 3666
Erie, PA 16508
814-455-6171

Lupus

The American Lupus Society
3914 Del Amo Boulevard, Suite 922
Torrance, CA 90503
310-542-8891

Mental Health

American Psychiatric Association
1400 K Street NW
Washington, DC 20005
202-682-6000

National Institute of Mental Health
Public Inquiries Branch
5600 Fishers Lane
Rockville, MD 20857
301-443-4536

National Mental Health Consumer's Self-Help
Clearinghouse
311 South Juniper Street, Suite 1000
Philadelphia, PA 19107
215-751-1810

Schizophrenics Anonymous
15920 W. Twelve Mile
Southfield, MI 48076
313-557-6777

Multiple Sclerosis

Multiple Sclerosis Foundation
6350 N. Andrews Avenue
Fort Lauderdale, FL 33309
305-776-6805

National Multiple Sclerosis Society
733 Third Avenue
New York, NY 10017-3288
212-986-3240
212-986-7981 (Fax)

Muscular Dystrophy

Muscular Dystrophy Association
3300 E. Sunrise Drive
Tucson, AZ 85718
602-529-2000

Osteoporosis

National Osteoporosis Foundation
1150 17th Street NW, Suite 500
Washington, DC 20036
202-223-2226

Pain

American Chronic Pain Association
P. O. Box 850
Rocklin, CA 95677
916-632-0922

Paralysis

American Paralysis Association
500 Morris Avenue
Springfield, NJ 07081
800-225-0292

National Spinal Cord Injury Association
545 Concord Avenue, Suite 29
Cambridge, MA 02138
800-962-9629

Parkinson's Disease

National Parkinson Foundation
122 East 42nd Street, Suite 2806
New York, NY 10168
212-374-1741

Parkinson's Disease Foundation
Wm. Black Medical Research Building
Columbia-Presbyterian Medical Center
650 W. 168th Street
New York, NY 10032
800-457-6676

Polio

International Polio Network
510 Oakland Avenue, Suite 206
St. Louis, MO 63110
314-361-0475

United Post-Polio Survivors
P. O. Box 273
Itasca, IL 60143-0273
800-526-0844

Stroke

Courage Stroke Network
c/o Courage Center
3915 Golden Valley Road
Golden Valley, MN 55422
800-553-6321

National Stroke Association
300 East Hampton Avenue, Suite 240
Englewood, CO 80110-2622
303-762-9922

Urinary

American Foundation for Urologic Disease, Inc.
1120 North Charles Street, Suite 401
Baltimore, MD 21201
800-242-2383

National Kidney and Urologic Diseases
  Information Clearinghouse
3 Information Way
Bethesda, MD 20892-3580
301-654-4415

Professional Organizations

American Art Therapy Association
1202 Allanson Road
Mundelein, IL 60060
708-949-6064

American Association of Homes and Services for
  the Aging
901 E Street NW
Suite 500
Washington, DC 20004-2037
202-783-2242
202-783-2255 (Fax)

American Association For Music Therapy
P. O. Box 80012
Valley Forge, PA 19484
215-265-4006

American Association of Pastoral Counselors
9504A Lee Highway
Fairfax, VA 22031-2303
703-385-6967
703-352-7725 (Fax)

American College of Health Care Administrators
  (ACHCA)
325 South Patrick Street
Alexandria, VA 22314-3571
703-549-5822
703-739-7901 (Fax)

American Dance Therapy Association
2000 Century Plaza, Suite 108
Columbia, MD 21044
410-997-4040

American Health Care Association (AHCA)
1201 L Street NW
Washington, DC 20005
202-842-4444

American Horticultural Therapy Association
362A Christopher Avenue
Gaithersburg, MD 20879
301-948-3010

The American Occupational Therapy Association
4720 Montgomery Lane
P. O. Box 31220
Bethesda, MD 20824-1220
301-652-2682

American Therapeutic Recreation Association
  (ATRA)
P.O. Box 15215
Hattiesburg, MS 39404-5215
800-553-0304

Association For Dance Movement Therapy UK
Arts Therapeutic Department
Springfield Hospital
Glenburnie Road
Tootong Bec, London SW17 7DJ

Association of Professional Music Therapists
Chestnut Cottage
38 Pierce Lane
Fulbourn, Cambs
CB1 5DL England
0223-880377

British Society For Music Therapy (BSMT)
25 Rosslyn Avenue
East Barnet
Herts
EN4 6DH
0181-368-8879

Canadian Association for Music Therapy
Wilfrid Laurier University
Waterloo, ON, Canada N2L 3C5
519-884-1970, Ext. 6828

Canadian Nurses Association
50 Driveway
Ottawa ON, Canada K2P 1E2
800-361-8404

Certification Board For Music Therapists
6336 N. Oracle Road, Suite 326
Box 345
Tucson, AZ 85704-5457
602-297-9892

Institute of Leisure and Amenity Management
ILAM Information
ILAM House
Lower Basildon, Reading, RG8 9NE
01491-874222
01491-874059 (Fax)

International Phototherapy Association
Photo Therapy Centre
1107 Homer Street, Suite 304
Vancouver, BC, Canada V6B 2Y1
604-689-9709

Joint Commission on Accreditation of Health
    Organizations (JCAHO)
1 Renaissance Boulevard
Oakbrook Terrace, IL 60181
708-916-5600

National Association of Activity Professionals
    (NAAP)
1401 Eye Street NW, Suite 900
Washington, DC 20005
202-218-4120
202-842-0621 (Fax)

National Association For Drama Therapy
2022 Cutter Drive
League City, TX 77573-6916
713-538-1689

National Association for Music Therapy, Inc.
8455 Colesville Road, Suite 930
Silver Spring, MD 20910-3392
301-589-3300

National Association For Poetry Therapy
P.O. Box 551
Port Washington, NY 11050
516-944-9791

National Certification Council For Activity
    Professionals (NCCAP)
526 King Street
Suite 423
Alexandria, VA 22314
703-706-9576

National Coalition of Arts Therapies Association
    (NCATA)
2000 Century Plaza, Suite 108
Columbia, MD 21044
410-997-4040

National Council for Therapeutic Recreation
    Certification (NCTRC)
P.O. Box 479
Thiells, NY 10984-0479
914-947-4346

National Federation For Biblio-Poetry Therapy
225 Lincoln Place, No. 2F
Brooklyn, NY 11217
718-636-0754

National Recreation and Parks Association
2775 South Quincy Street, Suite 300
Arlington, VA 22206-2204
703-820-4940

National Remotivational Therapy
    Organization, Inc.
P.O. Box 361
Andover, MA 01810-0007
207-351-1075

National Therapeutic Recreation Society
3101 Park Center Drive
Alexandria, VA 22302
703-820-4940

Therapy Dogs International, Inc.
6 Hilltop Road
Mendham, NJ 07945
201-543-0888

World Confederation for Physical Therapy
4a Abbots Place
London NW6 4NP
0710328 5448
071-624 7579 (Fax)

World Leisure and Recreation Association
P.O. Box 309
Sharbot Lake, Ontario
Canada K0H 2P0
613-279-3172

Miscellaneous Organizations

Adventures In Caring Foundation
P.O. Box 3859
Santa Barbara, CA 99130
805-687-5803
805-563-7678 (Fax)

Aim For The Handicapped, Inc.
945 Danbury Road
Dayton, OH 45420
800-332-8210
513-294-3783 (Fax)

American Association for Continuity of Care
1730 North Lynn Street
Suite 502
Arlington, VA 22209
703-525-1191)
703-276-8196 (Fax)

Broome County Child Development Council, Inc.
29 Fayette Street
P.O. Box 880
Binghamton, NY 13902-0880
607-723-8313

Bureau of Nursing
Ohio Department of Health
246 North High Street
Columbus, OH 43266-0588
614-466-2205

Centers for Disease Control and Prevention
  (CDC)
1600 Clifton Road NE
Atlanta, GA 30333
404-639-3311

Clearinghouse on Disability Information
United States Dept. of Education
Rm. 3132
Switzer Building.
Washington, DC 20202-2524
202-205-8241
202-205-8723

Eden Alternative
c/o Chase Memorial Nursing Home
1 Terrace Heights
New Berlin, NY 13411
607-847-6117

Generations Together
University Center for Social and Urban Research
University of Pittsburgh
121 University Place, Suite 300
Pittsburgh, PA 15260-5907
412-648-7150
412-624-4810 (Fax)

Horticultural Therapy Services
Chicago Biotanic Garden
P.O. Box 400
Glencoe, IL 60022
708-835-8248

The Humor Project
110 Spring Street
Saratoga Springs, NY 12866
518-587-8770

Laughter Therapy
P.O. Box 827
Monterey, CA 93942

National Federation Of Interfaith Care Givers
368 Broadway, Suite 103
P.O. Box 1939
Kingston, NY 12401
914-331-1358
914-331-4177 (Fax)

National Gardening Association
180 Flynn Avenue
Burlington, VT 05401
802-863-1308
802-863-5962 (Fax)

National Hospice Organization
1901 North Moore Street, Suite 901
Arlington, VA 22209
703-243-5900
703-525-5762 (Fax)

National Rehabilitation Information Center
8455 Colesville Road, Suite 935
Silver Spring, MD 20910
800-246-2742

Onlok Senior Health Services
1333 Bush Street
San Francisco, CA 94109
414-292-8888

Points of Light Foundation
1737 H Street NW
Washington, DC 20006
202-223-9186
202-223-9256 (Fax)

Project Magic
The Kansas Rehabilitation Hospital
1504 SW 8th Street
Topeka, Kansas 66606
913-235-6600
913-232-8545 (Fax)

Public Health Service
Region II
Federal Building
26 Federal Plaza
New York, NY 10278
212-264-2560

Sexuality In Middle And Later Life (SIECUS)
130 West 42nd Street, Suite 350
New York, NY 10036
212-819-9770

Special Olympics International
1325 G Street NW, Suite 500
Washington, DC 20005-3104
202-628-3630
202-824-0200 (Fax)

Touch for Health Association
6955 Fernhill Drive
Malibu, CA 90265
800-466-TFHA

U.S. Department of Health and Human Services
26 Federal Plaza
Room 3312
New York, NY 10278
212-264-4040

Volunteers of America
National Office
3939 North Causeway Boulevard
Suite 400
Metaire, LA 70002-1784
504-837-2652

A P P E N D I X E
Answers to the Review Questions/Self-Assessment Examination

ANSWERS TO THE REVIEW QUESTIONS

Chapter 1

1. Peckham and Peckham define an activity as "all the action and interaction the resident experiences during the day" whereas Peterson and Gunn characterize therapeutic recreation as "a process which utilizes recreation services for purposive intervention in some physical, emotional and/or social behavior to bring about a desired change in that behavior and to promote the growth and development of the individual."

2. The continuum of care is an illustrated guide to the range of services in the long-term care delivery system. Service options on the lower end include home care and increased needs that may require community services. The greatest needs are for those requiring institutional care.

3. The three components of long-term care are home services, community services, and institutional services.

4. Medicare is a federally funded insurance program for individuals over sixty-five and has two parts: A & B. Part A covers portions of an individual's hospital and long-term care stay when a person qualifies, whereas Part B covers partial physician costs and other expenses. Medicaid is a federal program administrated by each state to assist indigent, disabled, or blind individuals. Medicaid will pay for room, board, and other care items in long-term care institutional settings for qualified individuals.

5. The definition of subacute care is the level of care that involves complex treatments or other interventions above traditional nursing facility care. It is usually part of an acute phase of an illness or may be part of an extended disease process.

Chapter 2

1. Organizational chart.
2. An exposure control plan provides specific guidelines to all departments as to how to handle potentially infectious materials in the facility.

3. In the Fire and Evacuation Plan outlined in the policy and procedure manual and posted throughout the facility.

4. Nosocomial infections are acquired in a health care environment through contact with equipment, staff, or residents. Examples include flu or cold germs.

5. Incident report.

Chapter 3

1. Chronological age is the number of years a person has been alive. Functional capacity refers to the indicators of age, such as mobility and appearance. Life stages refers to physical and social attributes used to classify people, such as "old age."

2. The crisis in the old age stage of development involves a critique of one's own life with preparation for and acceptance of death.

3. Decline in visual ability and intolerance of glare, hearing, taste and smelling abilities decrease, greater unsteadiness seen along with cataracts, glaucoma, and tinnitus.

4. The nervous system. Alzheimer's disease has an unknown cause whereas multi-infarct dementia is related to strokes and a build up of damage in the brain.

5. Diabetes mellitus is caused by an inability of the pancreas to supply the body with the proper amount of insulin to adequately control blood sugar levels in the blood. Type I diabetes often begins in early life and reflects the necessity for insulin injections. Type II diabetes usually occurs in adults and may be controlled by diet and medications.

6. Normal aging

7. Depression. With drug therapy, psychotherapy or both, seventy percent of patients note an improvement.

8. Denial, anger, bargaining, depression, and acceptance.

9. Pharmacokinetics are changes in the body's ability to handle medications. Important factors in the elderly concern absorption, distri-

bution throughout the body, metabolism, and excretion.

10. A psychotropic drug is a psychiatric medication for the alleviation of symptoms or behavior. Psychotropic drugs may be anti-anxiety, anti-psychotic, and anti-depressant.

Chapter 4

1. Resident and family conversations, resident and family observations, review of medical record, meetings with the interdisciplinary care team, assessing documentation, and MDS initial assessment.
2. Resident satisfaction is the level of perceived quality of services. Quality indicators are factors, which when present, predict a positive experience for residents.
3. Role reversal, juggling many responsibilities, shift in dependency needs, guilt, anxiety, loneliness, and depression.
4. Each department receives notification of new and updated information about residents that effect programming and other factors.
5. Special celebrations, ethnic volunteers, materials in native language, traditional foods, and religious observations.

Chapter 5

1. Quality of work activities, industry competence, and control.
2. Allow adequate time, prepare questions, ask questions, describe job, allow candidates time for questions, give copy of job description, get permission for reference check, and host a facility tour.
3. When policies have not been adhered to on a regular basis or an employee has not been maintaining a consistent job performance.
4. A performance appraisal is a written summary of performance during a particular period of time. By sharing the information between supervisor and employee, the employee has an opportunity to modify behavior.
5. Body language.

Chapter 6

1. Community resource file, informational files, resident room list, volunteer and employee applications, consumable craft and supply items, activity calendars, and newsletters.
2. Material Safety Data Sheets, in-service education records, and policies and procedures.

3. Use of many spaces around the facility for programming with no primary or central location.
4. Wayfinding is a method of locating one's self in a space through use of landmarks, cues, and signage. It is important in reducing confusion and providing a comfortable environment.
5. Nursing helps the activity department by transporting residents to programs, offering training in health issues, encouraging participation in shift reports, and helping with ambulatory programs.

Chapter 7

1. A fiscal year is a twelve-month period of time, such as May 1 of one year to April 30 of the following year, in which financial records of revenue and expenses are maintained.
2. Payroll budget, activity supply budget, and capital expense budget.
3. Using federal and state regulations that apply to your facility as a guide, the owner and/or administrator determines the amount of staff hours per day allotted to your department. The hours are translated into a number of full- and part-time employees that will be needed to provide the necessary coverage.
4. Petty cash is a method of managing your activity supply budget by using a designated cash allotment per month backed up by receipts for purchases.
5. A check request form allows planned purchases outside of the petty cash system and is a good method of written communication on expenditures between administration, bookkeeping, and the activity department.
6. Fewer medications may be necessary and increased resident satisfaction may cause a decrease in the necessary staff interventions.

Chapter 8

1. Maslow's hierarchy of needs is a progressive list of human needs, ranging from the most basic (food, water) to the highest (esteem). The hierarchy is important to activity planning because it relates to motivation and participation factors.
2. Companionship, socialization, encouragement, engagement in the community, improved health, release of tension, and establishment of a feeling of purpose.
3. Setting purposes and goals, designing a program, planning delivery, implementation, and evaluation.
4. Treatment, leisure education, and recreation participation.

5. An interest checklist is a list of the hobbies, interests, occupations, and other resident information that assists in designing programs tailored to resident interests and needs.

Chapter 9

1. De Bolt and Kastner suggest: avoid rushing, do not act superior, share, use humor, be confidential and respectful, and use active listening.
2. Active stimulation refers to an activity established to promote reaction or participation. Passive stimulation makes reference to activity programs that require little in the way of participation.
3. Affective needs involve the yearning for emotional outlets or expressions of feeling. Reminiscence or art therapy are examples of activities to satisfy affective needs.
4. NAAP activity classifications are supportive activities, maintenance activities, and empowerment activities.
5. Cognitive impairments would benefit from use of environmental modifications and life-long activity skills or interests. Determine cognitive functioning and program to strengths. Use programs that are continuation of life roles and present diversional activities.

Chapter 10

1. Individual rather than group programs may be more important because of therapy schedules. Evening programs may also be beneficial
2. The benefits of dance/movement therapy include encouragement of self-expression, control of emotions, enhanced self-awareness, and a form of nonverbal communication.
3. Originally, reality orientation was thought to be an intervention for all dementia residents, but recent research shows that certain forms of dementia and cognitive impairments are irreversible and will not benefit from reality orientation.
4. NCATA is a coalition of The American Art Therapy Association, The American Association For Music Therapy, The American Dance Therapy Association, The American Society for Group Psychotherapy and Psychodrama, The National Association For Drama Therapy, and The National Association For Poetry Therapy.
5. Music is considered a universal language and reaches many residents on some level, despite physical, mental, and social problems.

Chapter 11

1. Developing a family atmosphere, improving knowledge, increasing performance, and re-

minding residents and staff about the activity program.
2. Reciprocal model, remedial model, and social goals model.
3. Cohesion, a part of group dynamics, is the binding or bonding of group members to a common goal.
4. Physical impairment, cognitive problems, social isolation, language or cultural difficulties, and environmental obstacles.
5. A catastrophic reaction is a behavior in cognitively impaired residents where a task becomes overwhelming and a reaction (a sudden mood change or extreme emotion) occurs.

Chapter 12

1. Assessment by MDS, Resident Assessment Protocols, and utilization guidelines.
2. It is a standardized system for assessment and measurement that leads users through a process that ends with care planning.
3. The MDS provides the means for assessment whereas the RAPs illustrate areas where intervention may need to occur. Without going through the assessment and problem identification steps, care planning would be difficult to accomplish.
4. A policy is a written statement that summarizes the standard of practice for a particular area in the facility. A procedure outlines the step-by-step process for meeting the objectives of the policy statement.
5. Integrated or focused charting is important because it links the interdisciplinary team together by having them use one area for documentation and progress of residents.

Chapter 13

1. OBRA stands for the Omnibus Budget Reconciliation Act of 1987 which changed the survey procedure to include a greater focus on residents' individuality and quality of life issues.
2. After a problem has been identified during the survey process, a remedy must be determined. In order to do this, the survey team must look at the scope of the deficiency and if the problem is isolated, occasional, or widespread. The severity refers to whether the problem causes no harm, potential for harm, immediate jeopardy, or serious safety issues.
3. Interventions you have used, on what basis programs were chosen, and resident participation patterns.
4. A resident sample is a selection of residents used by survey teams to give them an idea of

the type of care and services being provided to all residents.

5. OSCAR data is information compiled and sent to facilities concerning their history of deficiencies, as well as a review of these deficiencies in comparison to national and regional data.

Chapter 14

1. Quality assurance is the identification of areas for improvement. Quality improvement is a management philosophy and practice that establishes quality as an organization's first priority.
2. Quality assurance.
3. Identification of potential accidents and planning interventions to minimize risk.
4. Focus, analyze, develop, and execute.
5. Unclear purpose, using short-term goals instead of long-term goals, changing management, difficulty defining customer, high medical cost, and varying educational levels of employees.

Chapter 15

1. Problem clarification, review of factors influencing the problem, brainstorming, looking at alternatives, assigning roles and responsibilities, and implementation and evaluation.
2. Use of inappropriate clothing, salutations such as "dearie" or "honey," and use of child-like accessories.
3. Identification of the problem, detailed individual assessment, system of support, and finding a mentor.
4. A cycle of repeated experiences an individual has that demonstrates to the person he or she had no effect on the outcome.
5. Speak to your administrator, meet with your residents, design a new program, allow time for changes, and contact a consultant, if available.

Chapter 16

1. Expand and enhance the activity program, bring additional nonstaff reinforcement to resident goals and program plans, and provide a continuous bond to the community for residents.
2. To do something useful, enjoy the work, socialization, opportunity for recognition and acceptance, chance to obtain new abilities, fulfill course requirements, and relieve loneliness or boredom.
3. Thank you notes, personal praise, articles in facility newsletter, and taking an interest in their personal lives.

4. Resident-centered programs, activity administrative projects, and special assignments.
5. Training: policies and procedures, resident rights, aging process, handling residents, medication, and restraints. Orientation: fire/safety, alarms, introductions, handwashing/universal precautions, resident restrictions and precautions, parking, incident reports, and tour.

Chapter 17

1. McMillan and Chavis suggest membership, influence, social integration, and emotional connection. Other ideas include shared experiences, availability of services, neighbors and friends, familiar places, and landmarks.
2. Bring community services in, take groups out into the community, and establish partnerships to design programs of interest to residents that also meet community needs.
3. Elderly act as resources for children and children act as a resource for the elderly. Partnering with mutual goals benefits elderly and children alike.

Chapter 18

1. Problems of aging, tailoring recreation programs to specific residents, learning about management, information on specific medical conditions, and working with families.
2. Staff communication increases, staff role differences diminish, and staff meetings are improved.
3. Respite care is a short-term program for caregivers in which they are relieved of caregiving duties while the resident is cared for in a facility. Informal caregivers need special training and information.
4. The four stages of adjustment to institutionalization, according to Soloman, are decision to enter a facility, admission to the facility, change to a higher level of care, and death.
5. Simulation programs give participants a chance to experience a situation that is, at times, a better teaching tool than a traditional lecture.

Chapter 19

1. NAAP, ATRA, and NTRS.
2. Dress for success, master effective speaking skills, come to meetings prepared, welcome responsibility, increase ethics, learn more, share with colleagues, assert yourself, seek new challenges, and accept defeat gracefully.
3. ADC stands for Activity Director Certified, a

title that meets the National Certification Council for Activity Professional's standards to direct, coordinate, and supervise an activity program, staff, and department, primarily in a geriatric facility. CTRS stands for Certified Therapeutic Recreation Specialist and is a title that meets the National Council for Therapeutic Recreation Certification's standards to select activity modalities and to treat or maintain physical, mental, or emotional well-being of patients.

ANSWERS TO THE SELF-ASSESSMENT EXAMINATION— CHAPTER 20

True/False

1. T
2. T
3. T
4. T
5. T
6. F
7. T
8. T
9. F
10. T
11. F
12. T
13. F
14. F
15. F
16. T
17. F
18. F
19. T
20. T
21. F
22. T
23. T
24. F
25. T
26. F
27. F
28. T
29. F
30. T
31. T
32. T
33. F
34. F
35. F
36. T
37. F
38. F
39. F
40. T

Fill in the Blank

1. quality
2. integumentary
3. sandwich generation
4. empowerment
5. life review
6. cultural diversity
7. cost-benefit analysis
8. proprietary
9. gerontologist
10. staffing pattern
11. burnout
12. quality of care assessment
13. volunteer log sheet
14. termination
15. intergenerational
16. function request form
17. triggers
18. activity
19. Activity Consultant Certified
20. capital budget
21. confidentiality
22. Omnibus Budget Reconciliation Act
23. dementia
24. face sheet
25. nervous
26. activity assessment
27. delegation
28. drama therapy
29. Material Safety Data Sheets
30. fifteen
31. documentation
32. recognition
33. ageism
34. centralized
35. press release
36. sensory stimulation
37. policy and procedure
38. ombudsman's
39. incontinence
40. MDS 2.0

Multiple Choice ....

1. b
2. c
3. d
4. b
5. d
6. c
7. c
8. e
9. e
10. c
11. d
12. c
13. b
14. e
15. a
16. b
17. a
18. f
19. d
20. f
21. d
22. c
23. c
24. c
25. a

26. b
27. f
28. d
29. b
30. a
31. f
32. a
33. a
34. a
35. c
36. b
37. b
38. b
39. e
40. d
41. e
42. a
43. a
44. e
45. f
46. d
47. b
48. b
49. a
50. a

A P P E N D I X   F

• •

MDS 2.0 Forms

Numeric Identifier _____

MINIMUM DATA SET (MDS) — *VERSION 2.0*
FOR NURSING HOME RESIDENT ASSESSMENT AND CARE SCREENING

BASIC ASSESSMENT TRACKING FORM

SECTION AA. IDENTIFICATION INFORMATION

1.	RESIDENT NAME®	a. (First) b. (Middle Initial) c. (Last) d. (Jr/Sr)
2.	GENDER®	1. Male 2. Female
3.	BIRTHDATE®	☐☐ — ☐☐ — ☐☐☐☐ Month / Day / Year
4.	RACE/ ETHNICITY	1. American Indian/Alaskan Native 4. Hispanic 2. Asian/Pacific Islander 5. White, not of 3. Black, not of Hispanic origin Hispanic origin
5.	SOCIAL SECURITY® AND MEDICARE NUMBERS® [C in 1ˢᵗ box if non med. no.]	a. Social Security Number ☐☐☐ — ☐☐ — ☐☐☐☐ b. Medicare number (or comparable railroad insurance number) ☐☐☐☐☐☐☐☐☐☐☐☐
6.	FACILITY PROVIDER NO.®	a. State No. ☐☐☐☐☐☐☐☐☐☐☐☐☐☐ b. Federal No. ☐☐☐☐☐☐☐☐☐☐
7.	MEDICAID NO. ["+" if pending, "N" if not a Medicaid recipient ®	☐☐☐☐☐☐☐☐☐☐☐☐☐
8.	REASONS FOR ASSESS-MENT	[Note—Other codes do not apply to this form] **a. Primary reason for assessment** 1. Admission assessment (required by day 14) 2. Annual assessment 3. Significant change in status assessment 4. Significant correction of prior assessment 5. Quarterly review assessment 0. *NONE OF ABOVE* *b. Special codes for use with supplemental assessment types in Case Mix demonstration states or other states where required* 1. 5 day assessment 2. 30 day assessment 3. 60 day assessment 4. Quarterly assessment using full MDS form 5. Readmission/return assessment 6. Other state required assessment
9.	SIGNATURES OF PERSONS COMPLETING THESE ITEMS:	

GENERAL INSTRUCTIONS

Complete this information for submission with all full and quarterly assessments (Admission, Annual, Significant Change, State or Medicare required assessments, or Quarterly Reviews, etc.)

a. Signatures	Title	Date
b.		Date

® = Key items for computerized resident tracking

☐ = When box blank, must enter number or letter   ☐ = When letter in box, check if condition applies

MDS 2.0 10/18/94N
October, 1995

Figure F-1   MDS 2.0 Basic Assessment Tracking Form.

MINIMUM DATA SET (MDS) — VERSION 2.0
FOR NURSING HOME RESIDENT ASSESSMENT AND CARE SCREENING

BACKGROUND (FACE SHEET) INFORMATION AT ADMISSION

SECTION AB. DEMOGRAPHIC INFORMATION

1.	DATE OF ENTRY	Date the stay began. Note — Does not include readmission if record was closed at time of temporary discharge to hospital, etc. In such cases, use prior admission date [ ][ ] — [ ][ ] — [ ][ ][ ][ ] Month Day Year
2.	ADMITTED FROM (AT ENTRY)	1. Private home/apt. with no home health services 2. Private home/apt. with home health services 3. Board and care/assisted living/group home 4. Nursing home 5. Acute care hospital 6. Psychiatric hospital, MR/DD facility 7. Rehabilitation hospital 8. Other
3.	LIVED ALONE (PRIOR TO ENTRY)	0. No 1. Yes 2. In other facility
4.	ZIP CODE OF PRIOR PRIMARY RESIDENCE	[ ][ ][ ][ ][ ]
5.	RESIDEN-TIAL HISTORY 5 YEARS PRIOR TO ENTRY	(Check all settings resident lived in during 5 years prior to date of entry given in item AB1 above) Prior stay at this nursing home	a. Stay in other nursing home	b. Other residential facility—board and care home, assisted living, group home	c. MH/psychiatric setting	d. MR/DD setting	e. NONE OF ABOVE	f.
6.	LIFETIME OCCUPA-TION(S) [Put "/" between two occupations]	[ ][ ][ ][ ][ ][ ][ ][ ][ ][ ][ ][ ][ ][ ][ ][ ][ ][ ][ ]
7.	EDUCATION (Highest Level Completed)	1. No schooling 5. Technical or trade school 2. 8th grade/less 6. Some college 3. 9-11 grades 7. Bachelor's degree 4. High school 8. Graduate degree
8.	LANGUAGE	(Code for correct response) a. Primary Language 0. English 1. Spanish 2. French 3. Other b. If other, specify [ ][ ][ ][ ][ ][ ][ ][ ]
9.	MENTAL HEALTH HISTORY	Does resident's RECORD indicate any history of mental retardation, mental illness, or developmental disability problem? 0. No 1. Yes
10.	CONDITIONS RELATED TO MR/DD STATUS	(Check all conditions that are related to MR/DD status that were manifested before age 22, and are likely to continue indefinitely) Not applicable—no MR/DD (Skip to AB11)	a. MR/DD with organic condition Down's syndrome	b. Autism	c. Epilepsy	d. Other organic condition related to MR/DD	e. MR/DD with no organic condition	f.
11.	DATE BACK-GROUND INFORMA-TION COMPLETED	[ ][ ] — [ ][ ] — [ ][ ][ ][ ] Month Day Year

SECTION AC. CUSTOMARY ROUTINE

1.	CUSTOMARY ROUTINE	(Check all that apply. If all information UNKNOWN, check last box only.)
	(In year prior to DATE OF ENTRY to this nursing home, or year last in community if now being admitted from another nursing home)	**CYCLE OF DAILY EVENTS**

Stays up late at night (e.g., after 9 pm)	a.
Naps regularly during day (at least 1 hour)	b.
Goes out 1+ days a week	c.
Stays busy with hobbies, reading, or fixed daily routine	d.
Spends most of time alone or watching TV	e.
Moves independently indoors (with appliances, if used)	f.
Use of tobacco products at least daily	g.
NONE OF ABOVE	h.
EATING PATTERNS	
Distinct food preferences	i.
Eats between meals all or most days	j.
Use of alcoholic beverage(s) at least weekly	k.
NONE OF ABOVE	l.
ADL PATTERNS	
In bedclothes much of day	m.
Wakens to toilet all or most nights	n.
Has irregular bowel movement pattern	o.
Showers for bathing	p.
Bathing in PM	q.
NONE OF ABOVE	r.
INVOLVEMENT PATTERNS	
Daily contact with relatives/close friends	s.
Usually attends church, temple, synagogue (etc.)	t.
Finds strength in faith	u.
Daily animal companion/presence	v.
Involved in group activities	w.
NONE OF ABOVE	x.
UNKNOWN—Resident/family unable to provide information	y.

[END]

SECTION AD. FACE SHEET SIGNATURES

SIGNATURES OF PERSONS COMPLETING FACE SHEET:

a. Signature of RN Assessment Coordinator				Date
b. Signatures	Title		Sections	Date
c.				Date
d.				Date
e.				Date
f.				Date
g.				Date

[ ] = When box blank, must enter number or letter   [a.] = When letter in box, check if condition applies

October, 1996

MDS 2.0   10/18/94N

Figure F-2   MDS 2.0 Background (Face Sheet) Information At Admission, Sections AB–AD.

Resident _____ CH 1: Overview _____ Numeric Identifier_____ HCFA's RAI Version 2.0 Manual

MINIMUM DATA SET (MDS) — *VERSION 2.0*
FOR NURSING HOME RESIDENT ASSESSMENT AND CARE SCREENING
FULL ASSESSMENT FORM
(Status in last 7 days, unless other time frame indicated)

SECTION A. IDENTIFICATION AND BACKGROUND INFORMATION

1.	RESIDENT NAME				
		a. (First)	b. (Middle Initial)	c. (Last)	d. (Jr/Sr)

2.	ROOM NUMBER	

3.	ASSESS-MENT REFERENCE DATE	a. Last day of MDS observation period
		Month — Day — Year
		b. Original (0) or corrected copy of form (enter number of correction)

4a.	DATE OF REENTRY	Date of reentry from most recent temporary discharge to a hospital in last 90 days (or since last assessment or admission if less than 90 days)
		Month — Day — Year

5.	MARITAL STATUS	1. Never married 3. Widowed 5. Divorced 2. Married 4. Separated

6.	MEDICAL RECORD NO.	

7. CURRENT PAYMENT SOURCES FOR N.H. STAY (Billing Office to indicate; check all that apply in last 30 days)

Medicaid per diem	a.	VA per diem	f.
Medicare per diem	b.	Self or family pays for full per diem	g.
Medicare ancillary part A	c.	Medicaid resident liability or Medicare co-payment	h.
Medicare ancillary part B	d.	Private insurance per diem (including co-payment)	i.
CHAMPUS per diem	e.	Other per diem	j.

8. REASONS FOR ASSESS-MENT
[Note—If this is a discharge or reentry assessment, only a limited subset of MDS items need be completed]

a. Primary reason for assessment
1. Admission assessment (required by day 14)
2. Annual assessment
3. Significant change in status assessment
4. Significant correction of prior assessment
5. Quarterly review assessment
6. Discharged—return not anticipated
7. Discharged—return anticipated
8. Discharged prior to completing initial assessment
9. Reentry
0. *NONE OF ABOVE*

b. Special codes for use with supplemental assessment types in Case Mix demonstration states or other states where required
1. 5 day assessment
2. 30 day assessment
3. 60 day assessment
4. Quarterly assessment using full MDS form
5. Readmission/return assessment
6. Other state required assessment

9. RESPONSI-BILITY/ LEGAL GUARDIAN (Check all that apply)

		Durable power attorney/financial	d.
Legal guardian	a.	Family member responsible	e.
Other legal oversight	b.	Patient responsible for self	f.
Durable power of attorney/health care	c.	*NONE OF ABOVE*	g.

10. ADVANCED DIRECTIVES (For those items with supporting documentation in the medical record, check all that apply)

Living will	a.	Feeding restrictions	f.
Do not resuscitate	b.	Medication restrictions	g.
Do not hospitalize	c.	Other treatment restrictions	h.
Organ donation	d.	*NONE OF ABOVE*	i.
Autopsy request	e.		

SECTION B. COGNITIVE PATTERNS

1.	COMATOSE	(Persistent vegetative state/no discernible consciousness) 0. No 1. Yes (If yes, skip to Section G)

2.	MEMORY	(Recall of what was learned or known)
		a. Short-term memory OK—seems/appears to recall after 5 minutes 0. Memory OK 1. Memory problem
		b. Long-term memory OK—seems/appears to recall long past 0. Memory OK 1. Memory problem

☐ = When box blank, must enter number or letter
☐a. = When letter in box, check if condition applies

3. MEMORY/RECALL ABILITY (Check all that resident was normally able to recall during last 7 days)

Current season	a.		
Location of own room	b.	That he/she is in a nursing home	d.
Staff names/faces	c.	*NONE OF ABOVE* are recalled	e.

4. COGNITIVE SKILLS FOR DAILY DECISION-MAKING (Made decisions regarding tasks of daily life)
0. INDEPENDENT—decisions consistent/reasonable
1. MODIFIED INDEPENDENCE—some difficulty in new situations only
2. MODERATELY IMPAIRED—decisions poor; cues/supervision required
3. SEVERELY IMPAIRED—never/rarely made decisions

5. INDICATORS OF DELIRIUM—PERIODIC DISOR-DERED THINKING/AWARENESS (Code for behavior in the last 7 days.) [Note: Accurate assessment requires conversations with staff and family who have direct knowledge of resident's behavior over this time].
0. Behavior not present
1. Behavior present, not of recent onset
2. Behavior present, over last 7 days appears different from resident's usual functioning (e.g., new onset or worsening)

a. EASILY DISTRACTED—(e.g., difficulty paying attention; gets sidetracked)
b. PERIODS OF ALTERED PERCEPTION OR AWARENESS OF SURROUNDINGS—(e.g., moves lips or talks to someone not present; believes he/she is somewhere else; confuses night and day)
c. EPISODES OF DISORGANIZED SPEECH—(e.g., speech is incoherent, nonsensical, irrelevant, or rambling from subject to subject; loses train of thought)
d. PERIODS OF RESTLESSNESS—(e.g., fidgeting or picking at skin, clothing, napkins, etc; frequent position changes; repetitive physical movements or calling out)
e. PERIODS OF LETHARGY—(e.g., sluggishness; staring into space; difficult to arouse; little body movement)
f. MENTAL FUNCTION VARIES OVER THE COURSE OF THE DAY—(e.g., sometimes better, sometimes worse; behaviors sometimes present, sometimes not)

6. CHANGE IN COGNITIVE STATUS Resident's cognitive status, skills, or abilities have changed as compared to status of 90 days ago (or since last assessment if less than 90 days)
0. No change 1. Improved 2. Deteriorated

SECTION C. COMMUNICATION/HEARING PATTERNS

1. HEARING (With hearing appliance, if used)
0. HEARS ADEQUATELY—normal talk, TV, phone
1. MINIMAL DIFFICULTY when not in quiet setting
2. HEARS IN SPECIAL SITUATIONS ONLY—speaker has to adjust tonal quality and speak distinctly
3. HIGHLY IMPAIRED/absence of useful hearing

2. COMMUNI-CATION DEVICES/TECH-NIQUES (Check all that apply during last 7 days)

Hearing aid, present and used	a.
Hearing aid, present and not used regularly	b.
Other receptive comm. techniques used (e.g., lip reading)	c.
NONE OF ABOVE	d.

3. MODES OF EXPRESSION (Check all used by resident to make needs known)

Speech	a.	Signs/gestures/sounds	d.
Writing messages to express or clarify needs	b.	Communication board	e.
American sign language or Braille	c.	Other	f.
		NONE OF ABOVE	g.

4. MAKING SELF UNDER-STOOD (Expressing information content—however able)
0. UNDERSTOOD
1. USUALLY UNDERSTOOD—difficulty finding words or finishing thoughts
2. SOMETIMES UNDERSTOOD—ability is limited to making concrete requests
3. RARELY/NEVER UNDERSTOOD

5. SPEECH CLARITY (Code for speech in the last 7 days)
0. CLEAR SPEECH—distinct, intelligible words
1. UNCLEAR SPEECH—slurred, mumbled words
2. NO SPEECH—absence of spoken words

6. ABILITY TO UNDER-STAND OTHERS (Understanding verbal information content—however able)
0. UNDERSTANDS
1. USUALLY UNDERSTANDS—may miss some part/intent of message
2. SOMETIMES UNDERSTANDS—responds adequately to simple, direct communication
3. RARELY/NEVER UNDERSTANDS

7. CHANGE IN COMMUNI-CATION/HEARING Resident's ability to express, understand, or hear information has changed as compared to status of 90 days ago (or since last assessment if less than 90 days)
0. No change 1. Improved 2. Deteriorated

MDS 2.0 10/18/94N October, 1995

Figure F-3 MDS 2.0 Full Assessment Form, Sections A–C.

Resident _____ HCFA's RAI Version 2.0 Manual   Numeric Identifier _____   CH 1: Overview

SECTION D. VISION PATTERNS

1.	VISION	(Ability to see in adequate light and with glasses if used) 0. ADEQUATE—sees fine detail, including regular print in newspapers/books 1. IMPAIRED—sees large print, but not regular print in newspapers/books 2. MODERATELY IMPAIRED—limited vision; not able to see newspaper headlines, but can identify objects 3. HIGHLY IMPAIRED—object identification in question, but eyes appear to follow objects 4. SEVERELY IMPAIRED—no vision or sees only light, colors, or shapes; eyes do not appear to follow objects	
2.	VISUAL LIMITATIONS/ DIFFICULTIES	Side vision problems—decreased peripheral vision (e.g., leaves food on one side of tray, difficulty traveling, bumps into people and objects, misjudges placement of chair when seating self)	a.
		Experiences any of following: sees halos or rings around lights; sees flashes of light; sees "curtains" over eyes	b.
		NONE OF ABOVE	c.
3.	VISUAL APPLIANCES	Glasses; contact lenses; magnifying glass 0. No 1. Yes	

SECTION E. MOOD AND BEHAVIOR PATTERNS

| 1. | INDICATORS OF DEPRES- SION, ANXIETY, SAD MOOD | (Code for indicators observed in last 30 days, irrespective of the assumed cause)
0. Indicator not exhibited in last 30 days
1. Indicator of this type exhibited up to five days a week
2. Indicator of this type exhibited daily or almost daily (6, 7 days a week) | |

VERBAL EXPRESSIONS OF DISTRESS

a. Resident made negative statements—e.g., "Nothing matters; Would rather be dead; What's the use; Regrets having lived so long; Let me die"

b. Repetitive questions—e.g., "Where do I go; What do I do?"

c. Repetitive verbalizations— e.g., calling out for help, ("God help me")

d. Persistent anger with self or others—e.g., easily annoyed, anger at placement in nursing home; anger at care received

e. Self deprecation—e.g., "I am nothing; I am of no use to anyone"

f. Expressions of what appear to be unrealistic fears—e.g., fear of being abandoned, left alone, being with others

g. Recurrent statements that something terrible is about to happen—e.g., believes he or she is about to die, have a heart attack

h. Repetitive health complaints—e.g., persistently seeks medical attention, obsessive concern with body functions

i. Repetitive anxious complaints/concerns (non-health related) e.g., persistently seeks attention/reassurance regarding schedules, meals, laundry, clothing, relationship issues

SLEEP-CYCLE ISSUES

j. Unpleasant mood in morning

k. Insomnia/change in usual sleep pattern

SAD, APATHETIC, ANXIOUS APPEARANCE

l. Sad, pained, worried facial expressions—e.g., furrowed brows

m. Crying, tearfulness

n. Repetitive physical movements—e.g., pacing, hand wringing, restlessness, fidgeting, picking

LOSS OF INTEREST

o. Withdrawal from activities of interest—e.g., no interest in long standing activities or being with family/friends

p. Reduced social interaction

| 2. | MOOD PERSIS- TENCE | One or more indicators of depressed, sad or anxious mood were not easily altered by attempts to "cheer up", console, or reassure the resident over last 7 days
0. No mood indicators   1. Indicators present, easily altered   2. Indicators present, not easily altered | |
| 3. | CHANGE IN MOOD | Resident's mood status has changed as compared to status of 90 days ago (or since last assessment if less than 90 days)
0. No change   1. Improved   2. Deteriorated | |

| 4. | BEHAVIORAL SYMPTOMS | (A) Behavioral symptom frequency in last 7 days
0. Behavior not exhibited in last 7 days
1. Behavior of this type occurred 1 to 3 days in last 7 days
2. Behavior of this type occurred 4 to 6 days, but less than daily
3. Behavior of this type occurred daily

(B) Behavioral symptom alterability in last 7 days
0. Behavior not present OR behavior was easily altered
1. Behavior was not easily altered | (A) (B) |

a. WANDERING (moved with no rational purpose, seemingly oblivious to needs or safety)

b. VERBALLY ABUSIVE BEHAVIORAL SYMPTOMS (others were threatened, screamed at, cursed at)

c. PHYSICALLY ABUSIVE BEHAVIORAL SYMPTOMS (others were hit, shoved, scratched, sexually abused)

d. SOCIALLY INAPPROPRIATE/DISRUPTIVE BEHAVIORAL SYMPTOMS (made disruptive sounds, noisiness, screaming, self-abusive acts, sexual behavior or disrobing in public, smeared/threw food/feces, hoarding, rummaged through others' belongings)

e. RESISTS CARE (resisted taking medications/ injections, ADL assistance, or eating)

| 5. | CHANGE IN BEHAVIORAL SYMPTOMS | Resident's behavior status has changed as compared to status of 90 days ago (or since last assessment if less than 90 days)
0. No change   1. Improved   2. Deteriorated | |

SECTION F. PSYCHOSOCIAL WELL-BEING

1.	SENSE OF INITIATIVE/ INVOLVE- MENT	At ease interacting with others	a.
		At ease doing planned or structured activities	b.
		At ease doing self-initiated activities	c.
		Establishes own goals	d.
		Pursues involvement in life of facility (e.g., makes/keeps friends; involved in group activities; responds positively to new activities; assists at religious services)	e.
		Accepts invitations into most group activities	f.
		NONE OF ABOVE	g.
2.	UNSETTLED RELATION- SHIPS	Covert/open conflict with or repeated criticism of staff	a.
		Unhappy with roommate	b.
		Unhappy with residents other than roommate	c.
		Openly expresses conflict/anger with family/friends	d.
		Absence of personal contact with family/friends	e.
		Recent loss of close family member/friend	f.
		Does not adjust easily to change in routines	g.
		NONE OF ABOVE	h.
3.	PAST ROLES	Strong identification with past roles and life status	a.
		Expresses sadness/anger/empty feeling over lost roles/status	b.
		Resident perceives that daily routine (customary routine, activities) is very different from prior pattern in the community	c.
		NONE OF ABOVE	d.

SECTION G. PHYSICAL FUNCTIONING AND STRUCTURAL PROBLEMS

1. **(A) ADL SELF-PERFORMANCE**—(Code for resident's PERFORMANCE OVER ALL SHIFTS during last 7 days—Not including setup)

   0. INDEPENDENT—No help or oversight —OR— Help/oversight provided only 1 or 2 times during last 7 days

   1. SUPERVISION—Oversight, encouragement or cueing provided 3 or more times during last 7 days —OR— Supervision (3 or more times) plus physical assistance provided only 1 or 2 times during last 7 days

   2. LIMITED ASSISTANCE—Resident highly involved in activity; received physical help in guided maneuvering of limbs or other nonweight bearing assistance 3 or more times — OR—More help provided only 1 or 2 times during last 7 days

   3. EXTENSIVE ASSISTANCE—While resident performed part of activity, over last 7-day period, help of following type(s) provided 3 or more times:
      — Weight-bearing support
      — Full staff performance during part (but not all) of last 7 days

   4. TOTAL DEPENDENCE—Full staff performance of activity during entire 7 days

   8. ACTIVITY DID NOT OCCUR during entire 7 days

   (B) ADL SUPPORT PROVIDED—(Code for MOST SUPPORT PROVIDED OVER ALL SHIFTS during last 7 days; code regardless of resident's self-performance classification)

   0. No setup or physical help from staff
   1. Setup help only
   2. One person physical assist
   3. Two+ persons physical assist
   8. ADL activity itself did not occur during entire 7 days

			(A) SELF-PERF	(B) SUPPORT
a.	BED MOBILITY	How resident moves to and from lying position, turns side to side, and positions body while in bed		
b.	TRANSFER	How resident moves between surfaces—to/from: bed, chair, wheelchair, standing position (EXCLUDE to/from bath/toilet)		
c.	WALK IN ROOM	How resident walks between locations in his/her room		
d.	WALK IN CORRIDOR	How resident walks in corridor on unit		
e.	LOCOMO- TION ON UNIT	How resident moves between locations in his/her room and adjacent corridor on same floor. If in wheelchair, self-sufficiency once in chair		
f.	LOCOMO- TION OFF UNIT	How resident moves to and returns from off unit locations (e.g., areas set aside for dining, activities, or treatments). If facility has only one floor, how resident moves to and from distant areas on the floor. If in wheelchair, self-sufficiency once in chair		
g.	DRESSING	How resident puts on, fastens, and takes off all items of street clothing, including donning/removing prosthesis		
h.	EATING	How resident eats and drinks (regardless of skill). Includes intake of nourishment by other means (e.g., tube feeding, total parenteral nutrition)		
i.	TOILET USE	How resident uses the toilet room (or commode, bedpan, urinal); transfer on/off toilet, cleanses, changes pad, manages ostomy or catheter, adjusts clothes		
j.	PERSONAL HYGIENE	How resident maintains personal hygiene, including combing hair, brushing teeth, shaving, applying makeup, washing/drying face, hands, and perineum (EXCLUDE baths and showers)		

Figure F-4   MDS 2.0 Full Assessment Form, Sections D–G (*continued on next page*).

CH 1: Overview
Resident

Numeric Identifier

2.	BATHING	How resident takes full-body bath/shower, sponge bath, and transfers in/out of tub/shower (EXCLUDE washing of back and hair.) *Code for most dependent in self-performance and support.* (A) BATHING SELF-PERFORMANCE codes appear below	(A)	(B)
		0. Independent—No help provided		
		1. Supervision—Oversight help only		
		2. Physical help limited to transfer only		
		3. Physical help in part of bathing activity		
		4. Total dependence		
		8. Activity itself did not occur during entire 7 days		
		(Bathing support codes are as defined in Item 1, code B above)		

3.	TEST FOR BALANCE (see training manual)	(Code for ability during test in the last 7 days) 0. Maintained position as required in test 1. Unsteady, but able to rebalance self without physical support 2. Partial physical support during test; or stands (sits) but does not follow directions for test 3. Not able to attempt test without physical help	
		a. Balance while standing	
		b. Balance while sitting—position, trunk control	

4.	FUNCTIONAL LIMITATION IN RANGE OF MOTION (see training manual)	(Code for limitations during last 7 days that interfered with daily functions or placed resident at risk of injury) (A) RANGE OF MOTION (B) VOLUNTARY MOVEMENT 0. No limitation 0. No loss 1. Limitation on one side 1. Partial loss 2. Limitation on both sides 2. Full loss	(A)	(B)
		a. Neck		
		b. Arm—Including shoulder or elbow		
		c. Hand—Including wrist or fingers		
		d. Leg—Including hip or knee		
		e. Foot—Including ankle or toes		
		f. Other limitation or loss		

5.	MODES OF LOCOMOTION	(Check all that apply during last 7 days)		
		Cane/walker/crutch	a.	Wheelchair primary mode of locomotion	d.
		Wheeled self	b.		
		Other person wheeled	c.	NONE OF ABOVE	e.

6.	MODES OF TRANSFER	(Check all that apply during last 7 days)		
		Bedfast all or most of time	a.	Lifted mechanically	d.
		Bed rails used for bed mobility or transfer	b.	Transfer aid (e.g., slide board, trapeze, cane, walker, brace)	e.
		Lifted manually	c.	NONE OF ABOVE	f.

7.	TASK SEGMENTATION	Some or all of ADL activities were broken into subtasks during last 7 days so that resident could perform them 0. No 1. Yes	

8.	ADL FUNCTIONAL REHABILITATION POTENTIAL	Resident believes he/she is capable of increased independence in at least some ADLs	a.
		Direct care staff believe resident is capable of increased independence in at least some ADLs	b.
		Resident able to perform tasks/activity but is very slow	c.
		Difference in ADL Self-Performance or ADL Support, comparing mornings to evenings	d.
		NONE OF ABOVE	e.

9.	CHANGE IN ADL FUNCTION	Resident's ADL self-performance status has changed as compared to status of 90 days ago (or since last assessment if less than 90 days) 0. No change 1. Improved 2. Deteriorated	

SECTION H. CONTINENCE IN LAST 14 DAYS

1.	CONTINENCE SELF-CONTROL CATEGORIES (Code for resident's PERFORMANCE OVER ALL SHIFTS)
	0. CONTINENT—Complete control [includes use of indwelling urinary catheter or ostomy device that does not leak urine or stool]
	1. USUALLY CONTINENT—BLADDER, incontinent episodes once a week or less; BOWEL, less than weekly
	2. OCCASIONALLY INCONTINENT—BLADDER, 2 or more times a week but not daily; BOWEL, once a week
	3. FREQUENTLY INCONTINENT—BLADDER, tended to be incontinent daily, but some control present (e.g., on day shift); BOWEL, 2-3 times a week
	4. INCONTINENT—Had inadequate control BLADDER, multiple daily episodes; BOWEL, all (or almost all) of the time

a.	BOWEL CONTINENCE	Control of bowel movement, with appliance or bowel continence programs, if employed	
b.	BLADDER CONTINENCE	Control of urinary bladder function (if dribbles, volume insufficient to soak through underpants), with appliances (e.g., foley) or continence programs, if employed	

2.	BOWEL ELIMINATION PATTERN	Bowel elimination pattern regular—at least one movement every three days	a.	Diarrhea	c.
				Fecal impaction	d.
		Constipation	b.	NONE OF ABOVE	e.

MDS 2.0 10/18/94N   October, 1995

3.	APPLIANCES AND PROGRAMS	Any scheduled toileting plan	a.	Did not use toilet room/ commode/urinal	f.
		Bladder retraining program	b.	Pads/briefs used	g.
		External (condom) catheter	c.	Enemas/irrigation	h.
		Indwelling catheter	d.	Ostomy present	i.
		Intermittent catheter	e.	NONE OF ABOVE	

4.	CHANGE IN URINARY CONTINENCE	Resident's urinary continence has changed as compared to status of 90 days ago (or since last assessment if less than 90 days) 0. No change 1. Improved 2. Deteriorated	

SECTION I. DISEASE DIAGNOSES

Check only those diseases that have a relationship to current ADL status, cognitive status, mood and behavior status, medical treatments, nursing monitoring, or risk of death. (Do not list inactive diagnoses.)

1.	DISEASES	(If none apply, CHECK the NONE OF ABOVE box)		
		ENDOCRINE/METABOLIC/ NUTRITIONAL		Hemiplegia/Hemiparesis	v.
				Multiple sclerosis	w.
		Diabetes mellitus	a.	Paraplegia	x.
		Hyperthyroidism	b.	Parkinson's disease	y.
		Hypothyroidism	c.	Quadriplegia	z.
		HEART/CIRCULATION		Seizure disorder	aa.
		Arteriosclerotic heart disease (ASHD)	d.	Transient ischemic attack (TIA)	bb.
				Traumatic brain injury	cc.
		Cardiac dysrhythmias	e.	PSYCHIATRIC/MOOD	
		Congestive heart failure	f.	Anxiety disorder	dd.
		Deep vein thrombosis	g.	Depression	ee.
		Hypertension	h.	Manic depression (bipolar disease)	ff.
		Hypotension	i.	Schizophrenia	gg.
		Peripheral vascular disease	j.	PULMONARY	
		Other cardiovascular disease	k.	Asthma	hh.
		MUSCULOSKELETAL		Emphysema/COPD	ii.
		Arthritis	l.	SENSORY	
		Hip fracture	m.	Cataracts	jj.
		Missing limb (e.g., amputation)	n.	Diabetic retinopathy	kk.
		Osteoporosis	o.	Glaucoma	ll.
		Pathological bone fracture	p.	Macular degeneration	mm.
		NEUROLOGICAL		OTHER	
		Alzheimer's disease	q.	Allergies	nn.
		Aphasia	r.	Anemia	oo.
		Cerebral palsy	s.	Cancer	pp.
		Cerebrovascular accident (stroke)	t.	Renal failure	qq.
		Dementia other than Alzheimer's disease	u.	NONE OF ABOVE	rr.

2.	INFECTIONS	(If none apply, CHECK the NONE OF ABOVE box)		
		Antibiotic resistant infection (e.g., Methicillin resistant staph)	a.	Septicemia	g.
				Sexually transmitted diseases	h.
		Clostridium difficile (c. diff.)	b.	Tuberculosis	i.
		Conjunctivitis	c.	Urinary tract infection in last 30 days	j.
		HIV infection	d.	Viral hepatitis	k.
		Pneumonia	e.	Wound infection	l.
		Respiratory infection	f.	NONE OF ABOVE	m.

3.	OTHER CURRENT OR MORE DETAILED DIAGNOSES AND ICD-9 CODES	a.		·
		b.		·
		c.		·
		d.		·

SECTION J. HEALTH CONDITIONS

1.	PROBLEM CONDITIONS	(Check all problems present in last 7 days unless other time frame is indicated)		
		INDICATORS OF FLUID STATUS		Dizziness/Vertigo	f.
		Weight gain or loss of 3 or more pounds within a 7 day period	a.	Edema	g.
				Fever	h.
				Hallucinations	i.
		Inability to lie flat due to shortness of breath	b.	Internal bleeding	j.
				Recurrent lung aspirations in last 90 days	k.
		Dehydrated; output exceeds input	c.	Shortness of breath	l.
				Syncope (fainting)	m.
		Insufficient fluid; did NOT consume all/almost all liquids provided during last 3 days	d.	Unsteady gait	n.
				Vomiting	o.
		OTHER		NONE OF ABOVE	p.
		Delusions	e.		

Figure F-5 MDS 2.0 Full Assessment Form, Sections G (continued)–J (continued on next page).

2.	PAIN SYMPTOMS	(Code the highest level of pain present in the last 7 days)		
		a. FREQUENCY with which resident complains or shows evidence of pain 0. No pain (skip to J4) 1. Pain less than daily 2. Pain daily		**b. INTENSITY** of pain 1. Mild pain 2. Moderate pain 3. Times when pain is horrible or excruciating	
3.	PAIN SITE	(If pain present, check all sites that apply in last 7 days)			
		Back pain	a.	Incisional pain	f.
		Bone pain	b.	Joint pain (other than hip)	g.
		Chest pain while doing usual activities	c.	Soft tissue pain (e.g., lesion, muscle)	h.
		Headache	d.	Stomach pain	i.
		Hip pain	e.	Other	j.
4.	ACCIDENTS	(Check all that apply)			
		Fell in past 30 days	a.	Hip fracture in last 180 days	c.
		Fell in past 31-180 days	b.	Other fracture in last 180 days	d.
				NONE OF ABOVE	e.
5.	STABILITY OF CONDITIONS	Conditions/diseases make resident's cognitive, ADL, mood or behavior patterns unstable—(fluctuating, precarious, or deteriorating)			a.
		Resident experiencing an acute episode or a flare-up of a recurrent or chronic problem			b.
		End-stage disease, 6 or fewer months to live			c.
		NONE OF ABOVE			d.

SECTION K. ORAL/NUTRITIONAL STATUS

1.	ORAL PROBLEMS	Chewing problem	a.
		Swallowing problem	b.
		Mouth pain	c.
		NONE OF ABOVE	d.
2.	HEIGHT AND WEIGHT	Record (a.) height in inches and (b.) weight in pounds. Base weight on most recent measure in last 30 days; measure weight consistently in accord with standard facility practice—e.g., in a.m. after voiding, before meal, with shoes off, and in nightclothes a. HT (in.) [ ][ ][ ] b. WT (lb.) [ ][ ][ ]	
3.	WEIGHT CHANGE	a. Weight loss—5 % or more in last 30 days; or 10 % or more in last 180 days 0. No 1. Yes	
		b. Weight gain—5 % or more in last 30 days; or 10 % or more in last 180 days 0. No 1. Yes	
4.	NUTRITIONAL PROBLEMS	Complains about the taste of many foods	a.	Leaves 25% or more of food uneaten at most meals	c.
		Regular or repetitive complaints of hunger	b.	NONE OF ABOVE	d.
5.	NUTRITIONAL APPROACHES	(Check all that apply in last 7 days)			
		Parenteral/IV	a.	Dietary supplement between meals	f.
		Feeding tube	b.	Plate guard, stabilized built-up utensil, etc.	g.
		Mechanically altered diet	c.	On a planned weight change program	h.
		Syringe (oral feeding)	d.		
		Therapeutic diet	e.	NONE OF ABOVE	i.
6.	PARENTERAL OR ENTERAL INTAKE	(Skip to Section L if neither 5a nor 5b is checked) a. Code the proportion of total calories the resident received through parenteral or tube feedings in the last 7 days 0. None 3. 51% to 75% 1. 1% to 25% 4. 76% to 100% 2. 26% to 50%	
		b. Code the average fluid intake per day by IV or tube in last 7 days 0. None 3. 1001 to 1500 cc/day 1. 1 to 500 cc/day 4. 1501 to 2000 cc/day 2. 501 to 1000 cc/day 5. 2001 or more cc/day	

SECTION L. ORAL/DENTAL STATUS

1.	ORAL STATUS AND DISEASE PREVENTION	Debris (soft, easily movable substances) present in mouth prior to going to bed at night	a.
		Has dentures or removable bridge	b.
		Some/all natural teeth lost—does not have or does not use dentures (or partial plates)	c.
		Broken, loose, or carious teeth	d.
		Inflamed gums (gingiva); swollen or bleeding gums; oral abcesses; ulcers or rashes	e.
		Daily cleaning of teeth/dentures or daily mouth care—by resident or staff	f.
		NONE OF ABOVE	g.

SECTION M. SKIN CONDITION

1.	ULCERS (Due to any cause)	(Record the number of ulcers at each ulcer stage—regardless of cause. If none present at a stage, record "0" (zero). Code all that apply during last 7 days. Code 9 = 9 or more.) [Requires full body exam.]	Number at Stage
		a. Stage 1. A persistent area of skin redness (without a break in the skin) that does not disappear when pressure is relieved.	
		b. Stage 2. A partial thickness loss of skin layers that presents clinically as an abrasion, blister, or shallow crater.	
		c. Stage 3. A full thickness of skin is lost, exposing the subcutaneous tissues - presents as a deep crater with or without undermining adjacent tissue.	
		d. Stage 4. A full thickness of skin and subcutaneous tissue is lost, exposing muscle or bone.	
2.	TYPE OF ULCER	(For each type of ulcer, code for the highest stage in the last 7 days using scale in item M1—i.e., 0=none; stages 1, 2, 3, 4)	
		a. Pressure ulcer—any lesion caused by pressure resulting in damage of underlying tissue	
		b. Stasis ulcer—open lesion caused by poor circulation in the lower extremities	
3.	HISTORY OF RESOLVED ULCERS	Resident had an ulcer that was resolved or cured in LAST 90 DAYS 0. No 1. Yes	
4.	OTHER SKIN PROBLEMS OR LESIONS PRESENT	(Check all that apply during last 7 days)	
		Abrasions, bruises	a.
		Burns (second or third degree)	b.
		Open lesions other than ulcers, rashes, cuts (e.g., cancer lesions)	c.
		Rashes—e.g., intertrigo, eczema, drug rash, heat rash, herpes zoster	d.
		Skin desensitized to pain or pressure	e.
		Skin tears or cuts (other than surgery)	f.
		Surgical wounds	g.
		NONE OF ABOVE	h.
5.	SKIN TREATMENTS	(Check all that apply during last 7 days)	
		Pressure relieving device(s) for chair	a.
		Pressure relieving device(s) for bed	b.
		Turning/repositioning program	c.
		Nutrition or hydration intervention to manage skin problems	d.
		Ulcer care	e.
		Surgical wound care	f.
		Application of dressings (with or without topical medications) other than to feet	g.
		Application of ointments/medications (other than to feet)	h.
		Other preventative or protective skin care (other than to feet)	i.
		NONE OF ABOVE	j.
6.	FOOT PROBLEMS AND CARE	(Check all that apply during last 7 days)	
		Resident has one or more foot problems—e.g., corns, callouses, bunions, hammer toes, overlapping toes, pain, structural problems	a.
		Infection of the foot—e.g., cellulitis, purulent drainage	b.
		Open lesions on the foot	c.
		Nails/calluses trimmed during last 90 days	d.
		Received preventative or protective foot care (e.g., used special shoes, inserts, pads, toe separators)	e.
		Application of dressings (with or without topical medications)	f.
		NONE OF ABOVE	g.

SECTION N. ACTIVITY PURSUIT PATTERNS

1.	TIME AWAKE	(Check appropriate time periods over last 7 days) Resident awake all or most of time (i.e., naps no more than one hour per time period) in the:			
		Morning	a.	Evening	c.
		Afternoon	b.	NONE OF ABOVE	d.
(If resident is comatose, skip to Section O)					
2.	AVERAGE TIME INVOLVED IN ACTIVITIES	(When awake and not receiving treatments or ADL care) 0. Most—more than 2/3 of time 2. Little—less than 1/3 of time 1. Some—from 1/3 to 2/3 of time 3. None			
3.	PREFERRED ACTIVITY SETTINGS	(Check all settings in which activities are preferred)			
		Own room	a.		
		Day/activity room	b.	Outside facility	d.
		Inside NH/off unit	c.	NONE OF ABOVE	e.
4.	GENERAL ACTIVITY PREFERENCES (adapted to resident's current abilities)	(Check all PREFERENCES whether or not activity is currently available to resident)			
		Cards/other games	a.	Trips/shopping	g.
		Crafts/arts	b.	Walking/wheeling outdoors	h.
		Exercise/sports	c.	Watching TV	i.
		Music	d.	Gardening or plants	j.
		Reading/writing	e.	Talking or conversing	k.
		Spiritual/religious activities	f.	Helping others	l.
				NONE OF ABOVE	m.

Figure F-6 MDS 2.0 Full Assessment Form, Sections J (continued)–N (continued on next page).

5.	PREFERS CHANGE IN DAILY ROUTINE	*Code for resident preferences in daily routines* 0. No change 1. Slight change 2. Major change	
		a. Type of activities in which resident is currently involved	
		b. Extent of resident involvement in activities	

SECTION O. MEDICATIONS

1.	NUMBER OF MEDICA-TIONS	*(Record the number of different medications used in the last 7 days; enter "0" if none used)*	
2.	NEW MEDICA-TIONS	*(Resident currently receiving medications that were initiated during the last 90 days)* 0. No 1. Yes	
3.	INJECTIONS	*(Record the number of DAYS injections of any type received during the last 7 days; enter "0" if none used)*	
4.	DAYS RECEIVED THE FOLLOWING MEDICATION	*(Record the number of DAYS during last 7 days; enter "0" if not used. Note—enter "1" for long-acting meds used less than weekly)*	

a. Antipsychotic	d. Hypnotic	
b. Antianxiety	e. Diuretic	
c. Antidepressant		

SECTION P. SPECIAL TREATMENTS AND PROCEDURES

1.	SPECIAL TREAT-MENTS, PROCE-DURES, AND PROGRAMS	a. SPECIAL CARE—*Check treatments or programs received during the last 14 days*

TREATMENTS		Ventilator or respirator	l.
Chemotherapy	a.	**PROGRAMS**	
Dialysis	b.	Alcohol/drug treatment program	m.
IV medication	c.		
Intake/output	d.	Alzheimer's/dementia special care unit	n.
Monitoring acute medical condition	e.	Hospice care	o.
Ostomy care	f.	Pediatric unit	p.
Oxygen therapy	g.	Respite care	q.
Radiation	h.	Training in skills required to return to the community (e.g., taking medications, house work, shopping, transportation, ADLs)	r.
Suctioning	i.		
Tracheostomy care	j.		
Transfusions	k.	NONE OF ABOVE	s.

b. THERAPIES - *Record the number of days and total minutes each of the following therapies was administered (for at least 15 minutes a day) in the last 7 calendar days (Enter 0 if none or less than 15 min. daily)*
[Note—count only post admission therapies]

(A) = # of days administered for 15 minutes or more (B) = total # of minutes provided in last 7 days	DAYS (A)	MIN (B)
a. Speech - language pathology and audiology services		
b. Occupational therapy		
c. Physical therapy		
d. Respiratory therapy		
e. Psychological therapy (by any licensed mental health professional)		

2.	INTERVEN-TION PROGRAMS FOR MOOD, BEHAVIOR, COGNITIVE LOSS	*(Check all interventions or strategies used in last 7 days—no matter where received)*	
		Special behavior symptom evaluation program	a.
		Evaluation by a licensed mental health specialist in last 90 days	b.
		Group therapy	c.
		Resident-specific deliberate changes in the environment to address mood/behavior patterns—e.g., providing bureau in which to rummage	d.
		Reorientation—e.g., cueing	e.
		NONE OF ABOVE	f.

3.	NURSING REHABILITA-TION/ RESTOR-ATIVE CARE	*Record the NUMBER OF DAYS each of the following rehabilitation or restorative techniques or practices was provided to the resident for more than or equal to 15 minutes per day in the last 7 days (Enter 0 if none or less than 15 min. daily.)*

a. Range of motion (passive)	f. Walking	
b. Range of motion (active)	g. Dressing or grooming	
c. Splint or brace assistance	h. Eating or swallowing	
TRAINING AND SKILL PRACTICE IN:	i. Amputation/prosthesis care	
d. Bed mobility	j. Communication	
e. Transfer	k. Other	

4.	DEVICES AND RESTRAINTS	*(Use the following codes for last 7 days:)* 0. Not used 1. Used less than daily 2. Used daily

Bed rails	
a. — Full bed rails on all open sides of bed	
b. — Other types of side rails used (e.g., half rail, one side)	
c. Trunk restraint	
d. Limb restraint	
e. Chair prevents rising	

5.	HOSPITAL STAY(S)	Record number of times resident was admitted to hospital with an overnight stay in last 90 days (or since last assessment if less than 90 days). (Enter 0 if no hospital admissions)	
6.	EMERGENCY ROOM (ER) VISIT(S)	Record number of times resident visited ER without an overnight stay in last 90 days (or since last assessment if less than 90 days). (Enter 0 if no ER visits)	
7.	PHYSICIAN VISITS	In the LAST 14 DAYS (or since admission if less than 14 days in facility) how many days has the physician (or authorized assistant or practitioner) examined the resident? (Enter 0 if none)	
8.	PHYSICIAN ORDERS	In the LAST 14 DAYS (or since admission if less than 14 days in facility) how many days has the physician (or authorized assistant or practitioner) changed the resident's orders? Do not include order renewals without change. (Enter 0 if none)	
9.	ABNORMAL LAB VALUES	Has the resident had any abnormal lab values during the last 90 days (or since admission)? 0. No 1. Yes	

SECTION Q. DISCHARGE POTENTIAL AND OVERALL STATUS

1.	DISCHARGE POTENTIAL	a. Resident expresses/indicates preference to return to the community 0. No 1. Yes	
		b. Resident has a support person who is positive towards discharge 0. No 1. Yes	
		c. Stay projected to be of a short duration— discharge projected within 90 days (do not include expected discharge due to death) 0. No 2. Within 31-90 days 1. Within 30 days 3. Discharge status uncertain	
2.	OVERALL CHANGE IN CARE NEEDS	Resident's overall self sufficiency has changed significantly as compared to status of 90 days ago (or since last assessment if less than 90 days) 0. No change 1. Improved—receives fewer supports, needs less restrictive level of care 2. Deteriorated—receives more support	

SECTION R. ASSESSMENT INFORMATION

1.	PARTICIPA-TION IN ASSESS-MENT	a. Resident: 0. No 1. Yes	
		b. Family: 0. No 1. Yes 2. No family	
		c. Significant other: 0. No 1. Yes 2. None	

2. SIGNATURES OF PERSONS COMPLETING THE ASSESSMENT:

a. Signature of RN Assessment Coordinator (sign on above line)

b. Date RN Assessment Coordinator signed as complete

	Month	Day	Year

c. Other Signatures	Title	Sections	Date
d.			Date
e.			Date
f.			Date
g.			Date
h.			Date

Figure F-7   MDS 2.0 Full Assessment Form, Sections N *(continued)*–R.

Resident _____   Numeric Identifier _____

SECTION T. SUPPLEMENT—CASE MIX DEMO

1.	SPECIAL TREAT-MENTS AND PROCE-DURES	**a. RECREATION THERAPY**—*Enter number of days and total minutes of recreation therapy administered (for at least 15 minutes a day) in the last 7 days (Enter 0 if none)*

			DAYS (A)	MIN (B)
		(A) = # of days administered for 15 minutes or more		
		(B) = total # of minutes provided in last 7 days		

Skip unless this is a Medicare 5 day or initial admission assessment.

b. ORDERED THERAPIES—*Has physician ordered any of following therapies to begin in FIRST 14 days of stay—physical therapy, occupational therapy, or speech pathology service?*
0. No   1. Yes

If not ordered, skip to Item 2

c. Through day 15, provide an estimate of the number of days when at least 1 therapy service can be expected to have been delivered.

d. Through day 15, provide an estimate of the number of therapy minutes (across the therapies) that can be expected to be delivered?

2.	WALKING WHEN MOST SELF SUFFICIENT	*Complete Item 2 if ADL self-performance score for TRANSFER (G.1.b.A) is 0,1,2, or 3 AND at least one of the following are present:*

  • Resident received physical therapy involving gait training (P.1.b.c)
  • Physical therapy was ordered for the resident involving gait training (T.2.b)
  • Resident received nursing rehabilitation for walking (P.3.f)
  • Physical therapy involving walking has been discontinued within the past 180 days

Skip to Item 3 if resident did not walk in last 7 days

(FOR FOLLOWING FIVE ITEMS, BASE CODING ON THE EPISODE WHEN THE RESIDENT WALKED THE FARTHEST WITHOUT SITTING DOWN. INCLUDE WALKING DURING REHABILITATION SESSIONS.)

a. Furthest distance walked without sitting down during this episode.

0. 150+ feet   3. 10-25 feet
1. 51-149 feet   4. Less than 10 feet
2. 26-50 feet

b. Time walked without sitting down during this episode.

0. 1-2 minutes   3. 11-15 minutes
1. 3-4 minutes   4. 16-30 minutes
2. 5-10 minutes   5. 31+ minutes

c. Self-Performance in walking during this episode.

0. *INDEPENDENT*—No help or oversight

1. *SUPERVISION*—Oversight, encouragement or cueing provided

2. *LIMITED ASSISTANCE*—Resident highly involved in walking; received physical help in guided maneuvering of limbs or other nonweight bearing assistance

3. *EXTENSIVE ASSISTANCE*—Resident received weight bearing assistance while walking

d. Walking support provided associated with this episode (code regardless of resident's self-performance classification).

0. No setup or physical help from staff
1. Setup help only
2. One person physical assist
3. Two+ persons physical assist

e. Parallel bars used by resident in association with this episode.

0. No   1. Yes

3.	CASE MIX GROUP	Medicare					State					

Figure F-8   MDS 2.0 Full Assessment Form, Section T.

MDS QUARTERLY ASSESSMENT FORM

A1.	**RESIDENT NAME**	a. (First) b. (Middle Initial) c. (Last) d. (Jr/Sr)
A2.	**ROOM NUMBER**	☐☐☐☐☐
A3.	**ASSESSMENT REFERENCE DATE**	a. Last day of MDS observation period ☐☐ — ☐☐ — ☐☐☐☐ Month Day Year b. Original (0) or corrected copy of form (enter number of correction)
A4a	**DATE OF REENTRY**	Date of reentry from most recent temporary discharge to a hospital in last 90 days (or since last assessment or admission if less than 90 days) ☐☐ — ☐☐ — ☐☐☐☐ Month Day Year
A6.	**MEDICAL RECORD NO.**	☐☐☐☐☐☐☐☐
B1.	**COMATOSE**	(Persistent vegetative state/no discernible consciousness) 0. No 1. Yes (Skip to Section G)
B2.	**MEMORY**	(Recall of what was learned or known) a. Short-term memory OK—seems/appears to recall after 5 minutes 0. Memory OK 1. Memory problem b. Long-term memory OK—seems/appears to recall long past 0. Memory OK 1. Memory problem
B4.	**COGNITIVE SKILLS FOR DAILY DECISION-MAKING**	(Made decisions regarding tasks of daily life) 0. INDEPENDENT—decisions consistent/reasonable 1. MODIFIED INDEPENDENCE—some difficulty in new situations only 2. MODERATELY IMPAIRED—decisions poor; cues/supervision required 3. SEVERELY IMPAIRED—never/rarely made decisions
B5.	**INDICATORS OF DELIRIUM— PERIODIC DISORDERED THINKING/ AWARENESS**	(Code for behavior in the last 7 days.) [Note: Accurate assessment requires conversations with staff and family who have direct knowledge of resident's behavior over this time]. 0. Behavior not present 1. Behavior present, not of recent onset 2. Behavior present, over last 7 days appears different from resident's usual functioning (e.g., new onset or worsening) a. EASILY DISTRACTED—(e.g., difficulty paying attention; gets sidetracked) b. PERIODS OF ALTERED PERCEPTION OR AWARENESS OF SURROUNDINGS—(e.g., moves lips or talks to someone not present; believes he/she is somewhere else; confuses night and day) c. EPISODES OF DISORGANIZED SPEECH—(e.g., speech is incoherent, nonsensical, irrelevant, or rambling from subject to subject; loses train of thought) d. PERIODS OF RESTLESSNESS—(e.g., fidgeting or picking at skin, clothing, napkins, etc; frequent position changes; repetitive physical movements or calling out) e. PERIODS OF LETHARGY—(e.g., sluggishness; staring into space; difficult to arouse; little body movement) f. MENTAL FUNCTION VARIES OVER THE COURSE OF THE DAY—(e.g., sometimes better, sometimes worse; behaviors sometimes present, sometimes not)
C4.	**MAKING SELF UNDERSTOOD**	(Expressing information content—however able) 0. UNDERSTOOD 1. USUALLY UNDERSTOOD—difficulty finding words or finishing thoughts 2. SOMETIMES UNDERSTOOD—ability is limited to making concrete requests 3. RARELY/NEVER UNDERSTOOD
C6.	**ABILITY TO UNDERSTAND OTHERS**	(Understanding verbal information content—however able) 0. UNDERSTANDS 1. USUALLY UNDERSTANDS—may miss some part/intent of message 2. SOMETIMES UNDERSTANDS—responds adequately to simple, direct communication 3. RARELY/NEVER UNDERSTANDS
E1.	**INDICATORS OF DEPRESSION, ANXIETY, SAD MOOD**	(Code for indicators observed in last 30 days, irrespective of the assumed cause) 0. Indicator not exhibited in last 30 days 1. Indicator of this type exhibited up to five days a week 2. Indicator of this type exhibited daily or almost daily (6, 7 days a week) **VERBAL EXPRESSIONS OF DISTRESS** a. Resident made negative statements—e.g., "Nothing matters; Would rather be dead; What's the use; Regrets having lived so long; Let me die" b. Repetitive questions—e.g., "Where do I go; What do I do?" c. Repetitive verbalizations—e.g., calling out for help, ("God help me") d. Persistent anger with self or others—e.g., easily annoyed, anger at placement in nursing home; anger at care received e. Self deprecation—e.g., "I am nothing; I am of no use to anyone"

E1.	**INDICATORS OF DEPRESSION, ANXIETY, SAD MOOD (cont.)**	**VERBAL EXPRESSIONS OF DISTRESS** f. Expressions of what appear to be unrealistic fears—e.g., fear of being abandoned, left alone, being with others g. Recurrent statements that something terrible is about to happen—e.g., believes he or she is about to die, have a heart attack h. Repetitive health complaints—e.g., persistently seeks medical attention, obsessive concern with body functions i. Repetitive anxious complaints/concerns (non-health related) e.g., persistently seeks attention/reassurance regarding schedules, meals, laundry, clothing, relationship issues
		SLEEP-CYCLE ISSUES j. Unpleasant mood in morning k. Insomnia/change in usual sleep pattern **SAD, APATHETIC, ANXIOUS APPEARANCE** l. Sad, pained, worried facial expressions—e.g., furrowed brows m. Crying, tearfulness n. Repetitive physical movements—e.g., pacing, hand wringing, restlessness, fidgeting, picking **LOSS OF INTEREST** o. Withdrawal from activities of interest—e.g., no interest in long standing activities or being with family/friends p. Reduced social interaction
E2.	**MOOD PERSISTENCE**	One or more indicators of depressed, sad or anxious mood were not easily altered by attempts to "cheer up", console, or reassure the resident over last 7 days 0. No mood indicators 1. Indicators present, easily altered 2. Indicators present, not easily altered
E4.	**BEHAVIORAL SYMPTOMS**	(A) Behavioral symptom frequency in last 7 days 0. Behavior not exhibited in last 7 days 1. Behavior of this type occurred 1 to 3 days in last 7 days 2. Behavior of this type occurred 4 to 6 days, but less than daily 3. Behavior of this type occurred daily (B) Behavioral symptom alterability in last 7 days 0. Behavior not present OR behavior was easily altered 1. Behavior was not easily altered (A) (B) a. WANDERING (moved with no rational purpose, seemingly oblivious to needs or safety) b. VERBALLY ABUSIVE BEHAVIORAL SYMPTOMS (others were threatened, screamed at, cursed at) c. PHYSICALLY ABUSIVE BEHAVIORAL SYMPTOMS (others were hit, shoved, scratched, sexually abused) d. SOCIALLY INAPPROPRIATE/DISRUPTIVE BEHAVIORAL SYMPTOMS (made disruptive sounds, noisiness, screaming, self-abusive acts, sexual behavior or disrobing in public, smeared/threw food/feces, hoarding, rummaged through others' belongings) e. RESISTS CARE (resisted taking medications/ injections, ADL assistance, or eating)
G1.	**(A) ADL SELF-PERFORMANCE**—(Code for resident's PERFORMANCE OVER ALL SHIFTS during last 7 days—Not including setup)	0. INDEPENDENT—No help or oversight —OR— Help/oversight provided only 1 or 2 times during last 7 days 1. SUPERVISION—Oversight, encouragement or cueing provided 3 or more times during last 7 days —OR— Supervision (3 or more times) plus physical assistance provided only 1 or 2 times during last 7 days 2. LIMITED ASSISTANCE—Resident highly involved in activity; received physical help in guided maneuvering of limbs or other nonweight bearing assistance 3 or more times — OR—More help provided only 1 or 2 times during last 7 days 3. EXTENSIVE ASSISTANCE—While resident performed part of activity, over last 7-day period, help of following type(s) provided 3 or more times: — Weight-bearing support — Full staff performance during part (but not all) of last 7 days 4. TOTAL DEPENDENCE—Full staff performance of activity during entire 7 days 8. ACTIVITY DID NOT OCCUR during entire 7 days (A)
a.	**BED MOBILITY**	How resident moves to and from lying position, turns side to side, and positions body while in bed
b.	**TRANSFER**	How resident moves between surfaces—to/from: bed, chair, wheelchair, standing position (EXCLUDE to/from bath/toilet)
c.	**WALK IN ROOM**	How resident walks between locations in his/her room.
d.	**WALK IN CORRIDOR**	How resident walks in corridor on unit.
e.	**LOCOMOTION ON UNIT**	How resident moves between locations in his/her room and adjacent corridor on same floor. If in wheelchair, self-sufficiency once in chair
f.	**LOCOMOTION OFF UNIT**	How resident moves to and returns from off unit locations (e.g., areas set aside for dining, activities, or treatments). If facility has only one floor, how resident moves to and from distant areas on the floor. If in wheelchair, self-sufficiency once in chair
g.	**DRESSING**	How resident puts on, fastens, and takes off all items of street clothing, including donning/removing prosthesis
h.	**EATING**	How resident eats and drinks (regardless of skill). Includes intake of nourishment by other means (e.g., tube feeding, total parenteral nutrition).

Figure F-9   MDS 2.0 Quarterly Assessment Form (*continued on next page*).

Appendix B
Resident_____

Numeric Identifier _____

I.	TOILET USE	How resident uses the toilet room (or commode, bedpan, urinal); transfer on/off toilet, cleanses, changes pad, manages ostomy or catheter, adjusts clothes
I.	PERSONAL HYGIENE	How resident maintains personal hygiene, including combing hair, brushing teeth, shaving, applying makeup, washing/drying face, hands, and perineum (EXCLUDE baths and showers)
G2.	BATHING	How resident takes full-body bath/shower, sponge bath, and transfers in/out of tub/shower (EXCLUDE washing of back and hair.) Code for most dependent in self-performance. (A) BATHING SELF PERFORMANCE codes appear below: (A) 0. Independent—No help provided 1. Supervision—Oversight help only 2. Physical help limited to transfer only 3. Physical help in part of bathing activity 4. Total dependence 8. Activity itself did not occur during entire 7 days
G4.	FUNCTIONAL LIMITATION IN RANGE OF MOTION	(Code for limitations during last 7 days that interfered with daily functions or placed residents at risk of injury) (A) RANGE OF MOTION (B) VOLUNTARY MOVEMENT 0. No limitation 0. No loss 1. Limitation on one side 1. Partial loss 2. Limitation on both sides 2. Full loss (A) (B) a. Neck b. Arm—Including shoulder or elbow c. Hand—Including wrist or fingers d. Leg—Including hip or knee e. Foot—Including ankle or toes f. Other limitation or loss
G6.	MODES OF TRANSFER	(Check all that apply during last 7 days) Bedfast all or most of time a. NONE OF ABOVE f. Bed rails used for bed mobility or transfer b.
H1.	CONTINENCE SELF-CONTROL CATEGORIES (Code for resident's PERFORMANCE OVER ALL SHIFTS) 0. CONTINENT—Complete control [includes use of indwelling urinary catheter or ostomy device that does not leak urine or stool] 1. USUALLY CONTINENT—BLADDER, incontinent episodes once a week or less; BOWEL, less than weekly 2. OCCASIONALLY INCONTINENT—BLADDER, 2 or more times a week but not daily; BOWEL, once a week 3. FREQUENTLY INCONTINENT—BLADDER, tended to be incontinent daily, but some control present (e.g., on day shift); BOWEL, 2-3 times a week 4. INCONTINENT—Had inadequate control BLADDER, multiple daily episodes; BOWEL, all (or almost all) of the time	
a.	BOWEL CONTI-NENCE	Control of bowel movement, with appliance or bowel continence programs, if employed
b.	BLADDER CONTI-NENCE	Control of urinary bladder function (if dribbles, volume insufficient to soak through underpants), with appliances (e.g., foley) or continence programs, if employed
H2.	BOWEL ELIMINATION PATTERN	Fecal impaction d. NONE OF ABOVE e.
H3.	APPLIANCES AND PROGRAMS	Any scheduled toileting plan a. Indwelling catheter d. Bladder retraining program b. Ostomy present i. External (condom) catheter c. NONE OF ABOVE j.
I2.	INFECTIONS	Urinary tract infection in last 30 days NONE OF ABOVE m.
I3.	OTHER CURRENT DIAGNOSES AND ICD-9 CODES	(Include only those diseases diagnosed in the last 90 days that have a relationship to current ADL status, cognitive status, mood or behavior status, medical treatments, nursing monitoring, or risk of death) a.					.		b.					.		
J1.	PROBLEM CONDITIONS	(Check all problems present in last 7 days) Dehydrated; output exceeds input c. Hallucinations l. NONE OF ABOVE p.
J2.	PAIN SYMPTOMS	(Code the highest level of pain present in the last 7 days) a. FREQUENCY with which resident complains or shows evidence of pain 0. No pain (skip to J4) 1. Pain less than daily 2. Pain daily b. INTENSITY of pain 1. Mild pain 2. Moderate pain 3. Times when pain is horrible or excruciating
J4.	ACCIDENTS	(Check all that apply) Fell in past 30 days a. Hip fracture in last 180 days c. Fell in past 31-180 days b. Other fracture in last 180 days d. NONE OF ABOVE e.

J5.	STABILITY OF CONDITIONS	Conditions/diseases make resident's cognitive, ADL, mood or behavior status unstable—(fluctuating, precarious, or deteriorating) a. Resident experiencing an acute episode or a flare-up of a recurrent or chronic problem b. End-stage disease, 6 or fewer months to live c. NONE OF ABOVE d.
K3.	WEIGHT CHANGE	a. Weight loss—5 % or more in last 30 days; or 10 % or more in last 180 days 0. No 1. Yes b. Weight gain—5 % or more in last 30 days; or 10 % or more in last 180 days 0. No 1. Yes
K5.	NUTRI-TIONAL APPROACH-ES	Feeding tube b. On a planned weight change program h. NONE OF ABOVE i.
M1.	ULCERS (Due to any cause)	(Record the number of ulcers at each ulcer stage—regardless of cause. If none present at a stage, record "0" (zero). Code all that apply during last 7 days. Code 9 = 9 or more.) [Requires full body exam.] Number at Stage a. Stage 1. A persistent area of skin redness (without a break in the skin) that does not disappear when pressure is relieved. b. Stage 2. A partial thickness loss of skin layers that presents clinically as an abrasion, blister, or shallow crater. c. Stage 3. A full thickness of skin is lost, exposing the subcutaneous tissues - presents as a deep crater with or without undermining adjacent tissue. d. Stage 4. A full thickness of skin and subcutaneous tissue is lost, exposing muscle or bone.
M2.	TYPE OF ULCER	(For each type of ulcer, code for the highest stage in the last 7 days using scale in item M1—i.e., 0=none; stages 1, 2, 3, 4) a. Pressure ulcer—any lesion caused by pressure resulting in damage of underlying tissue b. Stasis ulcer—open lesion caused by poor circulation in the lower extremities
N1.	TIME AWAKE	(Check appropriate time periods over last 7 days) Resident awake all or most of time (i.e., naps no more than one hour per time period) in the: Morning a. Evening c. Afternoon b. NONE OF ABOVE d.
(If resident is comatose, skip to Section O)		
N2.	AVERAGE TIME INVOLVED IN ACTIVITIES	(When awake and not receiving treatments or ADL care) 0. Most—more than 2/3 of time 2. Little—less than 1/3 of time 1. Some—from 1/3 to 2/3 of time 3. None
O1.	NUMBER OF MEDICA-TIONS	(Record the number of different medications used in the last 7 days; enter "0" if none used)
O4.	DAYS RECEIVED THE FOLLOWING MEDICATION	(Record the number of DAYS during last 7 days; enter "0" if not used. Note—enter "1" for long-acting meds used less than weekly) a. Antipsychotic d. Hypnotic b. Antianxiety e. Diuretic c. Antidepressant
P4.	DEVICES AND RESTRAINTS	Use the following codes for last 7 days: 0. Not used 1. Used less than daily 2. Used daily Bed rails a. — Full bed rails on all open sides of bed b. — Other types of side rails used (e.g., half rail, one side) c. Trunk restraint d. Limb restraint e. Chair prevents rising
Q2.	OVERALL CHANGE IN CARE NEEDS	Resident's overall level of self sufficiency has changed significantly as compared to status of 90 days ago (or since last assessment if less than 90 days) 0. No change 1. Improved—receives fewer 2. Deteriorated—receives supports, needs less more support restrictive level of care
R2.	SIGNATURES OF PERSONS COMPLETING THE ASSESSMENT:	a. Signature of RN Assessment Coordinator (sign on above line) b. Date RN Assessment Coordinator signed as complete □□ - □□ - □□□□ Month Day Year c. Other Signatures Title Sections Date d. Date e. Date f. Date g. Date

MDS 2.0 10/18/94ℕ October, 1995

Figure F-10 MDS 2.0 Quarterly Assessment Form, (continued).

MDS QUARTERLY ASSESSMENT FORM
(OPTIONAL VERSION FOR RUG III)

A1.	RESIDENT NAME	a. (First) b. (Middle Initial) c. (Last) d. (Jr/Sr)
A2.	ROOM NUMBER	
A3.	ASSESSMENT REFERENCE DATE	a. Last day of MDS observation period Month — Day — Year b. Original (0) or corrected copy of form (enter number of correction)
A4.	DATE OF READMISSION	Date of readmission from most recent temporary discharge due to hospitalization in last 90 days (or since last assessment or admission if less than 90 days) Month — Day — Year
A6.	MEDICAL RECORD NO.	
B1.	COMATOSE	(Persistent vegetative state/no discernible consciousness) 0. No 1. Yes (Skip to Section G)

B2.	MEMORY	(Recall of what was learned or known)
		 a. Short-term memory OK—seems/appears to recall after 5 minutes
		    0. Memory OK 1. Memory problem
		 b. Long-term memory OK—seems/appears to recall long past
		    0. Memory OK 1. Memory problem

B3.	MEMORY/ RECALL ABILITY	(Check all that resident was normally able to recall during last 7 days) Current season a. That he/she is in a nursing home d. Location of own room b. Staff names/faces c. NONE OF ABOVE are recalled e.
B4.	COGNITIVE SKILLS FOR DAILY DECISION-MAKING	(Made decisions regarding tasks of daily life) 0. INDEPENDENT—decisions consistent/reasonable 1. MODIFIED INDEPENDENCE—some difficulty in new situations only 2. MODERATELY IMPAIRED—decisions poor; cues/supervision required 3. SEVERELY IMPAIRED—never/rarely made decisions
B5.	INDICATORS OF DELIRIUM— PERIODIC DISORDERED THINKING/ AWARENESS	(Code for behavior in the last 7 days.) [Note: Accurate assessment requires conversations with staff and family who have direct knowledge of resident's behavior over this time]. 0. Behavior not present 1. Behavior present, not of recent onset 2. Behavior present, over last 7 days appears different from resident's usual functioning (e.g., new onset or worsening) a. EASILY DISTRACTED—(e.g., difficulty paying attention; gets sidetracked) b. PERIODS OF ALTERED PERCEPTION OR AWARENESS OF SURROUNDINGS—(e.g., moves lips or talks to someone not present; believes he/she is somewhere else; confuses night and day) c. EPISODES OF DISORGANIZED SPEECH—(e.g., speech is incoherent, nonsensical, irrelevant, or rambling from subject to subject; loses train of thought) d. PERIODS OF RESTLESSNESS—(e.g., fidgeting or picking at skin, clothing, napkins, etc; frequent position changes; repetitive physical movements or calling out) e. PERIODS OF LETHARGY—(e.g., sluggishness; staring into space; difficult to arouse; little body movement) f. MENTAL FUNCTION VARIES OVER THE COURSE OF THE DAY—(e.g., sometimes better, sometimes worse; behaviors sometimes present, sometimes not)
C4.	MAKING SELF UNDERSTOOD	(Expressing information content—however able) 0. UNDERSTOOD 1. USUALLY UNDERSTOOD—difficulty finding words or finishing thoughts 2. SOMETIMES UNDERSTOOD—ability is limited to making concrete requests 3. RARELY/NEVER UNDERSTOOD
C6.	ABILITY TO UNDERSTAND OTHERS	(Understanding verbal information content—however able) 0. UNDERSTANDS 1. USUALLY UNDERSTANDS—may miss some part/intent of message 2. SOMETIMES UNDERSTANDS—responds adequately to simple, direct communication 3. RARELY/NEVER UNDERSTANDS
E1.	INDICATORS OF DEPRESSION, ANXIETY, SAD MOOD	(Code for indicators observed in last 30 days, irrespective of the assumed cause) 0. Indicator not exhibited in last 30 days 1. Indicator of this type exhibited up to five days a week 2. Indicator of this type exhibited daily or almost daily (6, 7 days a week)

E1.	INDICATORS OF DEPRESSION, ANXIETY, SAD MOOD	VERBAL EXPRESSIONS OF DISTRESS	
		a. Resident made negative statements—e.g., "Nothing matters; Would rather be dead; What's the use; Regrets having lived so long; Let me die"	h. Repetitive health complaints—e.g., persistently seeks medical attention, obsessive concern with body functions
		b. Repetitive questions—e.g., "Where do I go; What do I do?"	i. Repetitive anxious complaints/concerns (non-health related) e.g., persistently seeks attention/ reassurance regarding schedules, meals, laundry, clothing, relationship issues
		c. Repetitive verbalizations—e.g., calling out for help, ("God help me")	**SLEEP-CYCLE ISSUES**
		d. Persistent anger with self or others—e.g., easily annoyed, anger at placement in nursing home; anger at care received	j. Unpleasant mood in morning
			k. Insomnia/change in usual sleep pattern
		e. Self deprecation—e.g., "I am nothing; I am of no use to anyone"	**SAD, APATHETIC, ANXIOUS APPEARANCE**
			l. Sad, pained, worried facial expressions—e.g., furrowed brows
		f. Expressions of what appear to be unrealistic fears—e.g., fear of being abandoned, left alone, being with others	m. Crying, tearfulness
		g. Recurrent statements that something terrible is about to happen—e.g., believes he or she is about to die, have a heart attack	n. Repetitive physical movements—e.g., pacing, hand wringing, restlessness, fidgeting, picking
			LOSS OF INTEREST
			o. Withdrawal from activities of interest—e.g., no interest in long standing activities or being with family/friends
			p. Reduced social interaction

E2.	MOOD PERSISTENCE	One or more indicators of depressed, sad or anxious mood were not easily altered by attempts to "cheer up", console, or reassure the resident over last 7 days 0. No mood indicators 1. Indicators present, easily altered 2. Indicators present, not easily altered

E4.	BEHAVIORAL SYMPTOMS	(A) Behavioral symptom frequency in last 7 days 0. Behavior not exhibited in last 7 days 1. Behavior of this type occurred 1 to 3 days in last 7 days 2. Behavior of this type occurred 4 to 6 days, but less than daily 3. Behavior of this type occurred daily (B) Behavioral symptom alterability in last 7 days 0. Behavior not present OR behavior was easily altered 1. Behavior was not easily altered	(A)	(B)
		a. WANDERING (moved with no rational purpose, seemingly oblivious to needs or safety)		
		b. VERBALLY ABUSIVE BEHAVIORAL SYMPTOMS (others were threatened, screamed at, cursed at)		
		c. PHYSICALLY ABUSIVE BEHAVIORAL SYMPTOMS (others were hit, shoved, scratched, sexually abused)		
		d. SOCIALLY INAPPROPRIATE/DISRUPTIVE BEHAVIORAL SYMPTOMS (made disruptive sounds, noisiness, screaming, self-abusive acts, sexual behavior or disrobing in public, smeared/threw food/feces, hoarding, rummaged through others' belongings)		
		e. RESISTS CARE (resisted taking medications/ injections, ADL assistance, or eating)		

G1.	(A) ADL SELF-PERFORMANCE—(Code for resident's PERFORMANCE OVER ALL SHIFTS during last 7 days—Not including setup)		
	0. INDEPENDENT—No help or oversight —OR— Help/oversight provided only 1 or 2 times during last 7 days		
	1. SUPERVISION—Oversight, encouragement or cueing provided 3 or more times during last 7 days —OR— Supervision (3 or more times) plus physical assistance provided only 1 or 2 times during last 7 days		
	2. LIMITED ASSISTANCE—Resident highly involved in activity; received physical help in guided maneuvering of limbs or other nonweight bearing assistance 3 or more times — OR—More help provided only 1 or 2 times during last 7 days		
	3. EXTENSIVE ASSISTANCE—While resident performed part of activity, over last 7-day period, help of following type(s) provided 3 or more times: — Weight-bearing support — Full staff performance during part (but not all) of last 7 days		
	4. TOTAL DEPENDENCE—Full staff performance of activity during entire 7 days		
	8. ACTIVITY DID NOT OCCUR during entire 7 days		
	(B) ADL SUPPORT PROVIDED—(Code for MOST SUPPORT PROVIDED OVER ALL SHIFTS during last 7 days; code regardless of resident's self-performance classification)	(A) SELF-PERF	(B) SUPPORT
	0. No setup or physical help from staff 1. Setup help only 2. One person physical assist 3. Two+ persons physical assist 8. ADL activity itself did not occur during entire 7 days		
a.	BED MOBILITY	How resident moves to and from lying position, turns side to side, and positions body while in bed		
b.	TRANSFER	How resident moves between surfaces—to/from: bed, chair, wheelchair, standing position (EXCLUDE to/from bath/toilet)		

October, 1995

MDS 2.0 10/18/94N

Figure F-11   MDS 2.0 Quarterly Assessment Form, (Optional Version for Rug III) (page 1 of 3) (continued on next page).

G1.			(A)	(B)
c.	**WALK IN ROOM**	How resident walks between locations in his/her room		
d.	**WALK IN CORRIDOR**	How resident walks in corridor on unit		
e.	**LOCOMO-TION ON UNIT**	How resident moves between locations in his/her room and adjacent corridor on same floor. If in wheelchair, self-sufficiency once in chair		
f.	**LOCOMO-TION OFF UNIT**	How resident moves to and returns from off unit locations (e.g., areas set aside for dining, activities, or treatments). If facility has only one floor, how resident moves to and from distant areas on the floor. If in wheelchair, self-sufficiency once in chair		
g.	**DRESSING**	How resident puts on, fastens, and takes off all items of **street** clothing, including donning/removing prosthesis		
h.	**EATING**	How resident eats and drinks (regardless of skill). Includes intake of nourishment by other means (e.g., tube feeding, total parenteral nutrition)		
i.	**TOILET USE**	How resident uses the toilet room (or commode, bedpan, urinal); transfer on/off toilet, cleanses, changes pad, manages ostomy or catheter, adjusts clothes		
j.	**PERSONAL HYGIENE**	How resident maintains personal hygiene, including combing hair, brushing teeth, shaving, applying makeup, washing/drying face, hands, and perineum (EXCLUDE baths and showers)		

G2.	**BATHING**	How resident takes full-body bath/shower, sponge bath, and transfers in/out of tub/shower (EXCLUDE washing of back and hair.) *Code for most dependent in self-performance.* (A) BATHING SELF PERFORMANCE codes appear below		(A)
		0. Independent—No help provided		
		1. Supervision—Oversight help only		
		2. Physical help limited to transfer only		
		3. Physical help in part of bathing activity		
		4. Total dependence		
		8. Activity itself did not occur during entire 7 days		

G3.	**TEST FOR BALANCE** (see training manual)	*(Code for ability during test in the last 7 days)* 0. Maintained position as required in test 1. Unsteady, but able to rebalance self without physical support 2. Partial physical support during test; or stands (sits) but does not follow directions for test 3. Not able to attempt test without physical help	
		a. Balance while standing	
		b. Balance while sitting—position, trunk control	

G4.	**FUNCTIONAL LIMITATION IN RANGE OF MOTION**	*(Code for limitations during last 7 days that interfered with daily functions or placed residents at risk of injury)*		
		(A) RANGE OF MOTION 0. No limitation 1. Limitation on one side 2. Limitation on both sides	(B) VOLUNTARY MOVEMENT 0. No loss 1. Partial loss 2. Full loss	(A) (B)
		a. Neck		
		b. Arm—Including shoulder or elbow		
		c. Hand—Including wrist or fingers		
		d. Leg—Including hip or knee		
		e. Foot—Including ankle or toes		
		f. Other limitation or loss		

G6.	**MODES OF TRANSFER**	*(Check all that apply during last 7 days)*		
		Bedfast all or most of time	a.	NONE OF ABOVE	f.
		Bed rails used for bed mobility or transfer	b.		

G7.	**TASK SEGMENTA-TION**	Some or all of ADL activities were broken into subtasks during last 7 days so that resident could perform them 0. No 1. Yes	

H1. CONTINENCE SELF-CONTROL CATEGORIES
(Code for resident's PERFORMANCE OVER ALL SHIFTS)

0. **CONTINENT**—Complete control *[includes use of indwelling urinary catheter or ostomy device that does not leak urine or stool]*

1. **USUALLY CONTINENT**—BLADDER, incontinent episodes once a week or less; BOWEL, less than weekly

2. **OCCASIONALLY INCONTINENT**—BLADDER, 2 or more times a week but not daily; BOWEL, once a week

3. **FREQUENTLY INCONTINENT**—BLADDER, tended to be incontinent daily, but some control present (e.g., on day shift); BOWEL, 2-3 times a week

4. **INCONTINENT**—Had inadequate control BLADDER, multiple daily episodes; BOWEL, all (or almost all) of the time

a.	**BOWEL CONTI-NENCE**	Control of bowel movement, with appliance or bowel continence programs, if employed	
b.	**BLADDER CONTI-NENCE**	Control of urinary bladder function (if dribbles, volume insufficient to soak through underpants), with appliances (e.g., foley) or continence programs, if employed	

H2.	**BOWEL ELIMINATION PATTERN**	Diarrhea	c.	NONE OF ABOVE	e.
		Fecal impaction	d.		

H3.	**APPLIANCES AND PROGRAMS**	Any scheduled toileting plan	a.	Indwelling catheter	d.
		Bladder retraining program	b.	Ostomy present	l.
		External (condom) catheter	c.	NONE OF ABOVE	

Check only those diseases that have a relationship to current ADL status, cognitive status, mood and behavior status, medical treatments, nursing monitoring, or risk of death. (Do not list inactive diagnoses)

I1.	**DISEASES**	*(If none apply, CHECK the NONE OF ABOVE box)*			
		MUSCULOSKELETAL		Hemiplegia/Hemiparesis	v.
		Hip fracture	m.	Multiple sclerosis	w.
		NEUROLOGICAL		PSYCHIATRIC/MOOD	
		Aphasia	r.	Depression	ee.
		Cerebral palsy	s.	Manic depressive (bipolar disease)	ff.
		Cerebrovascular accident (stroke)	t.	OTHER	
		Quadriplegia	z.	NONE OF ABOVE	rr.

I2.	**INFECTIONS**	*(If none apply, CHECK the NONE OF ABOVE box)*			
		Antibiotic resistant infection (e.g., Methicillin resistant staph)	a.	Septicemia	g.
				Sexually transmitted diseases	h.
		Clostridium difficile (c. diff.)	b.	Tuberculosis	i.
		Conjunctivitis	c.	Urinary tract infection **in last 30 days**	j.
		HIV infection	d.	Viral hepatitis	k.
		Pneumonia	e.	Wound infection	l.
		Respiratory infection	f.	NONE OF ABOVE	m.

I3.	**OTHER CURRENT DIAGNOSES AND ICD-9 CODES**	*(Include only those diseases diagnosed in the last 90 days that have a relationship to current ADL status, cognitive status, mood or behavior status, medical treatments, nursing monitoring, or risk of death)*	
		a. _____	|||•|
		b. _____	|||•|

J1.	**PROBLEM CONDITIONS**	*(Check all problems present in last 7 days unless other time frame is indicated)*			
		INDICATORS OF FLUID STATUS		OTHER	
		Weight gain or loss of 3 or more pounds within a 7 day period	a.	Delusions	e.
				Edema	g.
		Inability to lie flat due to shortness of breath	b.	Fever	h.
				Hallucinations	i.
		Dehydrated; output exceeds input	c.	Internal bleeding	j.
				Recurrent lung aspirations in last 90 days	k.
		Insufficient fluid; did NOT consume all/almost all liquids provided during last 3 days	d.	Shortness of breath	l.
				Unsteady gait	n.
				Vomiting	o.
				NONE OF ABOVE	p.

J2.	**PAIN SYMPTOMS**	*(Code the highest level of pain present in the last 7 days)*	
		a. FREQUENCY with which resident complains or shows evidence of pain 0. No pain *(skip to J4)* 1. Pain less than daily 2. Pain daily	b. INTENSITY of pain 1. Mild pain 2. Moderate pain 3. Times when pain is horrible or excrutiating

J4.	**ACCIDENTS**	*(Check all that apply)*			
		Fell in past 30 days	a.	Hip fracture in last 180 days	c.
		Fell in past 31-180 days	b.	NONE OF ABOVE	e.

J5.	**STABILITY OF CONDITIONS**	Conditions/diseases make resident's cognitive, ADL, mood or behavior status unstable—(fluctuating, precarious, or deteriorating)	a.
		Resident experiencing an acute episode or a flare-up of a recurrent or chronic problem	b.
		End-stage disease, 6 or fewer months to live	c.
		NONE OF ABOVE	d.

K1.	**ORAL PROBLEMS**	Chewing problem	a.
		Swallowing problem	b.
		NONE OF ABOVE	d.

K2.	**HEIGHT AND WEIGHT**	Record (a.) **height in inches** and (b.) **weight in pounds**. Base weight on most recent measure in last 30 days; measure weight consistently in accord with standard facility practice—e.g., in a.m. after voiding, before meal, with shoes off, and in nightclothes	
		a. HT (in.) _____ b. WT (lb.) _____	

K2.	**HEIGHT AND WEIGHT**	Record (a.) **height in inches** and (b.) **weight in pounds**. Base weight on most recent measure in last 30 days; measure weight consistently in accord with standard facility practice—e.g., in a.m. after voiding, before meal, with shoes off, and in nightclothes	
		a. HT (in.) _____ b. WT (lb.) _____	

K3.	**WEIGHT CHANGE**	a. Weight loss—5 % or more in last 30 days; or 10 % or more in last 180 days 0. No 1. Yes	

MDS 2.0 10/18/94N   **October, 1995**

Figure F-12 MDS 2.0 Quarterly Assessment Form (Optional Version for Rug III) (page 2 of 3) *(continued on next page)*.

K3.	WEIGHT CHANGE	b. Weight gain—5 % or more in last 30 days; or 10 % or more in last 180 days 0. No　　　　　1. Yes	

K5.	NUTRI-TIONAL APPROACH-ES	(Check all that apply in last 7 days)	
		Parenteral/IV　　a.	On a planned weight change program　h.
		Feeding tube　　b.	NONE OF ABOVE　i.

M1.	ULCERS (Due to any cause)	(Record the number of ulcers at each ulcer stage—regardless of cause. If none present at a stage, record "0" (zero). Code all that apply during last 7 days. Code 9 = 9 or more.) [Requires full body exam.]	Number at Stage
		a. Stage 1. A persistent area of skin redness (without a break in the skin) that does not disappear when pressure is relieved.	
		b. Stage 2. A partial thickness loss of skin layers that presents clinically as an abrasion, blister, or shallow crater.	
		c. Stage 3. A full thickness of skin is lost, exposing the subcutaneous tissues - presents as a deep crater with or without undermining adjacent tissue.	
		d. Stage 4. A full thickness of skin and subcutaneous tissue is lost, exposing muscle or bone.	

M2.	TYPE OF ULCER	(For each type of ulcer, code for the highest stage in the last 7 days using scale in item M1—i.e., 0=none; stages 1, 2, 3, 4)	
		a. Pressure ulcer—any lesion caused by pressure resulting in damage of underlying tissue	
		b. Stasis ulcer—open lesion caused by poor circulation in the lower extremities	

M4.	OTHER SKIN PROBLEMS OR LESIONS PRESENT	(Check all that apply during last 7 days)	
		Abrasions, bruises	a.
		Burns (second or third degree)	b.
		Open lesions other than ulcers, rashes, cuts (e.g., cancer lesions)	c.
		Rashes—e.g., intertrigo, eczema, drug rash, heat rash, herpes zoster	d.
		Skin desensitized to pain or pressure	e.
		Skin tears or cuts (other than surgery)	f.
		Surgical wounds	g.
		NONE OF ABOVE	h.

M5.	SKIN TREAT-MENTS	(Check all that apply during last 7 days)	
		Pressure relieving device(s) for chair	a.
		Pressure relieving device(s) for bed	b.
		Turning/repositioning program	c.
		Nutrition or hydration intervention to manage skin problems	d.
		Ulcer care	e.
		Surgical wound care	f.
		Application of dressings (with or without topical medications) other than to feet	g.
		Application of ointments/medications (other than to feet)	h.
		Other preventative or protective skin care (other than to feet)	i.
		NONE OF ABOVE	j.

M6.	FOOT PROBLEMS AND CARE	(Check all that apply during last 7 days)	
		Resident has one or more foot problems—e.g., corns, callouses, bunions, hammer toes, overlapping toes, pain, structural problems	a.
		Infection of the foot—e.g., cellulitis, purulent drainage	b.
		Open lesions on the foot	c.
		Nails/calluses trimmed during last 90 days	d.
		Received preventative or protective foot care (e.g., used special shoes, inserts, pads, toe separators)	e.
		Application of dressings (with or without topical medications)	f.
		NONE OF ABOVE	g.

N1.	TIME AWAKE	(Check appropriate time periods over last 7 days) Resident awake all or most of time (i.e., naps no more than one hour per time period) in the:	
		Morning　a.	Evening　c.
		Afternoon　b.	NONE OF ABOVE　d.

(If resident is comatose, skip to Section O)

N2.	AVERAGE TIME INVOLVED IN ACTIVITIES	(When awake and not receiving treatments or ADL care) 0. Most—more than 2/3 of time　　2. Little—less than 1/3 of time 1. Some—from 1/3 to 2/3 of time　　3. None	

O1.	NUMBER OF MEDICA-TIONS	(Record the number of different medications used in the last 7 days; enter "0" if none used)	

O3.	INJECTIONS	(Record the number of DAYS injections of any type received during the last 7 days; enter "0" if none used)	

O4.	DAYS RECEIVED THE FOLLOWING MEDICATION	(Record the number of DAYS during last 7 days; enter "0" if not used. Note—enter "1" for long-acting meds used less than weekly)	
		a. Antipsychotic	d. Hypnotic
		b. Antianxiety	e. Diuretic
		c. Antidepressant	

P1.	SPECIAL TREAT-MENTS, PROCE-DURES, AND PROGRAMS	a. SPECIAL CARE—Check treatments or programs received during the last 14 days	

TREATMENTS			
Chemotherapy	a.	Ventilator or respirator	l.
Dialysis	b.	**PROGRAMS**	
IV medication	c.	Alcohol/drug treatment program	m.
Intake/output	d.	Alzheimer's/dementia special care unit	n.
Monitoring acute medical condition	e.	Hospice care	o.
Ostomy care	f.	Pediatric unit	p.
Oxygen therapy	g.	Respite care	q.
Radiation	h.	Training in skills required to return to the community (e.g., taking medications, house work, shopping, transportation, ADLs)	r.
Suctioning	i.		
Tracheostomy care	j.		
Transfusions	k.	NONE OF ABOVE	s.

b. THERAPIES - Record the number of days and total minutes each of the following therapies was administered (for at least 15 minutes a day) in the last 7 calendar days (Enter 0 if none or less than 15 min. daily) [Note—count only post admission therapies]
(A) = # of days administered for 15 minutes or more
(B) = total # of minutes provided in last 7 days

	DAYS (A)	MIN (B)
a. Speech - language pathology and audiology services		
b. Occupational therapy		
c. Physical therapy		
d. Respiratory therapy		
e. Psychological therapy (by any licensed mental health professional)		

P3.	NURSING REHABILITA-TION/ RESTOR-ATIVE CARE	Record the NUMBER OF DAYS each of the following rehabilitation or restorative techniques or practices was provided to the resident for more than or equal to 15 minutes per day in the last 7 days (Enter 0 if none or less than 15 min. daily.)	
		a. Range of motion (passive)	f. Walking
		b. Range of motion (active)	g. Dressing or grooming
		c. Splint or brace assistance	h. Eating or swallowing
		TRAINING AND SKILL PRACTICE IN:	i. Amputation/prosthesis care
		d. Bed mobility	j. Communication
		e. Transfer	k. Other

P4.	DEVICES AND RESTRAINTS	Use the following codes for last 7 days: 0. Not used 1. Used less than daily 2. Used daily	
		Bed rails	
		a. — Full bed rails on all open sides of bed	
		b. — Other types of side rails used (e.g., half rail, one side)	
		c. Trunk restraint	
		d. Limb restraint	
		e. Chair prevents rising	

P7.	PHYSICIAN VISITS	In the LAST 14 DAYS (or since admission if less than 14 days in facility) how many days has the physician (or authorized assistant or practitioner) examined the resident? (Enter 0 if none)	

P8.	PHYSICIAN ORDERS	In the LAST 14 DAYS (or since admission if less than 14 days in facility) how many days has the physician (or authorized assistant or practitioner) changed the resident's orders? Do not include order renewals without change. (Enter 0 if none)	

Q2.	OVERALL CHANGE IN CARE NEEDS	Resident's overall level of self sufficiency has changed significantly as compared to status of 90 days ago (or since last assessment if less than 90 days) 0. No change　1. Improved—receives fewer supports, needs less restrictive level of care　2. Deteriorated—receives more support	

R2. SIGNATURES OF PERSONS COMPLETING THE ASSESSMENT:

a. Signature of RN Assessment Coordinator (sign on above line)

b. Date RN Assessment Coordinator signed as complete

	Month	Day	Year

c. Other Signatures	Title	Sections	Date
d.			Date
e.			Date
f.			Date
g.			Date
h.			Date

Figure F-13　MDS 2.0 Quarterly Assessment Form (Optional Version for Rug III) (page 3 of 3) (continued).

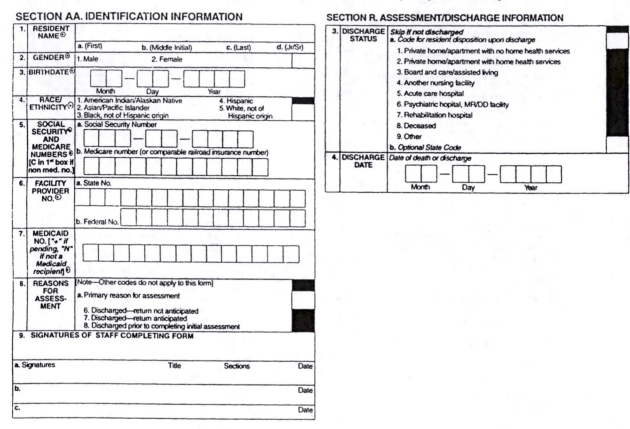

Numeric Identifier_____

MINIMUM DATA SET (MDS) — *VERSION 2.0*
FOR NURSING HOME RESIDENT ASSESSMENT AND CARE SCREENING

DISCHARGE TRACKING FORM [do not use for temporary visits home]

⊖ = Key items for computerized resident tracking

☐ = When box blank, must enter number or letter   [a.] = When letter in box, check if condition applies

MDS 2.0 10/18/94ₙ

October, 1995

Figure F-14   MDS 2.0 Discharge Tracking Form.

Numeric Identifier_____

MINIMUM DATA SET (MDS) — *VERSION 2.0*
FOR NURSING HOME RESIDENT ASSESSMENT AND CARE SCREENING

REENTRY TRACKING FORM

SECTION AA. IDENTIFICATION INFORMATION

1.	RESIDENT NAME ⓦ	
		a. (First) b. (Middle Initial) c. (Last) d. (Jr/Sr)
2.	GENDER ⓦ	1. Male 2. Female
3.	BIRTHDATE ⓦ	Month — Day — Year
4.	RACE/ ETHNICITY ⓦ	1. American Indian/Alaskan Native 4. Hispanic 2. Asian/Pacific Islander 5. White, not of 3. Black, not of Hispanic origin Hispanic origin
5.	SOCIAL SECURITY ⓦ AND MEDICARE NUMBERS ⓦ [C In 1st box If non med. no.]	a. Social Security Number b. Medicare number (or comparable railroad insurance number)
6.	FACILITY PROVIDER NO. ⓦ	a. State No. b. Federal No.
7.	MEDICAID NO. ["+" If pending, "N" If not a Medicaid recipient] ⓦ	
8.	REASONS FOR ASSESS-MENT	[Note—Other codes do not apply to this form] a. Primary reason for assessment 9. Reentry
9.	SIGNATURES OF PERSONS COMPLETING FORM	

a. Signatures	Title	Sections	Date
b.			Date
c.			Date

SECTION A. IDENTIFICATION AND BACKGROUND INFORMATION

4a.	DATE OF REENTRY	Date of reentry Month — Day — Year
4b.	ADMITTED FROM (AT REENTRY)	1. Private home/apt. with no home health services 2. Private home/apt. with home health services 3. Board and care/assisted living/group home 4. Nursing home 5. Acute care hospital 6. Psychiatric hospital, MR/DD facility 7. Rehabilitation hospital 8. Other
6.	MEDICAL RECORD NO.	

ⓦ = Key Items for computerized resident tracking

☐ = When box blank, must enter number or letter   [a.] = When letter in box, check if condition applies

MDS 2.0 10/18/94N

October, 1995

Figure F-15   MDS 2.0 Reentry Tracking Form.

A P P E N D I X   G
Glossary

abuse reporting a procedure, specific in each state, in which guidelines are given to notify state agencies of potential physical or verbal abuse of the elderly

accident a situation involving resident, staff, or visitors' injury

accountability responsibility for a particular function or duty

accumulation theory a cellular theory of aging that suggests that dangerous or toxic materials accumulate in cells over time and eventually cause death

Acquired Immunodeficiency Syndrome (AIDS) a disease in which the immune system is damaged and the host is left vulnerable to many secondary infections

action plans quality methods that look at possible solutions

active stimulation refers to an activity established to promote a reaction or participation from a resident

activities of daily living (ADLs) skills that must be conducted daily such as eating, dressing, bathing, and so forth

activity a specified time spent in pursuits from which the person receives personal benefits

activity analysis: defined by Crepeau as the process by which an activity is broken down into component parts to determine the skills required to do it.

activity assessment a method of information-gathering about a resident's background, interests, medical condition, and limitations that assist in planning therapeutic interventions

activity assessment/data collection form a form to assist the activity professional fill out the information required on the MDS

Activity Assistant Certified (AAC) one who meets NCCAP standards to carry out a supervised activity program

Activity Consultant Certified (ACC) one who meets the NCCAP standards to be a consultant, trainer, and instructor for an activity program, staff, department, or course

Activity Director Certified (ADC) an individual who meets the NCCAP guidelines to direct, coordinate, and supervise an activity program, staff, and department in a geriatric setting

Activity Director Provisional Certified a person who is working toward the NCCAP guidelines for ADC qualifications

activity photo release form a form in which residents give permission to use their photograph in the facility or for publicity purposes

activity pursuit patterns Section N of the MDS 2.0 Full Assessment Form, which deals with the residents' patterns of activity pursuits

activity supply budget the yearly or monthly amount of money allocated to the activity department for expenses

activity supply expenses the amount of money spent on a regular basis to purchase activity supply items

activity theory a social aging theory suggesting that high amounts of social involvement in valued roles can produce feelings of self-satisfaction and increased esteem

activity trip release form a sheet for residents to sign that states their consent to leave the facility for outings

acute care the treatment for a medical condition normally given over a short period of time through direct medical intervention

acute illness an illness of a short duration; usually less than six months.

Addison's disease a disease marked by a deficiency of hormones produced by the adrenal cortex, resulting in weakness and fatigue

ad hoc committee a group of facility employees appointed to meet on a short-term basis to resolve a particular issue

administration responsible for the overall operation of the facility; can be composed of the administrator, assistant administrator, department heads, and office staff

admissions director a staff member who handles tours, inquiries, marketing, and admissions of new residents

adult day care centers free-standing or attached to other health facilities, these centers offer alternatives to individuals living at home who need diversion or medical supervision during day-time hours

advance directive a living will, durable power of attorney, or health care proxy designation that states a person's written wishes for medical treatment should they become unable to state their wishes.

affective needs the yearning for emotional outlets or expressions of feelings.

ageism a term coined by Butler to mean a process of stereotyping people because of their age.

aging defined by Atchley as the physical, psychological, and social changes that occur during life

aging in place a theoretical concept suggesting that elderly clients should be provided with adequate services during their current stage in the long-term care continuum to prevent the need for moving on to another level

agitation a disturbed state; restlessness or excitement

agnosia a functional disorder that causes an individual to perceive an object or person incorrectly

Alzheimer's Disease a primary dementia of the elderly with an unknown cause, marked by a slow deterioration of cognitive function

Americans With Disabilities Act (ADA) a law that gives protection to disabled individuals in the areas of employment, transportation, public accommodations, and services

American Therapeutic Recreation Association (ATRA) a national organization dedicated to uphold the principles of therapeutic recreation

amnesia a functional disorder resulting in partial or total memory loss

anger a high level of displeasure

angina a term for the painful attacks that result when the heart does not receive the proper amount of oxygen

anniversary date an annual date that marks the original date of employment for an individual or marks years of service

anxiety an overwhelming feeling of nervousness or apprehension

aphasia a functional disorder in which loss of language exists and understanding and communication are impaired

approaches an intervention or plan used to achieve a goal

apraxia a functional disorder in which a deficit in gross or fine motor skills causes an inability to perform previously learned functions despite desire or capacity

aromatherapy a process where healing is supposed to occur through the inhalation of aromatic oils

arteriosclerosis a disease in which the arteries harden; caused by diet, genetics, obesity, smoking, or hypertension

art therapy a modality in which feelings are communicated, expressed, and interpreted through artwork

assessment the process of collecting data about a particular resident to plan and conduct appropriate medical care

assisted living facilities a facility similar to boarding or personal care homes except that more services may be available to clients, and participants may have more independence because of the facility or room layout, including kitchen areas

attending physician the physician designated by the resident as responsible for their primary care

auxiliary a board-of-directors-appointed committee of members given particular volunteer duties in support of the organization

background (face sheet) information at admission form completed on admission, the form contains information about prior patterns and living conditions of the resident

basic assessment tracking form part of the RAI process, this form contains vital information on residents such as birth date, race, social security number, and the reason for the assessment

behavior modification   a methodology for modifying or handling behaviors

benchmarking   measuring and comparing results against exemplary performances in a similar field

bibliotherapy   a process that assists individuals by sharing examples of similar situations found in reading materials

bioethics   a study of the ethical issues involved in delivering health care

biological theories   those theories having to do with the body and its processes

bloodborne pathogens   any disease elements transmitted by contact with blood

boarding homes   another term for personal-care homes

brainstorming   a group process in which numerous ideas are suggested to solve a problem without judgement on their merit

bronchitis   an inflammation of the bronchi that causes mucus secretions and a cough

budget   a written plan that projects how money will be allocated and spent

budget committee   a meeting of selected individuals held at least annually between the administrator and other staff to develop, review, and finalize the budget for the facility

burnout   exhaustion and loss of energy or commitment to a job or project

business office   a department composed of an office manager and clerical or bookkeeping staff who handle facility communication, correspondence, financial services, and payroll

cancer   a medical condition in which destructive cells multiply and invade healthy tissue areas

capital budget   a yearly financial allotment made against a larger item, such as equipment, that depreciates over time

cardiovascular system   a body system composed of the heart, arteries, capillaries, veins, blood, and lymph glands; responsible for transporting food and oxygen through the body and exchanging them for wastes

case management system   a method of coordinating medical services to make them easier to access

cataracts   a murky or opaque lens, caused by protein changes that forms over the eye and causes impaired vision

catastrophic reaction   a behavior defined by Burnside in which an individual is overwhelmed by a task or exercise that cannot be performed

cellular genetic theory   a genetic aging theory that purports DNA molecules have been damaged or changed, resulting in misinformation about body enzymes leading to aging

Centers For Disease Control and Prevention (CDC)   an Atlanta, Georgia-based federal office that monitors and tracks disease and epidemics throughout the United States and abroad

centralized system   an activity program system using one main activity room as a base of operations

cerebrovascular accident (CVA)   a condition in which the supply of blood to the brain is cut off, resulting in impairments in muscles, vision, speech, and memory; a stroke

certification process   a survey procedure used by Medicare and Medicaid at facilities to determine if compliance with regulations continues to be met

Certified Leisure Associate (CLA)   a certification category within the NCB and NTRS

Certified Leisure Professional (CLP)   a person with sufficient education and experience to receive certification from the NCB of the NTRS

Certified Therapeutic Recreation Specialist (CTRS)   a person who has completed the required coursework and passed an examination by the NCTRC to function as a therapeutic recreation specialist

cervical cancer   a disease caused by the production of abnormal cancer cells in the cervix

chain of command   a procedure dictating that issues must be resolved in a systematic way, beginning at the lowest levels of authority

checklists   a quality data collection technique

check request   a written request for a check for a specific purchase

chemical restraints   any drug with the capacity to restrict a resident's movement or behavior

chronic illness   an extended pattern of illness, lasting from a number of months to years

chronic obstructive pulmonary disease (COPD) A chronic condition, the combination of obstructive bronchitis and emphysema, resulting in restriction and obstruction in breathing; this condition is found frequently in elderly clients with asthma

chronological age the number of years a person has lived, according to birth records

cirrhosis a disease in which deterioration and inflammation in the liver is caused by alcoholism or nutritional problems

clothing and possessions inventory a list of the clothing and possessions that residents bring into the facility at admission

cognitive and educational needs requirements for stimulation of the mind, and mental growth through learning

Commission On Accreditation of Rehabilitation Facilities (CARF) offers accreditation to rehabilitation facilities

communication a written, verbal, or physical means of alerting others of thoughts and feelings

community a group of individuals who share a common purpose and exist in a particular location

community-based services assistance offered by a community in the form of services, such as nutrition and meals, housing (senior living complex), and in-home services (meals and transportation)

community resource file a file listing all the area resources and contacts that residents may require

compliance adherence to standards or legal regulations

confidentiality the handling of resident information in a professional, discrete, and respectful manner

congestive heart failure (CHF) an inability of the heart to supply blood and oxygen to areas of the body

consultant an expert in a field of study

continuing care retirement communities (CCRC) a system that offers services in a community complex to seniors; services range from apartment living to skilled nursing care for a one-time fee and monthly maintenance costs

continuity theory: a social theory of aging that speculates adults make choices of adaptation to maintain their existing structure and role in society

continuous quality improvement (CQI) also called total quality management, this term refers to quality as the primary goal of the organization

continuum of care a concept of care that shows a gradual increase in needs with care and services that range from home care through institutionalization

coronary artery disease a frequent disease among the elderly that occurs when the blood supply is blocked or slowed by clots or deposits to arteries surrounding the heart

cost-benefit analysis a quality tool used during the development process.

cross-linkage theory a cellular theory of aging hypothesizes that alterations in the properties of molecules are changed over time, causing malfunctions

critical pathways a list of interventions expected to achieve standardized results

cues vision, smells, or other sensory information that guides someone to a destination

Cushing's syndrome a condition in which an over abundance of adrenal cortex hormones are produced

daily census form a sheet that reports changes in the facility population in the last twenty-four hours through information on discharges, admissions, room changes, bed holds, and financial eligibility

dance therapy use of movement to promote emotional, cognitive, and physical integration of an individual

decentralized system activity programming in which sessions are held in numerous rooms or on various floors with no central location

decubitus ulcer a skin breakdown caused by pressure or friction and worsened by poor dietary intake

defense mechanisms coping devices, such as withdrawal or rationalizing, used to handle excess stress

deficiency a statement of noncompliance with federal or state regulations

delegate a management technique that allows a manager to assign work to a subordinate, then follow up to monitor completion

delusion a belief not based in reality

dementia a commonly seen medical condition characterized by a declining cognitive level

denial a defense mechanism in which a person refuses to admit a problem exists

department head meeting a regular meeting of the heads of each department, usually chaired by a member from administration

depreciate a decrease in the value of an item over time

depression a common psychiatric problem marked by hopelessness, sadness, and loss of interest in normal activities

developmentally disabled refers to individuals with one of the following conditions autism, mental retardation, cerebral palsy, or neurological afflictions

diabetes mellitus an inability of the body to produce an adequate amount of insulin to control sugar levels in the blood. Type I begins early in life and requires insulin injections. Type II is usually adult-onset, and can be controlled with a modified diet or medication

diagnosis categories or classifications assigned by a physician to describe a resident's medical condition

dietary a department composed of a dietary manager, cooks, and dietary aides who provide three meals a day and snacks to residents

digestive system a system of the body comprised of the stomach, small intestine, large intestine, and mouth; this system digests food, helps the body absorb nutrients, and disposes of waste

disciplinary action a scheduled procedure for alerting an employee to problem areas and seeking specific action

disengagement theory a social theory of aging that suggests as roles in society decline, aging individuals begin to disengage from society and plan for death

displacement a defense mechanism in which an individual blames another person or situation for the sources of problems

diversional activity zones an intervention program that focuses on life skills and functional abilities for programming

diverticulosis a condition in which a weakened wall of the intestine allows sacs to protrude

documentation the act of an interdisciplinary team member writing an assessment, evaluation, order, progress, or episodic note onto the medical record of a particular resident

drama therapy use of creative drama techniques toward goals of self-improvement

durable power of attorney a written document with the name of an individual who is permitted to make health care decisions on behalf of another

eloping/exiting continued attempts to leave a secure or safe area

emphysema a chronic respiratory condition that results when the lungs are unable to expand and contract properly; resulting in cell destruction and poor quality oxygen intake

empowerment activities attainment of self-respect by receiving opportunities for self-expression and responsibility

endocrine system a system of the body made up of glands that release hormones to control and regulate body processes

enhanced diner a resident who requires minimal to moderate assistance with dining. Resident may require cuing or physical intervention with eating

error theory a genetic aging theory that proposes a build up of errors in sending or receiving DNA information overloads the cells

episodic notes periodic documentation noting changes in resident behavior or moods

ergonomic rules a set of guidelines proposed by OSHA to protect employees from signal risk factors, such as repetitive motion

ethnicity the expression of a person's cultural background or heritage

ethics committee a group of facility employees and outside designees charged by the administrator to monitor facility, resident, and family compliance with bioethical issues

evacuation plan   a conspicuously visible outline of the means of evacuation from the facility. All employees receive orientation and repeated review of the proper evacuation procedures in case of an emergency

evaluation   obtaining data to assess the quality or progress toward goals

exchange theory   a social theory of aging that assumes older adults will continue interactions as long as the benefits of the exchange are greater than the negative

exit conference   a brief meeting of the survey team and selected facility staff, held at the end of a survey

expenses   the amount of money spent in a facility for its operation

exposure control plan   a written plan that outlines the job classifications in the facility that have exposure to bloodborne pathogens, and lists guidelines for employees to minimize risks and control exposure

extended survey   a survey increased by a number of days to allow more time to investigate noted problems

face sheet   the first sheet on the medical record that includes resident information such as personal data, diagnosis, from what location the resident was transferred, medical insurance numbers, last address, responsible party, advance directive information, and funeral home designation

FADE process   quality improvement steps; focus, analyze, develop, and execute

family council   a formal or informal meeting of family members to support or offer ideas to administration

feeder   a discriminatory term used in some facilities to designate a resident who requires minimal to total assistance with feeding. *See* "enhanced diner"

fiscal year   a twelve-month period of time during which financial information is compiled

fishbone diagram   a quality tool used during the analysis process

flowcharts   tools to use during the quality data collection process

focused charting   a documentation method done collectively by all disciplines. Also called integrated charting

force-field analysis   a quality method used to study possible solutions

fracture   a break in a bone caused by weakening, stress, accident, or trauma

free radical theory   a cellular theory of aging that suggests certain chemicals (free radicals) have high levels of oxygen and react to other body processes, altering their structure

functional capacity   using mobility, appearance, and mental capacity as indicators of age

functional disorders   disruptions in nervous system functioning in areas such as memory, orientation, and comprehension

function request form   a form used by all departments to request facility services for a function

general staff meeting   a meeting of all staffing levels in the facility to discuss issues and problems

generic drug   a drug that contains the exact same ingredients as a brand name drug

genetic   based on inherited factors

geriatric medicine   the study of illness or disability in the aged or elderly population

geroethics   the view of ethical and moral issues as they relate to the elderly population

gerontologist   a person who studies or practices gerontology. *See* gerontology

gerontology   the study of the aging process

glaucoma   a slow progressive disease, caused by a build-up of pressure in the eye, and in which blindness occurs

global deterioration scale   seven stages of cognitive impairment, determined by clinical characteristics such as memory loss or confusion

goals   measurable objectives with specific time frames for completion

Grave's disease   also called hyperthyroidism, this condition is caused by an increase in the production of the thyroid hormone

grieving process   the response to a loss such as death

group dynamics   a process whereby a group takes on a singular identity

governing body   the group of people who own and/or set the policy for the operation of the facility; it may be a board of directors, individuals owners, or a corporation

government-owned a facility or medical building owned and operated by the local, state, or federal government

handwashing an important procedure using soap and water in a scrubbing action to cleanse the hands and arms of dirt and potential germs

hazard communication an OSHA-mandated system for identifying potentially dangerous chemicals and materials

head trauma a serious head injury that requires a long period of recovery or long-term care

Health Care Financing Administration (HCFA) a division of the U.S. Department of Health and Human Services with responsibilities for nursing home surveys and certification

health care proxy a person designated by an individual to make medical decisions for him or her if and when the person is medically unable to do so

hepatitis B virus (HBV) a disease of the liver spread by blood, body secretions, or excremental contact

hiatal hernia a painful condition in which the stomach is pushed into the diaphragm

hoarding the activity of searching and collecting miscellaneous objects.

home care services services brought into the home, such as chore and personal care assistance, maintenance help, and telephone reassurance

horticultural therapy a technique that involves using plants and other horticulture activities to improve social, educational, psychological, and physical well-being

hospice an organization that caters to the needs of a dying patient and his or her family in the areas of physical, mental, social, and spiritual support

hostility a mild to moderate degree of displeasure

housekeeping a department that includes a housekeeping supervisor, housekeepers, porters, and other aides who provide the cleaning of all facility areas on a regular basis

human immunodeficiency virus (HIV) an infection, which can be transmitted by blood and body fluid contact, and can develop into AIDS (Acquired Immunodeficiency Syndrome)

humor applying joy and laughter in the treatment of illnesses

hypertension elevated blood pressure that is continuous or persistent, and can result in many other serious medical situations

hypothyroidism a lack of the thyroid hormone that causes weakness, fatigue, and depression

I-9 Form a required pre-employment form that mandates employers to verify certain documents related to immigration and naturalization status

immunological theory a physiological theory of aging that assumes an older person may have a weakened immune system and cannot properly fend off disease

incident an unusual occurrence involving residents, staff, or visitors in a facility

incident report a detailed written account of an accident or unusual occurrence involving residents, staff, or visitors

incontinence the inability to control bladder or bowel functions because of physical or cognitive changes

infantilization a situation in which child-like qualities are attributed to an elderly adult

infection bacterial or viral conditions in the skin, body tissues, or organs

infection control methods and procedures that outline the proper way to prevent the spread of infection

in-service/quality assurance and improvement employees who handle staff education and planning and implement quality improvement programs

in-service education on-the-job programs to increase workers' education

inspection a process of observation, interviews, and record reviews conducted by a state or federal agency that takes place over a specified period of time for the purpose of determining compliance with regulations

institutional care medical and other services provided in a facility setting to long-term care clients twenty-four hours a day

integrated charting a documentation method used collectively by all disciplines. Also called focused charting

integration or awareness needs involves being observant or having knowledge of something that can result in increased self-esteem or self-acceptance

integumentary system a system of the body composed of the skin, hair, and nails; this system protects the body against infection and regulates body temperature

interdisciplinary care plan meeting a regularly scheduled meeting of health care team members, such as the activity professional, dietician, charge nurse, social worker, occupational therapist, speech therapist, and physical therapist to discuss and set care goals for residents

interest checklist a method of consolidating the interests of all residents to assist in program planning

intergenerational programs planned between two or more generations

intern a student assigned to a field of study for the purpose of gaining experience

interpretive guidelines detailed written explanations to surveyors on the way to determine if compliance with certain regulations has been met

intravenous therapy a mode of treatment whereby medicines or other fluids enter the body through veins on a prescribed basis

irreversible dementia brain dysfunction characterized by a progressive disease in which no secondary cause is known

job description a written list of duties, responsibilities and physical/educational requirements for a particular position

job title the name given to a specific position in a facility such as Activity Director, Recreation Therapist, or Activities Coordinator

Joint Commission of Accreditation of Healthcare Organizations (JCAHO) Promotes quality care and offers accreditation to healthcare organizations

landmarks obvious and identifiable objects used for directions

laundry a department composed of a laundry supervisor and aides who provide the pick-up, cleaning, and delivery of linens and personal clothing in the facility

leadership the ability and skill to take charge and have others follow your directives

learned helplessness a cycle of repeated experiences an individual has that eventually teaches them they have no impact on the outcome of a situation

leisure time spent away from work; pursuing interests

leisure awareness as part of the leisure education process proposed by Peterson & Gunn, it refers to the development of an understanding of the benefits of leisure and the choice to begin involvement

leisure counseling an intervention technique to help clients become aware of their leisure attitudes and needs

leisure education one of the areas within the therapeutic recreation service delivery model proposed by Peterson & Gunn, this area assists clients with information and helps in the formation of new skills and feelings toward leisure

leisure resources as part of the leisure education process proposed by Peterson & Gunn, this area focuses on the client being aware and utilizing all available information to maximize leisure potential

leisure skills development as part of the leisure education process proposed by Peterson & Gunn, this area involves helping the client choose and enhance skills to increase enjoyment and satisfaction

lesson plan a written guideline to assist in teaching or for an in-service presentation

life expectancy the average amount of time that people are expected to live

life review the process of reviewing one's life to resolve outstanding conflicts

life satisfaction a term to designate a person's feeling of general well-being

life span the longest length of biological time that a person is expected to live

life stage breaking the key time periods of life into stages to look for similarities

living will a written instruction compiled by a resident explaining his or her medical wishes in case of physical or mental incapacitation

loneliness a reaction to social losses and adjustments, characterized by a feeling of emptiness and isolation

longitudinal study   a study over an extended period of time using the same participants

long-term care   three levels of care that require assistance for prolonged periods of illness, recovery, or chronic conditions; long-term care can be home-based, community-based, or institutional

long-term care insurance   special insurance policies set up to offer coverage for room and board charges for admission to skilled nursing care facilities

long-term care model   objectives in this recreation service delivery model involve providing ongoing care while assisting the resident to meet goals in physical, emotional, social, and spiritual areas

lung cancer   abnormal growth of cells in the lungs normally caused by smoking or exposure to hazardous materials

maintenance   a supervisor and staff who ensure that facility property and equipment are in good working order

maintenance activities   residents are provided with events that help maintain physical, cognitive, social, spiritual, and emotional health

management   a method of supervision that allows work to be accomplished

marketing   the act of selling or promoting a product or service

Material Safety Data Sheet (MSDS)   an OSHA-mandated form requiring manufacturers to list potential hazards and risks in the chemicals and related products that they sell; facilities are required to properly notify and train staff in the proper use of hazardous materials

Medicaid/Medical   a federal program, administered by each state that provides health care services and benefits to those who are indigent or have low incomes

Medical Device Reporting Act   a procedure enacted to require facilities to report resident accidents and injuries that come as a result of defective medical equipment

medical-clinical model   an illness-focused approach to treatment whereby the disease guides the type of service delivery

medical director   a consultant physician responsible for planning and directing the overall medical care in the facility

medical record   a written compilation of all medical data, reports, progress notes, and so forth, on a resident from the date of admission to the date of discharge

medical terminology   abbreviations, symbols, and words that assist the health care professional in documenting care

medical waste   garbage that is considered dangerous or could cause a potential spread of infection, disposed of by a special arrangement

Medicare   a federal insurance program that offers medical benefits to individuals over the age of sixty-five

Medicare Part A   the hospitalization portion of Medicare that covers limited amounts of room and board and other expenses in hospitals and skilled nursing facilities to individuals who meet certain qualifying criteria

Medicare Part B   the medical services portion of Medicare that covers limited amounts of physician and other practitioner services on an outpatient basis

medication orders   a prescription by a physician for drugs to treat a particular illness

medi-gap insurance   medical benefits insurance designed to bridge the gap between services that Medicare does not cover

mentor   an established and experienced colleague who lends guidance and support

methicillin-resistant staphyloccus aureus (MRSA)   a particular strain of the staph aureus bacteria, resistant to the antibiotic methicillin

milieu therapy   therapeutic interventions planned to decrease the negative effects of the institutional environment

mini-mental state examination   an eleven-question test used by health care professionals to quickly determine mental status

Minimum Data Set (MDS) 2.0   a federally required document that includes an overview or assessment, medical, and other information for a particular resident. A core set of screening and assessment elements including common definitions and coding categories form the foundation of the comprehensive resident assessment

MDS 2.0 Full Assessment Form   the main MDS form used at the time of admission and annually thereafter to determine the functional abilities of a resident and to identify problems

mission statement a written plan for the organization that indicates goals and objectives

mortality rates the current life expectancy ranges for men and women

motivation the reason for an action or choice

multi-infarct dementia caused by strokes, this dementia results from a build up of damage to the brain

multiple sclerosis a slow developing disease that causes difficulties in brain and spinal cord functioning and results in motor and sensory problems

musculoskeletal system a system of the body composed of the muscles, bones, and joints that holds the body together and allows it to move

music therapy using music to promote therapeutic values and restore or improve physical and mental health

myocardial infarction a situation in which the heart rhythm stops or becomes erratic when the blood supply from the coronary arteries to the heart muscle is stopped or reduced; a heart attack

National Association of Activity Professionals (NAAP) a national organization formed in 1982 with the goal of educating and upgrading the activity profession

National Certification Council for Activity Professionals (NCCAP) a certification organization that oversees the certification process for activity professionals

National Council for Therapeutic Recreation Certification (NCTRC) a certification organization that monitors the certification process for therapeutic recreation personnel

National Therapeutic Recreation Society (NTRS) a branch of the National Recreation and Parks Association dedicated to therapeutic recreation issues

need a psychosocial factor that relates to a person's ability to adjust; needs range from physiological needs for food and shelter to safety needs, love, and self actualization

negative outcome the result of an action that may be detrimental or harmful to a resident

negative reinforcement ignoring negative or destructive behavior as a means of changing behavior

nervous system a system of the body comprised of the brain, spinal cord, and nerves to help coordinate all body functions

newsletter a written or pictorial publication with specific goals and objectives

nonprofit facilities medical establishments operated on a tax-exempt basis

noise-making excessive and disruptive talking or yelling

nosocomial infections an infection acquired in a hospital or similar setting and not carried into the facility from an outside source

nursing a department composed of registered nurses, licensed practical nurses, and certified nursing assistants and headed by a director of nursing who provides personal and skilled care twenty-four hours a day

nursing facility an organization which offers nursing services and care assistance to individuals with health concerns

Occupational Safety and Health Administration (OSHA) Federal Act of 1970 that mandates states to enact standards for occupational safety and health for employees

occupational therapy a field of study that focuses on the physical and social aspects of achieving independence in daily living activities

Older Americans Act an act of Congress passed in 1965 and revised in 1973, 1978, and 1981; it specified the formation of the ombudsman's offices as part of each state's office on aging, among other legislation

ombudsman a state-designated office that forms policies to uphold the rights of the elderly and other vulnerable populations

Omnibus Budget Reconciliation Act (OBRA) legislation enacted originally in 1987 to reform the regulations and survey process for assessing nursing home care

operating budget the expected expenses required to run a facility on a yearly basis

OnLine Survey Certification And Reporting Data (OSCAR) historical survey information compiled by state and federal agencies for use by a specific facility

organizational chart a written chart illustrating the overall reporting structures of the facility

organ system theory a physiological theory of aging that assumes one system of the body deteriorates through disease and leads to aging

orientation an on-the-job process of receiving necessary information from a supervisor or co-worker to perform the functions of a position successfully

orientation checklist a written list of items that an employee is required to complete during an initial period of time on the job. When complete, the list is signed by the employee and the supervisor

osteoarthritis also called degenerative joint disease (DJD), this condition is a form of arthritis marked by a loss of cartilage that causes the bones to be exposed to pain

osteoporosis a bone disease in which bone tissue is absorbed at a higher rate than new bone can be formed, resulting in a reduction of bone tissue that causes fractures and alignment problems

over-the-counter drug (OTC) a drug purchased without orders or prescription from a physician

pacing an interchangeable term for wandering

Pareto analysis one of the quality tools used during an analysis phase

Parkinson's disease a progressive disease in which muscle rigidity, shaking, and slow movements occur because of a chemical imbalance in the information transmission area of the brain

passive stimulation refers to activity programs that require little or no participation

payment source the method that an individual employs to pay for room, board, and other services in a facility

payroll expenses the cost of employing labor in a facility; includes salary and benefits

peptic ulcer a break in the skin of the stomach, esophagus, or duodenum because of an excess of stomach acids or other factors

performance appraisal a written summary of an employee's overall performance during a particular time period

performance objectives measurable and observable areas to assess for quality standards

periodontal disease an inflammation or deterioration of the tissues surrounding the teeth

personal-care homes facilities or homes set up to provide services such as meals, light housekeeping, and minimal supervision to elderly clients

pet therapy the use of animals to gain positive responses and other therapeutic effects

petty cash available cash for minor expenses

pharmacy an in-house or outside company that fills prescriptions for residents based on physician's orders

pharmacokinetics changes in the body effecting its ability to tolerate medications resulting in problems with absorption, distribution, metabolism, and excretion

philanthropy an act of humanitarianism or a donation of service or time

phlebitis an inflammation of the veins, commonly found in the legs

phototherapy the use of snapshots and family photo albums to stimulate feelings and therapeutic discussions

physical needs desires for exercise, movement, and general stimulation of body parts

physical therapy a field of study that focuses on the physical aspects of rehabilitation, such as walking

physician's orders written or verbal designations about residents' care, such as medications or limitations

physiological theories aging theories concerned with the breakdown of the control mechanisms in living matter

plan of correction a written approach to rectify problems found during a facility survey

pneumonia caused by bacteria or viruses, this lung inflammation may be a result of other chronic conditions

poetry therapy use of poetry to probe thoughts and feelings in a therapeutic manner

policy a written statement of the standards of practice in a particular area of a department or discipline

policies and procedures documentation to support the purpose, function, and implementation methods of the practices in your department

policy and procedure manual   a binder or collection of guidelines describing in detail how the operation of a facility and its specific departments are to be handled

positive reinforcement   the rewarding of positive behaviors as part of the group process

power of attorney   a legal document that gives authority to an individual in specific situations

practitioner behavior or conduct   the level of competency and standards expected in a position or a job title

prefix   a word part added in front of another word to denote a different meaning

presentation   quality methods such as group meetings that are part of the execution stage

press release   a written method for releasing information to the news media for publication

private insurance   medical benefits coverage for long-term care room and board that may be part of a regular insurance package

private payment   payment for medical services, such as room and board in a nursing home, through out-of-pocket funds instead of through medical insurance

probationary period   a span of time immediately following employment in which an employee receives orientation, training, and evaluation

procedure   a written step-by-step process to meet the objectives of the policy statement

program   a specific intervention plan or a method for service delivery

program theory   a genetic aging theory that suggests a finite amount of DNA material exists in each cell. Aging causes DNA to be removed and the cell dies

progress notes   medical notes recorded by all disciplines in the medical record and used to log changes in a resident's condition and achievement of goals

projection   a defense mechanism in which one person transfers troubled feelings onto another

proprietary facilities   medical facilities operated to realize a profit at the end of each year

prostate cancer   an abnormal cell growth in the prostate gland

provider agreement   a contract between a facility (the provider) and a program (Medicare or Medicaid) to provide services

psychotropic drugs   drugs designated for use in psychiatric situations

quality   a measure of the amount of services actually meeting resident expectations

quality assurance   an organized, facility-wide plan to monitor the level of services provided by each department

quality indicators   warning signs or flags that note areas where quality improvement is needed

Quarterly Minimum Data Set 2.0   a reduced version of the Full Assessment Form; it monitors resident changes on a quarterly basis in between full assessments

quality monitoring   collection of data to evaluate quality

quarterly board of directors meeting   a meeting of the owners or board of directors every three months; they make recommendations to the administrator concerning the operations of the facility

quarterly quality assurance/therapeutics meeting   meeting held at least four times a year to discuss issues that concern every department in the facility

Rancho Los Amigos Scale of Cognitive Functioning   a scale which ranks the levels of cognitive impairments in individuals from level one to level eight

RAP Keys for Activities   a summary of the situations and guidelines for Resident Assessment Protocol use for Activity Services

rationalization   a defense mechanism in which an individual gives reasons why something has or has not happened

reality orientation   a treatment designed in 1959 for moderate to severe cognitively impaired residents to stress information as to time, place, and person

reciprocal model of leadership   a group process that assumes group members need to be restored to full capacity

recognition   an informal or formal way of rewarding and thanking volunteers or others for their efforts

recreation   leisure time for pleasurable activities

recreation participation   one of the areas in the therapeutic recreation service delivery model proposed by Peterson & Gunn; it involves organized choices for enjoyment and fun

regulations   a written mandate of performance for state or federal facilities

rehabilitation services.   physical therapy, occupational therapy, and speech therapy services

release forms   any of a number of sheets, which when signed, release the facility from responsibility in certain situations

remedial model of leadership   a group process that uses the group's concerns as a method for sharing and support

remedy   a mandated method of correcting deficiencies

reminiscence   a process of recalling past memories that has therapeutic value for families and residents

remotivation   a method of providing opportunities to stimulate areas of an individual's personality

renal failure   acute or chronic condition in which the kidney(s) cannot effectively remove waste from the body

reproductive system   the body system involved in the recreation of the species and sexual function

resident assessment instrument (RAI)   a set of standardized tools to measure resident needs, identify problems, and plan for meaningful interventions

resident assessment protocol (RAP)   triggers that indicate areas in need of intervention; the RAPs outline a series of steps for resolving each situation

Resident Assessment Protocol Summary Form   a form summarizing the status of the Resident Assessment Protocols for a particular resident

resident concern form   a written method of recording and handling resident problems

resident council   a group of residents who meet regularly to participate in facility life

resident sample   a cross section of current facility residents who are observed and interviewed during a survey visit to determine compliance with regulations for all residents

resident satisfaction   a term that describes a resident's satisfaction with the care and services a facility offers

residents' rights   federally mandated list of the minimal entitlement of residents living in a long-term care facility. These rights include guidelines on basic services such as mail, privacy, and choice of physician

resident status form   a form describing resident changes such as room, admission status, or financial eligibility

respiratory system   a system of the body made up of the lungs, nose, trachea, larynx, and so forth. The respiratory system brings oxygen into the lungs and expels carbon dioxide from them

respite care   a short-term break for caregivers from the responsibilities of caring for someone

responsible party   a person accountable for assisting a resident with bills and other duties

restraints   a chemical (i.e., a medication) or physical application (i.e., tray table hooked onto a wheelchair) used for safety, to prevent injury, and to prevent extremely destructive behaviors

revenue   the amount of money received by a facility for room and board and other charges

reversible dementia   brain dysfunction which may improve over time

rheumatoid arthritis   a chronic, painful condition in which an inflammation of connective tissues or joint membranes occurs because of an antibody attack in the connective tissues

risk awareness profile   a summary of all the limitations or cautionary risk information on residents to assist in program planning

risk management   a study to monitor the vulnerability that exists in a facility in security and safety for residents, staff, and visitors

rummaging   repeated attempts to search for lost or missing items

safety committee   a group of facility employees who regularly review incident reports, safety issues, and policies, and make recommendations to administration

sandwich generation   a group of individuals balancing the care responsibilities of children and parents; they are "sandwiched" in the middle

scope   a determining factor used to select a remedy for deficiencies. The scope of a problem may be isolated, a pattern, or widespread

selection grid   a method used to select quality techniques

senior centers   a building or complex operated in a town or city to serve elderly clients by offering activities, support services, and minimal medical services

sensory stimulation   a method of activating one or more of the five senses to cause a positive reaction

sensory system   a body system composed of processes such as taste, smell, touch, balance, and muscle sensation

sequencing analysis   analyzing events for antecedents and consequences of behavior

service delivery   the way in which activity or recreation services are brought to long-term care residents

severity   a factor used to select a remedy for deficiencies. Severity ranges from no actual harm with potential for only minimal harm to immediate jeopardy to resident health or safety

sharps   medical instruments that can puncture the skin and spread infection (i.e., hypodermic needles)

signage   signs or guides to assist individuals in locating something

signal risk factors   job elements monitored by the proposed OSHA ergonomics rule that involve repetitive motions, awkward positions, and continuous pushing or lifting

significant change   changes in resident status, such as changes that are not self-limiting or impact on more than one area of a resident's health that require a new Full Assessment Form be completed to reflect the change

single point of entry   a concept to attempt to make access of long-term care services easier for clients by providing a single access point in which to enter the system

skilled nursing care   medical care normally performed under the supervision of a registered nurse twenty-four hours a day. A skilled nursing care facility could be Medicare certified

skilled nursing facility (SNF)   a facility that offers skilled nursing care twenty-four hours a day under the supervision of a registered nurse

social goals model of leadership   a group technique that has the group work toward raising social consciousness and responsibility

social interaction skills   leisure participation through conversation, cooperation, and competition in group activities

social needs   a longing to be part of a group or have companionship with others

social services   a social worker or others who work as resident advocates and ensure that basic needs of residents are met

speaker's bureau   a group of organized individuals who are available to speak to groups

speech therapy   a field of study concerned with speaking, swallowing, and uttering sounds

special survey   a visit by a member or members of the survey team for purposes of investigating a particular problem or complaint

spiritual needs   desire for fulfillment in religious or other values that effect the disposition or outlook that a person may have

staffing patterns   the amount of staff members needed by a particular department to operate adequately

standard survey   an annual, unannounced facility visit from a survey team that has a time frame based on the size of the facility.

standing orders   a routine set of orders, usually agreed on by the facility and the medical staff

state licensure   laws within each individual state dictate guidelines for operation of institutions. Once the guidelines have been met, a state license is issued

stress theory   a physiological theory of aging that suggests the stresses and strains of life leave a collection of impaired material in the cell structure after each episode. Over a lifetime, harmful matter accumulates.

subacute care   specialized treatment that replaces acute hospital care or takes place following a hospitalization to treat medical conditions such as wounds, head trauma, and so forth

suffix   a word part added to the end of words to form different meanings

sundowning agitation noted at particular times of the day; thought to be associated with darkness

supplemental security income (SSI) a federal program that offers income assistance to individuals who are aged or disabled

supportive activities for those residents who have a lower tolerance for traditional activities, these activities provide a comfortable environment while providing stimulation or solace

survey a visit to a facility to determine compliance; also one of the quality measurement tools

survey and inspection process a procedure that occurs on the state level; facilities are observed to determine if compliance with state and federal regulations continues

suspicion a feeling of distrust for others

symptoms the evidence of disease, such as fever, pain, or nausea

tag number the identification prefix to any federal regulation

tardive dyskinesia a condition which is a permanent side effect of prolonged use of antipsychotic drugs

termination a separation from employment, usually initiated by the employer

therapeutic diets a specifically written directive that designates the preparation of food to meet nutritional and medical needs of a particular resident. Therapeutic diets may be recommended by the dietician and then ordered by the attending physician

therapeutic milieu model developed originally in mental illness settings, this service delivery model for recreation looks at all components of the delivery team

therapeutic recreation using leisure time to help fill a person's emotional, physical, cognitive, spiritual, and intellectual needs

therapeutic recreation process a step-by-step process described by O'Morrow and Reynolds as a goal to move an individual from the role of a nonparticipant in the environment to the highest participation level possible

therapeutic recreation service model a popular service delivery option developed by Peterson and Gunn; it is client-centered and in-cludes treatment, leisure education, and recreation participation

therapeutic touch a controversial therapy that relaxes patients, but is proposed to relieve pain and promote healing simply through touch

third-party payers a group of payment sources, such as long-term insurance, medigap insurance, and others that are billable sources for services such as room and board

tinnitus disorder of the ear marked by ringing or buzzing sounds that may impair hearing

total quality management (TQM) also called continuous quality improvement, this philosophy suggests quality as the primary goal of the organization

touch a tactile method of communicating

training the formal education and previous experiences that an individual has in a particular field

transfer sheet a form that gives a brief accounting of a resident at the time of transfer from one facility to another

trauma a forceful injury to the body

treatment part of the therapeutic recreation service model; a specifically planned process of bringing about a change in behavior or pathology

triage a staging area used during a facility disaster or emergency that provides direction to facility staff to safely manage the emergency

triggers indicators of areas of the assessment process where interventions should occur

transfer agreement a written declaration between two health care facilities or organizations to permit temporary transfers of residents in case of emergency

transient ischemic attack (TIA) called mini-strokes, these attacks are caused when the supply of blood to the brain is suddenly stopped or interrupted

tuberculosis exposure a situation in which an individual may accidentally reside or work near a person with a confirmed case of tuberculosis, and come in contact with the infection by way of respiratory secretions

universal precautions a system to protect employees; it is assumed that contact with all areas, surfaces, and resident blood and body fluids are potentially hazardous and proper protection and hygiene should be practiced.

urinary system a system of the body comprised of the bladder, kidneys, and urethra that process and eliminate liquid waste from the body

urinary tract infection (UTI) an infection of the bladder, kidney, or other part of the urinary tract caused by bacteria

utilization guidelines instructional directions for the use of parts of the Resident Assessment Instrument (RAI)

utilization review committee a committee composed of physicians, therapists, and other health care team members in a skilled nursing home or rehabilitation center, charged with the responsibility of seeing that Medicare benefits are used properly

validation survey an infrequent survey conducted by HCFA to determine a state agency's performance when conducting a survey

validation therapy a technique developed by Naomi Fell for communicating with "old-old" residents suffering from dementia

ventilator a respirator that provides breathing assistance

Veterans Administration an organization that manages and overseas the delivery of benefits and services to veterans

volunteer a person who donates time or services for the benefit of people or programs

volunteer log sheet a daily, weekly, or monthly record of time given by a volunteer

volunteer needs sheet a form used to calculate the number and type of volunteers needed for a particular program

wandering the act of repeatedly walking in nonpurposeful ways

warning notice a written corrective measure which notifies an employee of a substandard performance

wayfinding a series of guides or hints that help a person get from one place to another

wear and tear theory a cellular theory of aging that assumes the cells of the human body "wear out" from stress through repeated use

welfare/general assistance a community system of payment for services for which indigent individuals may qualify, including room and board in nursing facilities if certain criteria are met

wellness model an approach to recreation service delivery that is holistic; the whole person is considered during the course of treatment

withdrawal a defense mechanism in which a person retreats from a stressful situation in order to cope

word root the building blocks of words

worker's compensation an employer's insurance plan that covers certain situations when employee on-the-job injury occurs

wound management the care and treatment of an individual with open areas of the skin

INDEX

●●●●●●●●●●

(An "*f*" in italics following a page number refers to material in a figure.